AF761413

MEDICAL PROCEDURES, TESTING AND TECHNOLOGY

TESTING AND CONTRACT TRACING FOR COVID-19

Medical Procedures, Testing and Technology

Additional books and e-books in this series can be found on Nova's website under the Series tab.

MEDICAL PROCEDURES, TESTING AND TECHNOLOGY

TESTING AND CONTRACT TRACING FOR COVID-19

ERNESTO M. BATISTA

EDITOR

snova
New York

Copyright © 2020 by Nova Science Publishers, Inc.

All rights reserved. No part of this book may be reproduced, stored in a retrieval system or transmitted in any form or by any means: electronic, electrostatic, magnetic, tape, mechanical photocopying, recording or otherwise without the written permission of the Publisher.

We have partnered with Copyright Clearance Center to make it easy for you to obtain permissions to reuse content from this publication. Simply navigate to this publication's page on Nova's website and locate the "Get Permission" button below the title description. This button is linked directly to the title's permission page on copyright.com. Alternatively, you can visit copyright.com and search by title, ISBN, or ISSN.

For further questions about using the service on copyright.com, please contact:
Copyright Clearance Center
Phone: +1-(978) 750-8400 Fax: +1-(978) 750-4470 E-mail: info@copyright.com.

NOTICE TO THE READER

The Publisher has taken reasonable care in the preparation of this book, but makes no expressed or implied warranty of any kind and assumes no responsibility for any errors or omissions. No liability is assumed for incidental or consequential damages in connection with or arising out of information contained in this book. The Publisher shall not be liable for any special, consequential, or exemplary damages resulting, in whole or in part, from the readers' use of, or reliance upon, this material. Any parts of this book based on government reports are so indicated and copyright is claimed for those parts to the extent applicable to compilations of such works.

Independent verification should be sought for any data, advice or recommendations contained in this book. In addition, no responsibility is assumed by the Publisher for any injury and/or damage to persons or property arising from any methods, products, instructions, ideas or otherwise contained in this publication.

This publication is designed to provide accurate and authoritative information with regard to the subject matter covered herein. It is sold with the clear understanding that the Publisher is not engaged in rendering legal or any other professional services. If legal or any other expert assistance is required, the services of a competent person should be sought. FROM A DECLARATION OF PARTICIPANTS JOINTLY ADOPTED BY A COMMITTEE OF THE AMERICAN BAR ASSOCIATION AND A COMMITTEE OF PUBLISHERS.

Additional color graphics may be available in the e-book version of this book.

Library of Congress Cataloging-in-Publication Data

ISBN: 978-1-53618-857-8

Published by Nova Science Publishers, Inc. † New York

CONTENTS

Preface		**ix**
Chapter 1	COVID-19 Testing: Key Issues *Amanda K. Sarata*	**1**
Chapter 2	COVID-19 Testing: Frequently Asked Questions *Amanda K. Sarata and Elayne J. Heisler*	**9**
Chapter 3	Development and Regulation of Domestic Diagnostic Testing for Novel Coronavirus (COVID-19): Frequently Asked Questions *Amanda K. Sarata*	**107**
Chapter 4	COVID-19 Testing *United States Government Accountability Office*	**123**
Chapter 5	Interim Guidance on Developing a COVID-19 Case Investigation and Contact Tracing Plan *U.S. Department of Health and Human Services Centers for Disease Control and Prevention*	**129**
Chapter 6	Case Investigation and Contact Tracing: Part of a Multipronged Approach to Fight the COVID-19 Pandemic *U.S. Department of Health and Human Services Centers for Disease Control and Preventions*	**217**

Chapter 7	Contact Tracing for COVID-19: Domestic Policy Issues *Kavya Sekar and Laurie A. Harris*	**227**
Chapter 8	Health Department Checklist: Developing a Case Investigation and Contact Tracing Plan for Coronavirus Disease 2019 (COVID-19) *U.S. Department of Health and Human Services, Centers for Disease Control and Prevention*	**235**
Chapter 9	COVID-19 Case Investigation and Contact Tracing Supervisor or Lead Training: Guidance, Resources, and Sample Training Plan *U.S. Department of Health and Human Services Centers for Disease Control and Prevention*	**249**
Chapter 10	Contact Tracing: Part of a Multipronged Approach to Fight the COVID-19 Pandemic *U.S. Department of Health and Human Services Centers for Disease Control and Prevention*	**305**
Chapter 11	Contact Tracing – CDC's Role and Approach *U.S. Department of Health and Human Services Centers for Disease Control and Prevention*	**313**
Chapter 12	Contact Tracing: Do Your Part to Keep Your Family, Friends, and Community Safe *U.S. Department of Health and Human Services, Centers for Disease Control and Prevention*	**319**
Chapter 13	Contact Tracing Apps *United States Government Accountability Office*	**321**
Chapter 14	Contact Tracing Workflow (COVID-19) *U.S. Department of Health and Human Services Centers for Disease Control and Prevention*	**327**

Chapter 15 CDC-Funded Training for the COVID-19 Contact Tracing Workforce **329**
U.S. Department of Health and Human Services Centers for Disease Control and Prevention

Chapter 16 Digital Contact Tracing Tools for COVID-19 **333**
U.S. Department of Health and Human Services Centers for Disease Control and Prevention

Chapter 17 Guidelines for the Implementation and Use of Digital Tools to Augment Traditional Contact Tracing **335**
U.S. Department of Health and Human Services Centers for Disease Control and Prevention

Chapter 18 Preliminary Criteria for the Evaluation of Digital Contact Tracing Tools for COVID-19 **345**
U.S. Department of Health and Human Services Centers for Disease Control and Prevention

Chapter 19 Digital Contact Tracing Technology: Overview and Considerations for Implementation **351**
Patricia Moloney Figliola

Chapter 20 COVID-19: Digital Contact Tracing and Privacy Law **359**
Eric N. Holmes and Chris D. Linebaugh

Chapter 21 "Tracing Papers": A Comparison of COVID-19 Data Privacy Bills **369**
Jonathan M. Gaffney

Chapter 22 Constitutional Authority to Regulate the Privacy of State-Collected Contact-Tracing Data **377**
Edward C. Liu

Index **383**

PREFACE

The United States is reporting some of the highest number of cases and deaths from the Coronavirus Disease 2019 (COVID-19) pandemic globally, and the disease is affecting communities nationwide. In response, federal, state, and local governments have undertaken containment and mitigation efforts to "flatten the curve"—that is, to slow widespread transmission that could overwhelm the nation's health care system and to reduce spread of the disease while treatments and vaccines are being developed that will lessen the health impact of the virus. This book provides answers to numerous questions related to COVID-19 testing, including types of testing available and their reliability. It also discusses basic principles of contact tracing to stop COVID-19 transmission.

Chapter 1 - The COVID-19 pandemic is affecting communities throughout the United States, with the country reporting the highest number of cases and deaths from the disease globally. Containment and mitigation efforts by federal, state, and local governments have been undertaken to "flatten the curve"—that is, to slow widespread transmission that could overwhelm the nation's health care system. Diagnostic testing is a critical part of the clinical management of COVID-19, caused by the SARS-CoV-2 virus. In addition, both diagnostic and serology testing at scale may be a key component of efforts to ease mitigation measures prior to the development, manufacture, and broad distribution of a vaccine or effective therapeutic.

Efforts in the United States to rapidly develop, scale up, and disseminate testing for COVID-19 have faced challenges, including supply chain issues; a shifting regulatory landscape; a lack of consensus around federal coordination of or strategy for testing; concerns with the accuracy of both molecular and serology tests; an early lack of data on test results and capacity; and a delayed ramp-up by commercial laboratories and test manufacturers of both centralized and point-of-care testing. In addition, manufacturing and quality issues with the nation's initial test—developed by the Centers for Disease Control and Prevention (CDC)—resulted in significant delay in early access to testing throughout the country.

Chapter 2 - The United States is reporting some of the highest number of cases and deaths from the Coronavirus Disease 2019 (COVID-19) pandemic globally, and the disease is affecting communities nationwide. In response, federal, state, and local governments have undertaken containment and mitigation efforts to "flatten the curve"—that is, to slow widespread transmission that could overwhelm the nation's health care system and to reduce spread of the disease while treatments and vaccines are being developed that will lessen the health impact of the virus. Diagnostic testing is a critical part of the clinical management of COVID-19, which is caused by the SARS-CoV-2 virus. Both diagnostic (i.e., testing for active infection) and serology testing (i.e., testing for the presence of antibodies, potentially indicating a previous infection) over a wide population may be a key component of efforts to ease mitigation measures and allow people to return safely to work and school. Ongoing testing can be used for public health purposes to identify and isolate positive cases of COVID-19, thereby reducing spread of the disease. However, the use of testing for public health purposes rather than for the clinical diagnosis of individuals poses legal and policy complications, because regulation and payment policies can differ based on how the test is used. Further, COVID-19 testing in the United States is provided in a number of health care and community-based settings. Insurance coverage and payment for a given COVID-19 test can depend on a number of factors, including the entity administering the test or processing test results, and the reason for which the test is administered. These factors can determine whether a certain payment mechanism may be used to pay for a given test. Congress, through several coronavirus legislative packages, has enacted various insurance coverage requirements along with other funding mechanisms to help pay for testing. This chapter provides answers to numerous questions related to COVID-19 testing, including

- types of testing available and their reliability;
- testing capacity and infrastructure;
- delivery of testing, including the settings where testing is available;
- payment for testing, including the provision by federally operated health systems and payment by federal and private payors and payment sources available for people who are uninsured;
- reporting of test results; and
- federal funding for testing infrastructure and for the clinical provision of COVID-19 testing.

Chapter 3 - On December 31, 2019, the World Health Organization (WHO) was informed of a cluster of pneumonia cases in Wuhan City, Hubei Province of China. Illnesses have since been linked to a disease caused by a previously unidentified strain of coronavirus, designated Coronavirus Disease 2019, or COVID-19. Despite containment efforts in China, the United States, and elsewhere, by late February there were indications that the COVID-19 outbreak may have entered a new phase, with community spread occurring or suspected in several countries other than China, including in the United States. Diagnostic testing is a critical part of the public health response to and clinical management of COVID-19, caused by the SARS-CoV-2 virus. Efforts in the United States to develop and disseminate a test for COVID-19 have faced challenges. Manufacturing and quality issues with the nation's test—developed by the Centers for Disease Control and Prevention (CDC)—resulted in significant delay in access to testing throughout the country. In this context, on February 29, 2020, in an effort to facilitate the expansion of testing capacity as the first cases of community spread were confirmed in the United States, the Food and Drug

Administration (FDA) announced a new policy, issued via agency guidance and effective immediately, that would allow certain laboratories—principally clinical and large commercial and reference laboratories—that have developed and validated their own COVID-19 diagnostic to begin to use the test prior to it receiving an Emergency Use Authorization (EUA) from the agency. FDA's February 29 guidance aims to facilitate the expansion of diagnostic testing from the public health setting into the clinical health care and commercial settings. Doing so may help the country meet the increasing and substantial demand for testing generated by community spread of the disease and expanded clinical testing guidelines issued by the CDC. This chapter does not address financing or coverage of diagnostic testing for COVID-19.

Chapter 4 - As the nation works to save lives and flatten the curve of COVID-19 cases, widespread testing could help reduce the death rate, help identify those who should self-isolate, and help businesses recover. There are challenges, however, associated with the use and availability of tests, as well as with determining their accuracy.

Chapter 5 - Case investigation and contact tracing are fundamental activities that involve working with a client (symptomatic and asymptomatic) who has been diagnosed with an infectious disease to identify and provide support to people (contacts) who may have been infected through exposure to the patient. This process prevents further transmission of disease by separating people who have (or may have) an infectious disease from people who do not. It is a core disease control measure that has been employed by public health agency personnel for decades. Case investigation and contact tracing are most effective when part of a multifaceted response to an outbreak. Case investigation is the identification and investigation of clients with confirmed and probable diagnoses of COVID-19, and contact tracing is the subsequent identification, monitoring, and support of their contacts who have been exposed to, and possibly infected with, the virus. Prompt identification, voluntary quarantine (hereby referred to as *self-quarantine* in this document unless otherwise noted), and monitoring of these COVID-19 contacts can effectively break the chain of disease transmission and prevent further spread of the virus in a community. While case investigation and contact tracing for COVID-19 may be new, health departments and frontline public health professionals who perform these activities have experience conducting these activities for tuberculosis, sexually transmitted infections, HIV, and other infectious diseases. *Case investigation and contact tracing are well-honed skills that adapt easily to new public health demands and are effective tools to slow the spread of COVID-19 in a community.* This guidance aims to provide a foundation for state, territorial, local, and tribal development of case investigation and contact tracing plans. It is important to note that COVID-19 case investigation and contact tracing activities will vary based on the level of community transmission, characteristics of the community and their populations, and the local capacity to implement case investigation, contact tracing, and COVID-19 testing.

Chapter 6 - This web page highlights basic principles of case investigation and contact tracing to stop COVID-19 transmission; detailed guidance for health departments is available. Case investigation and contact tracing, a core disease control measure employed by local and state health department personnel for decades, is a key strategy for preventing further spread of COVID-19. Immediate action is needed. Communities must scale up and train a large workforce and work collaboratively across public and private agencies to stop the transmission of COVID-19.

Chapter 7 - Contact tracing is a classic tool of public health investigation used to identify the close contacts of persons infected with a communicable disease, notify themof potential exposure, and enable control measures such as quarantining exposed persons. Contact tracing programs are generally subjectto state, territorial, tribal, and local laws and policies. The U.S. Centers for Disease Control and Prevention (CDC) assists jurisdictions' programs by providing guidance, technical assistance, and funding. Several public health experts affiliated with universities (e.g., Johns Hopkins University), policy research organizations (e.g., American Enterprise Institute), and state associations (e.g., National Governors Association) have positedthat contact tracing (combined with adequate diagnostic testing) could help prevent surges in infections, particularly when case counts are low. Contact tracing to control Coronavirus Disease 2019 (COVID-19) has been used with arguable success in countries such as South Korea, Taiwan, Iceland, and New Zealand—many attribute their relatively low reported case counts, in part, to successfulcontact tracing. However, several experts assert that a successful contact tracing effort in the United States would require additional workforce and possibly the use of new technologies by jurisdictions. Federalismhas led to heterogeneous contact tracing efforts across states. As the pandemic progresses, Congress may consider whether and how to guide U.S. contact tracing efforts.

Chapter 8 - Case investigation and contact tracing are well-honed skills that adapt easily to new public health demands and are effective tools to slow the spread of COVID-19 in a community. Thoughtful planning can help ensure that these activities facilitate compassionate care for the people affected by COVID-19 and also prevent community transmission of the virus. This checklist is a supplement to CDC's Health Departments: Interim Guidance on Developing a COVID-19 Case Investigation & Contact Tracing Plan and is a tool that can assist health departments in developing a comprehensive plan. This tool does not describe mandatory requirements or standards; rather, it highlights important areas for consideration. For additional information, users can access the corresponding section of the guidance document listed in each header (i.e., *Guidance Section #*). COVID-19 case investigation and contact tracing activities will vary based on the level of community transmission, characteristics of the community and their populations, and the local capacity to implement both case investigation and contact tracing.

Chapter 9 - This document contains a sample training plan including training topics that may be helpful for state and local public health jurisdictions to consider when designing their own training plan for COVID-19 case investigation and contract tracing supervisors or leads. Each heading represents the learning objective for that section. Suggested training modalities/formats are provided, as well as information about sample existing trainings and resources. This document may be updated as new resources become available. For the purposes of this document, a case investigation and contact tracing supervisor or lead directly oversees the work of the case investigator and/or contact tracer and others who may work as part of a team. The supervision or leadership of these teams is combined into one position for the purposes of this sample training plan. This position coordinates between case investigators and contact tracers as an essential component of the quality oversight of the contact tracing program as part of the public health response.

Chapter 10 - This document highlights basic principles of *contact tracing* to stop COVID-19 transmission; detailed guidance for health departments and potential contact tracers is forthcoming. *Contact tracing*, a core disease control measure employed by local and state health department personnel for decades, is a key strategy for preventing further spread of COVID-19. Immediate action is needed. Communities must scale up and train a large contact tracer workforce and work collaboratively across public and private agencies to stop the transmission of COVID-19. Certain core principles of contact tracing must always be adhered to:

- Contact tracing is part of the process of supporting patients with suspected or confirmed infection.
- In contact tracing, public health staff work with a patient to help them recall everyone with whom they have had close contact during the timeframe while they may have been infectious.
- Public health staff then warn these exposed individuals (contacts) of their potential exposure as rapidly and sensitively as possible.
- To protect patient privacy, contacts are only informed that they may have been exposed to a patient with the infection. They are not told the identity of the patient who may have exposed them.
- Contacts are provided with education, information, and support to understand their risk, what they should do to separate themselves from others who are not exposed, monitor themselves for illness, and the possibility that they could spread the infection to others even if they themselves do not feel ill.
- Contacts are encouraged to stay home and maintain social distance from others (at least 6 feet) until 14 days after their last exposure, in case they also become ill. They should monitor themselves by checking their temperature twice daily and watching for cough or shortness of breath. To the extent possible, public health staff should

check in with contacts to make sure they are self-monitoring and have not developed symptoms. Contacts who develop symptoms should promptly isolate themselves and notify public health staff. They should be promptly evaluated for infection and for the need for medical care.

Chapter 11 - Contact tracing is an effective disease control strategy that involves investigating cases and their contacts and then interrupting disease transmission—typically by asking cases to isolate and contacts to quarantine at home voluntarily. *Contact tracing is a key strategy to prevent the further spread of COVID-19. Case investigation* is the identification and investigation of patients with confirmed and probable diagnoses of COVID-19 (cases). *Contact tracing*, also referred to as contact investigation, is the identification, monitoring, and support of the individuals (contacts) who have been exposed to the patient and possibly infected themselves. This process prevents further transmission of disease by separating people who have (or may have) an infectious disease from people who do not.

Chapter 12 - This is an edited, reformatted and augmented version of U.S. Department of Health and Human Services, Centers for Disease Control and Prevention publication CS317837-A.

Chapter 13 - Contact tracing can help reduce transmission rates for infectious diseases like COVID-19 by identifying and notifying people who may have been exposed. Contact tracing apps, notably those using proximity tracing, could expedite such efforts. However, there are challenges, including accuracy, adoption rates, and privacy concerns.

Chapter 14 - This is an edited, reformatted and augmented accessible version of Department of Health and Human Services publication, No. CS 317008-A, dated 06/15/2020.

Chapter 15 - Contact tracing is a key strategy to prevent the further spread of COVID-19. Contact tracing in the United States requires states, tribes, localities, and territories to recruit, hire, and train adequate levels of case investigators and contact tracers. Successful case investigation and contact tracing for COVID-19 depends on a robust and well-trained public health workforce, with staff who have excellent and tactful interpersonal skills, cultural sensitivity, and language and interviewing skills that help them to build and maintain trust with clients and contacts. The CDC COVID-19 Response and the CDC Division of STD Prevention are supporting two cooperative agreements to train the COVID-19 contact tracing workforce. The newly funded National Network Disease Intervention Training Centers (NNDITC) and the Association of State and Territorial Health Officials (ASTHO) in partnership with the National Coalition of STD Directors (NCSD) are leading a nationwide, coordinated training effort to build a well-trained public health COVID-19 contact tracing workforce, including case investigators, contact tracers, and contact tracing supervisors.

Chapter 16 - This is an edited, reformatted and augmented version of Department of Health and Human Services publication CS 316626-A 04/20/2020.

Chapter 17 - This document describes two broad categories of digital contact tracing tools, how and where they can improve timeliness and efficiency in the contact tracing process, and defines their minimum and preferred features. This document is based on research and ongoing discussions with contact tracing and informatics experts across local, state, territorial, tribal, and federal government agencies; national public health associations; academic consortia; and nongovernmental organizations. This document builds on previous guidance; it is a living body of knowledge and will be revised frequently in response to new information and the evolving needs of state, local, tribal, and territorial health departments. Use of trade names and commercial sources is for identification only and does not imply endorsement by the U.S. Department of Health and Human Services or the Centers for Disease Control and Prevention.

Chapter 18 - The following preliminary criteria define minimum and preferred characteristics of digital contact tracing tools to help health departments overcome one or more obstacles in the COVID-19 contact tracing workflow. They are based on preliminary research and targeted discussions with contact tracing and informatics experts across county, state, and federal government; national public health associations; academic consortia; and nongovernmental organizations.

Chapter 19 - "Contact tracing" is a public health measure used to control disease spread. Trained public health workers assist patients with an infectious disease recall their close contacts within a given timeframe, notify them of potential exposure, and provide advice to patients and contacts. Given the scale of the COVID-19 pandemic, some public health authorities are automating part of the tracing process with smartphone applications (apps). Some apps take advantage of Bluetooth signals to track individuals proximity to one another, otherwise known as "digital exposure notification (DEN)" Bluetooth allows short-range wireless communications between electronic devices. Apps may also be used by public health authorities to enable "digital contact tracing" (DCT), which may also use location data.

Chapter 20 - Many states, territories, and localities have implemented public health orders to limit the spread of Coronavirus Disease 2019 (COVID-19) in their respective communities, including stay-at-home orders, orders temporarily closing schools and businesses, and orders limiting the size of public gatherings. In preparation for the eventual relaxation and lifting of these orders, the Centers for Disease Control and Prevention (CDC) have advocated that public health authorities use robust "contact tracing" procedures to prevent the reoccurrence of widespread infections after communities reopen. While federal entities may advise on these procedures, state and local authorities are responsible for contact tracing operations, as provided by state law. The term "contact tracing" generally refers to identifying and monitoring people who have been in contact with someone diagnosed with an infectious disease, in order to locate other potentially infected individuals quickly and take targeted control measures (such as quarantines) to prevent the broader spread of the illness. Contact tracing is standard procedure in public health investigations, and historically involves officials interviewing and contacting infected and potentially-exposed persons. However, some of the contact tracing proposals aimed at controlling the spread of COVID-19 suggest supplementing traditional contact tracing procedures with technology to collect data electronically. These proposals raise questions about how federal laws governing health information privacy may apply to electronic or digital contact tracing. One such provision is the "HIPAA Privacy Rule," which refers collectively to regulations promulgated by the Department of Health and Human Services (HHS) under the Health Insurance Portability and Accountability Act (HIPAA). This Sidebar discusses the HIPAAPrivacy Rule's application to digital contact tracing and briefly discusses other federal laws that regulate data privacy.

Chapter 21 - As COVID-19 continues to spread, many public health authorities are turning to contact tracing— measures to identify, notify, and monitor infected individuals' contacts—to track potential COVID-19 exposure. Along with conventional techniques, technology companies, including Google and Apple, are developing digital contact-tracing and exposure notification tools. In addition, Congress has appropriated emergency funds to help facilitate contact-tracing efforts. But the idea of using personal information— including cell phone and location data—to track COVID-19 exposure has prompted groups such as the ACLU to raise privacy concerns and call for the protection of individuals' privacy and anonymity. In response, Members of Congress have introduced four data privacy bills addressing digital contact- tracing and exposure notification:

- the COVID-19 Consumer Data Protection Act of 2020 (CCDPA), S. 3663, introduced by Senators Roger Wicker, John Thune, Jerry Moran, Marsha Blackburn, and Deb Fischer on May 7, 2020;
- the Public Health Emergency Privacy Act (PHEPA), companion bills S. 3749 and H.R. 6866, introduced, respectively, by Senators Richard Blumenthal and Mark Warner and Representatives Anna Eshoo, Janice Schakowsky, Suzan DelBene, Yvette Clarke, G.K. Butterfield, and Tony Cardenas on May 14, 2020; and
- the Exposure Notification Privacy Act (ENPA), S. 3861, introduced by Senators Maria Cantwell and Bill Cassidy on June 1, 2020.

This chapter describes the main components of each bill and examines key differences among the proposals before identifying several issues for Congress.

Chapter 22 - Amid the ongoing COVID-19 pandemic, several states have developed and promoted contact-tracing mobile device apps to identify individuals who may have had contact with infected persons. Additionally, the two largest manufacturers of mobile device operating systems, Apple (iOS) and Google (Android), have announced plans to release application programming interfaces (APIs) to "enable interoperability between Android and iOS devices using apps from public health authorities."

Several bills in the 116th Congress would regulate the privacy of information collected through such contact-tracing apps.

- S. 3663, the COVID-19 Consumer Data Protection Act of 2020, would (1) require certain covered entities that collect contact-tracing information to provide individuals with prior notice of such collection and the opportunity to opt-in to such collection; (2) prohibit the use of such information for purposes unrelated to tracking the spread of COVID-19; and (3) require covered entities to publicize their privacy and data security practices.
- S. 3749 and H.R. 6866, the Public Health Emergency Privacy Act (PHEPA), would prohibit certain entities from disclosing contact-tracing information for purposes unrelated to public health. The bill would also prohibit such information from being used for commercial advertising or marketing purposes, or to discriminate against individuals with respect to "goods, services, facilities, privileges, advantages, or places of accommodations." Covered entities include state governmental entities, although PHEPA specifically exempts public health authorities.
- S. 3861, the Exposure Notification Privacy Act (ENPA), requires operators of "automated exposure notification systems" (AENS) to limit enrollment in such systems to individuals who have provided affirmative express consent, to publicize the system's privacy policy, and to limit transfers of covered data to the minimum necessary to notify other users or a public health authority of potential exposures. ENPA also requires operators of an AENS to establish data security practices to protect the confidentiality, integrity, availability, and accessibility of covered data.

In general, the bills above limit coverage to entities subject to the jurisdiction of the Federal Trade Commission or explicitly exempt state public health authorities. Nevertheless, during the debate surrounding this legislation, questions may arise over Congress's authority to regulate state governments' collection and dissemination of the relevant information. As context for that potential debate, this Legal Sidebar examines constitutional limitations on Congress's regulation of state activity, particularly in the context of applying federal privacy protections to state-held information.

In: Testing and Contract Tracing …
Editor: Ernesto M. Batista
ISBN: 978-1-53618-857-8
© 2020 Nova Science Publishers, Inc.

Chapter 1

COVID-19 TESTING: KEY ISSUES*

Amanda K. Sarata

The COVID-19 pandemic is affecting communities throughout the United States, with the country reporting the highest number of cases and deaths from the disease globally. Containment and mitigation efforts by federal, state, and local governments have been undertaken to "flatten the curve"—that is, to slow widespread transmission that could overwhelm the nation's health care system.

Diagnostic testing is a critical part of the clinical management of COVID-19, caused by the SARS-CoV-2 virus. In addition, both diagnostic and serology testing at scale may be a key component of efforts to ease mitigation measures prior to the development, manufacture, and broad distribution of a vaccine or effective therapeutic. Efforts in the United States to rapidly develop, scale up, and disseminate testing for COVID-19 have faced challenges, including supply chain issues; a shifting regulatory landscape; a lack of consensus around federal coordination of or strategy for testing; concerns with the accuracy of both molecular and serology tests; an early lack of data on test results and capacity; and a delayed ramp-up by

* This is an edited, reformatted and augmented version of Congressional Research Service Publication, No. IF11516 , dated April 23, 2020.

commercial laboratories and test manufacturers of both centralized and point-of-care testing. In addition, manufacturing and quality issues with the nation's initial test—developed by the Centers for Disease Control and Prevention (CDC)—resulted in significant delay in early access to testing throughout the country.

U.S. Laboratory Infrastructure

Public health testing may be used to help identify and contain the spread of a novel pathogen early in its introduction into the country, as well as to detect and monitor ongoing outbreaks. This testing relies on the CDC and the U.S. network of state and local public health laboratories, including some Department of Defense and international laboratories. In contrast, clinical diagnostic testing is carried out by a number of facilities, including private commercial laboratories (e.g., LabCorp); hospital and other clinical laboratories; and laboratories in academic medical centers and universities. These two systems, while overlapping and connected, have distinct purposes. Clinical testing may be centralized—a sample is collected and sent to a central laboratory for testing—or decentralized, or occurring at or near the patient or point of care, commonly referred to as point-of-care testing.

Diagnostic testing for COVID-19, in part because it is caused by a novel pathogen, was initially carried out by the country's network of public health laboratories. However, it is generally not the role of the public health laboratories to carry out the large-scale clinical diagnostic testing needed during a pandemic response, and demand outstripped supply quickly as the country transitioned to community spread. The commercial sector—including commercial laboratories and commercial test kit manufacturers—as well as clinical laboratories in hospitals and at universities are seen as critical to achieving the scope of testing needed during the COVID-19 public health emergency. Despite ramping up capacity across U.S. laboratories of all types, the country's network of laboratories continues to face challenges meeting the unprecedented demand for testing, in terms of volume, speed, and accuracy. Currently the country performs approximately 150,000 tests per day, and a significant increase in capacity would likely require additional infrastructure (more testing platforms, standing up additional laboratory facilities), in addition to maintaining testing at full current capacity.

TYPES OF COVID-19 TESTS

Testing for COVID-19 currently involves both molecular tests and immunoassays. Diagnostic testing for COVID-19 generally relies on *molecular* tests that use nucleic acid amplification techniques such as polymerase chain reaction (PCR) to detect viral genetic material. These tests identify viral nucleic acid in samples taken from individuals' noses or throats using swabs. This type of test is technically complex but well-characterized, generally requiring both specific instruments and highly trained laboratory personnel. PCR tests may be high-throughput, so many samples may be run simultaneously, but the run time is generally several hours. PCR tests may be laboratory- developed tests (LDTs), test kits, or point-of-care tests.Point-of-care tests are usually faster and simpler to run, but often only run a single or a few samples at one time.

COVID-19 testing may also be carried out using *immunoassays*. This type of test detects immune system proteins made by the host (antibodies) or viral components that stimulate the host's immune response (antigens). Tests that detect antibodies in the blood are called serology tests, and they generally indicate either late active infection or exposure to and recovery from prior infection. Serology tests are not generally used alone for diagnosis of disease; rather, they may sometimes be used in combination with a molecular test for diagnosis. Serology testing also may be used to identify individuals who can donate convalescent plasma as a possible therapeutic; to help guide development of a vaccine; and to determine the extent and spread of COVID-19 in the general population, as well as the infection fatality rate. Rapid antigen tests—which have not yet been authorized for use in the United States for COVID- 19—can detect viral antigens, generally in a throat or nose swab. These tests are usually point-of-care, low-cost, easy to use, and used for diagnostic purposes. However, these tests in particular tend to have lower accuracy than molecular diagnostic tests.

FDA Emergency Use Authorization (EUA) Guidance for COVID-19 Testing

Through guidance, the Food and Drug Administration (FDA) has allowed for modifications to the usual EUA process to facilitate a more rapid scale-up of testing. On February 29, FDA announced a policy which allows laboratories that have developed and validated their own COVID-19 diagnostics to begin using the tests prior to receiving Emergency Use Authorization, as long as the laboratory notifies FDA and submits EUA materials within 15 days. This guidance was updated on March 16 to apply similarly to commercial test kit manufacturers, allowing them to market test kits prior to receiving EUA. The agency also allowed tests to be used and marketed without EUA in two cases: (1) where states have authorized laboratories to carry out testing within the state and (2) for serology tests where the manufacturer notifies the agency and labels the test as required by the guidance. The agency reports that more than 100 serology tests are currently being marketed without EUA; serology tests may also be brought to market under an EUA, and several have been. In addition, any at- home test or self-collection of a specimen at home would need to have authorization prior to marketing. The agency has not yet authorized any at-home COVID-19 test. It did grant authorization for the first at-home self-collection kit for use with LabCorp's PCR test.

CLIA and the COVID-19 Pandemic

All clinical laboratories in the U.S. need to receive CLIA (Clinical Laboratory Improvement Amendments) certification in order to test human samples for purposes of clinical diagnosis and treatment. Many questions have arisen during the COVID-19 public health emergency about possible flexibilities in CLIA requirements, for example, with respect to the certification process or personnel qualifications, as well as the use of temporary testing sites. The Centers for Medicare & Medicaid Services (CMS) has issued guidance to provide some flexibility with respect to CLIA requirements using its enforcement discretion. In particular, CMS clarifies that testing may be performed at designated overflow sites and that laboratories may begin testing upon receiving a CLIA number, but prior to receiving a paper certificate.

ACCURACY CONCERNS WITH COVID-19 TESTING

Accuracy concerns have arisen with respect to both molecular diagnostic and serological COVID-19 testing. It has been reported that PCR tests for COVID-19 may return as many as 30% false negatives (a negative result, where the individual is a true positive). While no diagnostic test performs with perfect accuracy, certain issues may result in lower accuracy. PCR-based tests are generally very accurate, but problems can occur with sampling technique, storage and transport, and the extraction step. In addition, viral load varies during the course of an infection and can affect the amount of virus in a collected sample. Serology tests authorized by FDA generally have high sensitivity (ability to detect a true positive) and specificity (ability to detect a true negative); their accuracy may vary based on the prevalence of the infection in the tested population. In addition, technical issues such as cross- reactivity with antibodies from commonly circulating coronaviruses can return false positives. Serology tests are allowed to be marketed and used without an EUA, creating further unknowns about performance of these tests. The FDA is working with other federal agencies to provide voluntary validation for these tests.

Supply Chain and COVID-19 Testing

Supply chain issues related to COVID-19 diagnostic testing have affected access to testing nationally. As the FDA has granted EUAs for more LDTs and test kits—including point-of-care tests—and testing volume has increased, laboratories across the country have reported shortages in necessary supplies. PCR testing involves sample collection, nucleic acid extraction, and testing to identify presence of the SARS-CoV-2 virus. Supplies needed for each of these steps have been in shortage, including swabs needed for sample collection; viral transport media needed to stabilize and store the sample after collection and during transport; RNA extraction kits and reagents needed to extract viral RNA from the sample prior to testing; and instruments, test kits, and testing reagents needed to amplify and detect viral nucleic acid. Personal protective equipment (PPE) needed during sample collection has similarly been in short supply.

These shortages have been anecdotally reported by laboratories, and were documented in an April 3 report by the Department of Health and Human Services Office of the Inspector General addressing hospitals' experience responding to COVID-19. The report notes that "severe shortages of testing supplies and extended waits for test results limited hospitals' ability to monitor the health of patients and staff." FDA has worked with industry to try to identify and mitigate shortages through modifications to test EUAs that allow for the use of alternate supplies when carrying out a test and the establishment of an industry hotline for device shortages. However, shortages reportedly persist due to global demand and the unprecedented level of testing, as well as a lack of coordinated ascertainment, production, and allocation of supplies, and the FDA does not have the authority to allocate or distribute supplies.

Serology Testing to Determine COVID-19 Spread in the United States

Many cases of COVID-19 are reportedly mild or asymptomatic, and therefore go undetected. As such, widespread serology testing would help to characterize the scope and extent of the disease in the United States. CDC reported in late March that the agency is in the early stages of beginning serosurveys—surveys that measure the proportion of a population that has antibodies to an infection—to gauge the spread of COVID-19. The first of these studies is already underway in six major metropolitan areas, including New York City and Seattle, and it aims to "monitor how many people develop SARS-CoV-2 antibodies over time." NIH also recently reported it has undertaken a large serosurvey to determine how many healthy adults have been exposed to COVID-19.

In: Testing and Contract Tracing … ISBN: 978-1-53618-857-8
Editor: Ernesto M. Batista © 2020 Nova Science Publishers, Inc.

Chapter 2

COVID-19 TESTING: FREQUENTLY ASKED QUESTIONS*

Amanda K. Sarata and Elayne J. Heisler

ABSTRACT

The United States is reporting some of the highest number of cases and deaths from the Coronavirus Disease 2019 (COVID-19) pandemic globally, and the disease is affecting communities nationwide. In response, federal, state, and local governments have undertaken containment and mitigation efforts to "flatten the curve"—that is, to slow widespread transmission that could overwhelm the nation's health care system and to reduce spread of the disease while treatments and vaccines are being developed that will lessen the health impact of the virus.

Diagnostic testing is a critical part of the clinical management of COVID-19, which is caused by the SARS-CoV-2 virus. Both diagnostic (i.e., testing for active infection) and serology testing (i.e., testing for the presence of antibodies, potentially indicating a previous infection) over a wide population may be a key component of efforts to ease mitigation measures and allow people to return safely to work and school. Ongoing

* This is an edited, reformatted and augmented version of Congressional Research Service, Publication No. R46481, dated August 11, 2020.

testing can be used for public health purposes to identify and isolate positive cases of COVID-19, thereby reducing spread of the disease. However, the use of testing for public health purposes rather than for the clinical diagnosis of individuals poses legal and policy complications, because regulation and payment policies can differ based on how the test is used.

Further, COVID-19 testing in the United States is provided in a number of health care and community-based settings. Insurance coverage and payment for a given COVID-19 test can depend on a number of factors, including the entity administering the test or processing test results, and the reason for which the test is administered. These factors can determine whether a certain payment mechanism may be used to pay for a given test. Congress, through several coronavirus legislative packages, has enacted various insurance coverage requirements along with other funding mechanisms to help pay for testing.

This chapter provides answers to numerous questions related to COVID-19 testing, including

- types of testing available and their reliability;
- testing capacity and infrastructure;
- delivery of testing, including the settings where testing is available;
- payment for testing, including the provision by federally operated health systems and payment by federal and private payors and payment sources available for people who are uninsured;
- reporting of test results; and
- federal funding for testing infrastructure and for the clinical provision of COVID-19 testing.

This chapter concludes with several appendices: Appendix A identifies acronyms used in this chapter, Appendix B lists CRS experts on the various testing topics discussed, and Appendix C provides testing-related resources.

INTRODUCTION

The United States is reporting some of the highest number of cases and deaths from the Coronavirus Disease 2019 (COVID-19) pandemic globally, and the disease is affecting communities nationwide. In response, federal, state, and local governments have undertaken containment and mitigation efforts to "flatten the curve"—that is, to slow widespread transmission that could overwhelm the nation's health care system and to reduce spread of the disease while treatments and vaccines are being developed that will lessen the health impact of the virus.

Diagnostic testing is a critical part of the clinical management of COVID-19, which is caused by the SARS-CoV-2 virus. Both diagnostic (i.e., testing for active infection) and serology testing (i.e., testing for the presence of antibodies, potentially indicating a previous infection) over a wide population may be a key component of efforts to ease mitigation measures and allow people to return safely to work and school. Ongoing testing can be used for public health purposes to identify and isolate positive cases of COVID-19, thereby reducing spread of the disease.

However, the use of testing for public health purposes rather than for the clinical diagnosis of individuals poses legal and policy complications, because regulation and payment policies can differ based on how the test is used.

Further, COVID-19 testing in the United States is provided in a number of health care and community-based settings. Insurance coverage and payment for a given COVID-19 test can depend on a number of factors, including the entity administering the test or processing test results, and the reason for which the test is administered. These factors can determine whether a certain funding source or payment mechanism may be used to pay for a given test. Congress, through several coronavirus legislative packages, has enacted various insurance coverage requirements along with other funding mechanisms to help pay for testing.

This chapter provides answers to numerous questions related to COVID-19 testing. These include, among others, questions about the types of tests and their uses, where individuals can access testing, funding for testing-related efforts, and how different payers will reimburse providers for testing. As testing has become more widely available, questions have arisen about the settings where people can access testing, and how payment for such testing and accompanying services occurs. In addition, in anticipation of serology testing becoming more frequent, questions have arisen about the availability of and payment for those tests. Appendix C provides a list of testing- related resources; it will be updated as additional information becomes available or additional issues arise.

COVID-19 Testing Overview

COVID-19 testing—including its development, regulation, accuracy, supply, capacity, infrastructure, availability, coverage, and payment—has been a central and ongoing issue throughout the COVID-19 public health emergency. Early efforts to develop a national test, led by the Centers for Disease Control and Prevention (CDC), encountered challenges.[1] Actions taken by the Food and Drug Administration (FDA) to increase the flexibility of COVID-19 in vitro diagnostics (IVDs) regulation[2] facilitated access to testing, but also created an environment of uncertainty for commercial manufacturers and clinical laboratories, as well as for health care providers and patients.[3] Issues have arisen around the accuracy of tests, their broad uses, and the settings in which they may be used for clinical purposes, as well as for nondiagnostic purposes such as screening. In addition, considerations regarding these issues may vary based on whether a test is diagnostic or serological.

What Are the Different Types of COVID-19 Tests?

Generally, coronavirus diagnostics (IVDs) may be molecular, serological, or antigen tests.[4] From a technical perspective, tests are characterized by their methods, as well as by the substance they directly

---

[1] See *Development and Regulation of Domestic Diagnostic Testing for Novel Coronavirus (COVID-19): Frequently Asked Questions*.

[2] See CRS In Focus IF11516, *COVID-19 Testing: Key Issues*.

[3] Medium, "Regulatory uncertainty made COVID responses difficult," April 6, 2020, https://medium.com/cgo-benchmark/regulatory-uncertainty-made-covid-responses-difficult-c7e6e5e8f7c3.

[4] FDA, "Coronavirus Testing Basics," https://www.fda.gov/consumers/consumer-updates/coronavirus-testing-basics.

identify: antigens,[5] antibodies,[6] or viral nucleic acid. To date, development of COVID-19 tests has largely focused on molecular tests, and specifically tests using a technique called Polymerase Chain Reaction (PCR), as well as on serology tests, those tests that identify the presence of antibodies to the SARS-CoV-2 virus. Only a handful of antigen tests have been authorized by the FDA, although more may be authorized in the future.[7] This type of test directly identifies the presence of a SARS-CoV-2 antigen, or protein, through the use of SARS-CoV-2 antibodies which preferentially bind to the SARS-CoV-2 antigen.

From a clinical perspective, tests may be used to diagnose an active infection (by detecting the virus directly) or a prior infection (by detecting antibodies to the virus). Molecular and antigen tests are used to diagnose current infection, whereas serology tests are used to determine prior infection.[8] Table 1 provides a summary of the types of tests, their uses, and accuracy.

Molecular Diagnostic Testing

Molecular diagnostic testing for COVID-19 generally relies on nucleic acid amplification techniques (NAATs), such as PCR, to detect viral genetic material. These tests identify viral nucleic acid in samples taken from individuals' noses or throats using swabs and are technically complex but well characterized, generally requiring both specific instruments and highly trained laboratory personnel. PCR-based testing involves sample collection (usually a swab, as noted), viral nucleic acid extraction, and direct testing to

---

[5] An antigen is defined by the National Cancer Institute (NCI) as follows: "Any substance that causes the body to make an immune response against that substance. Antigens include toxins, chemicals, bacteria, viruses, or other substances that come from outside the body," https://www.cancer.gov/publications/dictionaries/cancer-terms/def/antigen.

[6] An antibody is defined by NCI as follows: "A protein made by plasma cells (a type of white blood cell) in response to an antigen (a substance that causes the body to make a specific immune response). Each antibody can bind to only one specific antigen. The purpose of this binding is to help destroy the antigen," https://www.cancer.gov/publications/ dictionaries/cancer-terms/def/antibody.

[7] Food and Drug Administration (FDA), "In Vitro Diagnostics EUAs," https://www.fda.gov/medical-devices/coronavirus-disease-2019-covid-19-emergency-use-authorizations-medical-devices/vitro-diagnostics-euas. EUA is an emergency use authorization.

[8] FDA, "FAQs on Testing for SARS-CoV-2," https://www.fda.gov/medical-devices/emergency-situations-medical- devices/faqs-testing-sars-cov-2.

identify the presence of the SARS-CoV-2 viral nucleic acid through reverse transcription, amplification, and detection techniques. PCR tests may be high-throughput, whereby many samples may be run simultaneously; in that case, the run time is generally several hours. PCR or other NAAT-based tests may also be point-of-care tests, which are typically faster and simpler to run, but often run only a single or a few samples at one time.

Antigen Testing

An antigen test uses antibodies to a specific antigen (e.g., SARS-CoV-2 virus) to identify the virus in a patient's sample. Unlike a COVID-19 serology test, which can determine prior infection, an antigen test can determine an active infection. This difference is accounted for by the fact that a serology test identifies antibodies, a product of the immune response whose generation lags infection, whereas an antigen test directly identifies the virus. Rapid antigen tests—of which only a handful have been authorized for use in the United States for COVID-19 to date[9]—can detect viral antigens, generally in a throat or nose swab. These tests, used for diagnostic purposes, are usually point-of-care, relatively low-cost, and easy to manufacture and use. However, they tend to be less accurate than molecular diagnostic tests.

Serology Testing

A COVID-19 serology test identifies antibodies to the SARS-CoV-2 virus, usually in an individual blood sample. Antibodies are proteins generated by the immune system in response to an antigen, or foreign substance, and their generation lags infection by a week or more. An antigen may be a pathogenic virus or bacteria, for example, or generally any substance recognized by the immune system as both foreign and harmful. Serology tests for SARS-CoV-2 indicate exposure to and recovery from prior infection with the virus. The FDA has stated that such tests are not

---

[9] FDA, "In Vitro Diagnostics EUAs," https://www.fda.gov/medical-devices/coronavirus-disease-2019-covid-19- emergency-use-authorizations-medical-devices/vitro-diagnostics-euas.

authorized to be used alone for the diagnosis of COVID-19.[10] However, serology testing may be used to identify individuals who can donate convalescent plasma[11] as a possible therapeutic, to help guide development of a vaccine, and to determine the extent and spread of COVID-19 in the general population, as well as the true infection fatality rate. In addition, as scientists learn more about the extent and duration of immunity that antibodies may confer after natural infection, serology testing could be informative about a given individual's immunity.

For What Purposes Is COVID-19 Testing Used?

Broadly, testing may be used for surveillance, screening, or diagnosis.[12] *Surveillance* may be used to provide information at a population or community level; it does not generally guide decisions at the individual level. Surveillance testing may guide decisions, for example, about public health mitigation or other measures. Such testing may employ serology testing to help determine what proportion of a given population or subpopulation has had and recovered from coronavirus infection, or it may use diagnostic testing to provide early indicators of emerging outbreaks or population-level estimates of the number of individuals with COVID-19 infections.

Screening is typically carried out in individuals who are asymptomatic and who have no reason to believe that they are currently infected (e.g., due to recent exposure or travel history). This type of testing is generally done in groups of individuals, such as students at a school or employees in a

---

[10] FDA, "FAQs on Testing for SARS-CoV-2," https://www.fda.gov/medical-devices/emergency-situations-medical- devices/faqs-testing-sars-cov-2.

[11] *Convalescent plasma* refers to blood plasma that is collected from an individual who has recovered (i.e., "convalesced") from a disease, in this case COVID-19, and then administered to a patient actively sick with COVID-19 for treatment. See CRS Report R46375, *The U.S. Blood Supply and the COVID-19 Response: In Brief*.

[12] For a high-level overview of these three types of testing, see FDA, "FAQs on Testing for SARS-CoV-2," "Q: What is the difference between surveillance, screening, and diagnostic testing for COVID-19 testing?," https://www.fda.gov/ medical-devices/emergency-situations-medical-devices/faqs-testing-sars-cov-2.

workplace, as a way to prevent the spread of disease to others rather than to inform treatment for an individual. Although screening in the case of COVID-19 in a setting such as a workplace or a school can guide decisions about individuals—for example, whether they should stay home or self-isolate for a period of time—it does not necessarily guide clinical decisions about an individual's care. Screening may use molecular- or antigen-based tests, rather than serology tests, to directly detect the presence of the virus, and this type of testing would generally be confirmed with additional testing were an individual to begin to show symptoms.

Finally, *diagnosis* involves a molecular or antigen test to directly test for the presence of the virus, either in the presence of signs or symptoms, or with a reason to suspect that an individual may be actively infected with SARS-CoV-2. Such testing would guide clinical decisions and disease management at the individual level. Serology tests are not currently used for clinical diagnostic purposes or to establish the exclusion of infection, per relevant FDA guidance on diagnostic testing for COVID-19 during the COVID-19 emergency period.[13]

When Is COVID-19 Testing Clinically Useful?

The answer to this question depends on the type of test and the circumstances of the testing. Serology testing at the current time is not generally clinically useful for the treatment or management of COVID-19 at an individual level.[14] Moreover, serology testing does not provide reliable information about an active, current infection, nor does it currently provide information about immunity to reinfection. The mechanism of the immune response to infection with SARS- CoV-2—whether antibodies provide immunity and, if so, for what duration, and what level of antibody might be required for this effect—is largely unknown at this time. In certain fact-

---

[13] FDA, "Policy for Coronavirus Disease-2019 Tests During the Public Health Emergency (Revised)," May 11, 2020, https://www.fda.gov/regulatory-information/search-fda-guidance-documents/policy-coronavirus-disease-2019-tests-during-public-health-emergency-revised.

[14] See for example, the American Medical Association, "Serological testing for SARS-CoV-2 antibodies," May 14, 2020, https://www.ama-assn.org/delivering-care/public-health/serological-testing-sars-cov-2-antibodies.

specific cases, serology testing results may inform clinical treatment or management, but these cases are not the norm.

Molecular diagnostic or rapid antigen testing is clinically useful in the presence of signs or symptoms, or in the context of a known or suspected exposure. This type of testing in the absence of any reason to suspect infection, or in the absence of signs or symptoms of illness, is generally not clinically useful. Individuals who receive a positive result in this case may be either asymptomatic (meaning they will not ever exhibit clinical disease) or presymptomatic (meaning they are infected but have not yet begun to show clinical signs or symptoms of the disease). In the case of an asymptomatic case, no clinical treatment will be needed, so the test result is not clinically useful. In the case of a presymptomatic case, once the tested individual begins to exhibit symptoms, clinical treatment may become necessary, but testing would likely be repeated at that time to confirm the diagnosis. At this time, there are no therapeutic options for individuals who have been exposed, but are asymptomatic or presymptomatic. In the future, it is possible that screening tests could be used to guide clinical decisions, such as giving an exposed individual treatment to prevent transmission to others and/or severe health outcomes.

How Accurate Are Diagnostic and Serology Tests?

The accuracy of diagnostic testing is primarily determined by assessing two test performance characteristics: (1) the ability of the test to identify true positives (people with disease) and (2) the ability of the test to identify true negatives (people without the disease). These are referred to as *sensitivity*—the ability to detect a true positive—and *specificity*—the ability to detect a true negative.[15] A test with high sensitivity will have a low rate of false negatives, whereas a test with high specificity will have a low rate of false positives. These distinctions have different implications in the context of an

---

[15] Cochrane UK, "Sensitivity and specificity explained: A Cochrane UK Trainees blog," https://uk.cochrane.org/news/sensitivity-and-specificity-explained-cochrane-uk-trainees-blog.

infectious disease; specifically, a false negative may result in the unknowing transmission of the disease to others, whereas a false positive may result in incorrect therapeutic treatment decisions or unnecessary use of Personal Protective Equipment (PPE), among other things.

Table 1. Summary of COVID-19 testing types, uses, and accuracy

Appropriate for						
Type of test	**What it tests for**	**Approval status**	**Diagnosis**	**Screening**	**Surveillance**	**Accuracy issues**
Molecular	Detects viral genetic material	More than 100 EUA authorized tests	Yes	Yes (e.g., workplace or school testing)	Yes (for outbreaks)	False negatives may occur where samples have low amounts of virus or due to poor sampling technique
Serological	Detects serum antibodies	More than 40 EUA authorized tests	No	No	Yes (for prevalence estimates)	False positives may occur from cross-reactivity of antibodies from non-SARS- CoV-2 common coronaviruses
Antigen	Detects viral antigen	Fewer than 5 EUA authorized tests	Yes	Yes (e.g., workplace or school testing)	Yes (for outbreaks)	False negatives or false positives may occur

Sources: CRS Analysis of "What Are the Different Types of COVID-19 Tests?," and FDA, "In Vitro Diagnostics EUAs," https://www.fda.gov/medical-devices/coronavirus-disease-2019-covid-19-emergency-use-authorizations- medical-devices/vitro-diagnostics-euas.

Note: EUA = emergency use authorization.

Accuracy concerns have arisen with respect to both diagnostic and serological COVID-19 testing.[16] With respect to molecular diagnostic testing for COVID-19, tests are generally highly specific (i.e., false positives are unlikely) but problems can occur with respect to sensitivity, or false

[16] S. Woloshin et al., "False Negative Tests for SARS-CoV-2 Infection—Challenges and Implications," *New England Journal of Medicine*, 383(6), August 6, 2020, https://www.nejm.org/doi/full/10.1056/NEJMp2015897.

negatives. Recent research indicates that the false negative rate varies based on the timing of the test, with the most accurate testing occurring approximately three days after the onset of symptoms.[17] Although no diagnostic test performs with perfect accuracy, certain issues may result in lower accuracy. PCR-based tests are usually very accurate and will generally reliably identify viral nucleic acid if it is present in amounts above the limit of detection for a given diagnostic. However, problems can occur with sampling technique, storage, and transport of the sample (e.g., over-dilution, temperature maintenance), and the extraction step.[18] In addition, viral load varies during the course of an infection by site (e.g., throat, nose), thereby affecting the amount of virus present in a collected sample, which can in turn affect the test results.

Serology tests authorized by the FDA are now required to meet specified thresholds for sensitivity and specificity, although the tests' accuracy can still vary based on the underlying prevalence of the infection in the tested population.[19] In terms of accuracy, serology tests may have the opposite problem that molecular diagnostics generally have—that is, they tend to have issues with specificity and the return of false positive results. This inaccuracy may occur because cross- reactivity with antibodies from commonly circulating coronaviruses or other viruses can return false positives (the result is not specific enough to SARS-CoV-2). Serology tests were initially allowed to be marketed and used without an Emergency Use Authorization (EUA), which contributed to uncertainty about how well these tests perform initially.[20] An EUA is an authorization granted by the FDA when certain conditions are met (e.g., a public health emergency) that allows

[17] LM Kucirka et al., "Variation in False-Negative Rate of Reverse Transcriptase Polymerase Chain Reaction–Based SARS-CoV-2 Tests by Time Since Exposure," *Annals of Internal Medicine*, May 13, 2020, https://www.acpjournals.org/doi/10.7326/M20-1495.

[18] FDA, "Coronavirus Testing Basics (Molecular Tests)," https://www.fda.gov/consumers/consumer-updates/coronavirus-testing-basics.

[19] FDA, "Medical Countermeasures Initiative Update," May 6, 2020, https://www.fda.gov/media/137706/download; and FDA, "In Vitro Diagnostics EUAs," Serology Template for Commercial Manufacturers, updated June 26, 2020, https://www.fda.gov/medical-devices/coronavirus-disease-2019-covid-19-emergency-use-authorizations-medical- devices/vitro-diagnostics-euas.

[20] FDA, "Insight into FDA's Revised Policy on Antibody Tests: Prioritizing Access and Accuracy," May 4, 2020, https://www.fda.gov/news-events/fda-voices/insight-fdas-revised-policy-antibody-tests-prioritizing-access-and- accuracy.

an unapproved medical product to be marketed and used clinically.[21] The FDA is currently working with other federal agencies (e.g., the National Institutes of Health (NIH)) to provide independent validation for these tests, and it has modified its guidance to require manufacturers to receive authorization for commercially manufactured and marketed serology tests.[22]

TESTING CAPACITY AND INFRASTRUCTURE

Testing for COVID-19—including for diagnostic, screening and surveillance purposes—is straining the clinical laboratory infrastructure in the United States and placing stress on the testing supply chain.[23] Clinical diagnostic testing is done by a network of private and public laboratories, as well as at the point of care by health care providers in health care settings. Clinical laboratories include large commercial reference laboratories (e.g., Quest); academic and university laboratories (e.g., University of Washington Medicine Virology Laboratory[24]); and hospital and other clinical laboratories. Testing is also carried out by CDC and other federal laboratories and the U.S. network of state and local public health laboratories, including some Department of Defense (DOD) and international laboratories.[25] Clinical laboratories report that the supply chain has been stressed at every point, and that access to testing and testing turn-around time continues to vary significantly across the country, with excess capacity in some areas and excess demand in others.[26] In late May, the

---

[21] For more information about the EUA mechanism, see CRS In Focus IF10745, *Emergency Use Authorization and FDA's Related Authorities*.

[22] FDA, "Immediately in Effect Guidance for Clinical Laboratories, Commercial Manufacturers, and Food and Drug Administration Staff," May 11, 2020, https://www.fda.gov/media/135659/download.

[23] American Association for Clinical Chemistry (AACC), "COVID-19 Survey Results," https://www.aacc.org/science-and-practice/aacc-covid-19-testing-survey/full-survey-results.

[24] University of Washington Medicine, "UW Virology COVID-19 Dashboard," http://depts.washington.edu/labmed/ covid19/.

[25] See CDC, "Introduction to Public Health Laboratories," https://www.cdc.gov/publichealth101/laboratories.html.

[26] Association of Molecular Pathology, "SARS-CoV-2 Molecular Testing, Summary of Recent SARS-CoV-2 Molecular Testing Survey," https://www.amp.org/AMP/assets/AMP_SARS-CoV-2_Survey_Report_FINAL.pdf?pass= 28.

Department of Health and Human Services (HHS) released a strategic plan compiling certain testing-related information pursuant to a requirement in the Paycheck Protection Program and Healthcare Enhancement Act (PPPHCEA, P.L. 116-139).[27] However, a uniform and centralized federal-level testing plan is not currently in place to establish and guide testing nationally.[28] A federal testing plan would likely involve assessing the amounts of each type of test needed and for what purpose; identifying existing and needed nationwide testing capacity; and completing an inventory of existing supplies, and tracking and overseeing their distribution, among other things. The HHS strategic plan defers to states to implement testing.[29] States and jurisdictions have developed strategies to test their populations, specifically with respect to the types and amount of tests needed, as well as their current capacity and plans for overall testing, including for diagnosis, contact tracing, surveillance, testing in congregate or high-risk health care and employment settings, and general workplace and school-based screening.[30]

What Is Point-of-Care vs. Centralized Testing?

Clinical testing may be *centralized*, in which a sample is collected and sent to a central laboratory for testing, or *decentralized*, in which the testing occurs entirely at or near the patient or point of care (POC), commonly referred to as point-of-care testing. The FDA notes that "point of care" includes patient care settings such as "hospitals, physician offices, urgent

---

[27] P.L. 116-139, Division B "Additional Emergency Appropriations for Coronavirus Response," Title I, "Department of Health and Human Services."

[28] See, for example, Politico, "A dangerous new chapter of the outbreak: Every state for itself," July 14, 2020, https://www.politico.com/news/2020/07/14/states-look-to-trump-for-a-national-plan-to-fight-coronavirus-361906.

[29] Department of Health and Human Services (HHS), "COVID Strategic Testing Plan," May 24, 2020, "The role of the Federal government is to enable innovation, help scale supplies, and provide strategic guidance. States, territories, and tribes are responsible for formulating and implementing testing plans; and the private sector will continue to develop and produce technologies, supplies, and services to meet the needs of the States," pp. 7, https://delauro.house.gov/sites/ delauro.house.gov/files/HHS_COVID_Testing_Report.pdf.

[30] HHS, "Coronavirus (COVID-19) Testing Plans by State and Jurisdiction," https://www.hhs.gov/coronavirus/testing- plans/index.html.

care, outreach clinics, pharmacies, and temporary patient care settings that have appropriately trained personnel to perform the test and are operating under a CLIA Certificate of Waiver or Certificate of Compliance."[31] In addition, the agency notes that, in general, "point of care" does not apply to at- home testing or at-home sample collection.[32] The FDA has authorized a handful of molecular diagnostic point-of-care tests (e.g., Abbott IDNow) and two antigen point-of-care tests to date, but the majority of EUA-authorized tests are not authorized for use in a point-of-care setting.[33] Sample collection alone may also occur in point-of-care settings (e.g., a drive-through testing site), with the test sample being collected at the site but sent to a central laboratory for processing and return of results.

POC tests are particularly important in cases where an individual is seriously ill and a test result is needed quickly to care for the individual and conserve PPE, as well as in places that are far away from centralized laboratories—particularly rural and remote areas. POC tests are generally noted for being faster, less expensive, less technically complex to run, and simpler to manufacture.[34] However, these tests are also often less accurate and, in particular, may be less sensitive, meaning they return more false negatives than a comparable non-POC molecular diagnostic would.[35] There have been accuracy issues with at least one of the FDA-authorized POC molecular diagnostics, which led the FDA to require confirmation of negative results with an authorized high-sensitivity molecular diagnostic.[36]

---

[31] CLIA refers to the Clinical Laboratory Improvement Amendments of 1988 (P.L. 100-578), a law that regulates all clinical laboratories in the United States. For more information, see https://www.cms.gov/Regulations-and-Guidance/ Legislation/CLIA.

[32] FDA, "FAQs on Testing for SARS-CoV-2," https://www.fda.gov/medical-devices/emergency-situations-medical- devices/faqs-testing-sars-cov-2.

[33] FDA, "In Vitro Diagnostics EUAs," https://www.fda.gov/medical-devices/coronavirus-disease-2019-covid-19-emergency-use-authorizations-medical-devices/vitro-diagnostics-euas.

[34] National Academy of Sciences, "Rapid Expert Consultation on SARS-CoV-2 Laboratory Testing for the COVID-19 Pandemic (April 8, 2020)," https://www.nap.edu/catalog/25775/rapid-expert-consultation-on-sars-cov-2-laboratory- testing-for-the-covid-19-pandemic-april-8-2020.

[35] See for example Office of the Assistant Secretary for Health, "Guidance – Proposed Use of Point-of-Care (POC) Testing Platforms for SARS-CoV-2 (COVID-19)," https://www.cdc.gov/coronavirus/2019-ncov/downloads/OASH-COVID-19-guidance-testing-platforms.pdf.

[36] FDA notes that "negative results should be treated as presumptive and, if inconsistent with clinical signs and symptoms or necessary for patient management, should be tested with

Consequently, the speed and cost- effectiveness associated with POC tests may potentially be offset if additional steps are needed to mitigate accuracy issues. However, POC diagnostics' sensitivity can be weighed against their turnaround time and frequency, particularly in the context of screening and surveillance. Specifically, research suggests that frequent testing with a faster turnaround time is more important than test sensitivity to effective control of virus spread. A recent article notes that "[t]esting frequency was found to be the primary driver of population-level epidemic control, with only a small margin of improvement provided by using a more sensitive test."[37]

Is There a Federal COVID-19 Testing Plan or Program?

There has been substantial discussion about how to coordinate and organize COVID-19 testing efforts in the United States. Numerous experts in public health and medicine have weighed in on this issue, with many preparing model testing strategies and recommending various approaches to a coordinated national plan.[38] Many experts have called for a national strategy coordinated and led by the federal government;[39] however, to date, the states have been generally tasked with carrying out their own testing programs and strategies, with strategic guidance from the federal

---

different authorized or cleared molecular tests." See Abbott IDNow Letter of Authorization, updated June 1, 2020, https://www.fda.gov/media/136522/download.

[37] Daniel B. Larremore et al., "Test sensitivity is secondary to frequency and turnaround time for COVID-19 surveillance," medRxiv, June 27, 2020, https://www.medrxiv.org/content/10.1101/2020.06.22.20136309v2.full.pdf.

[38] See for example: (1) Rockefeller Foundation, "National Covid-19 Testing & Tracing Action Plan," July 2020, https://www.rockefellerfoundation.org/national-covid-19-testing-and-tracing-action-plan/; (2) Harvard Center for Ethics, "ROADMAP TO PANDEMIC RESILIENCE: Massive Scale Testing, Tracing, and Supported Isolation (TTSI) as the Path to Pandemic Resilience for a Free Society," April 20, 2020, https://ethics.harvard.edu/files/center-for-ethics/files/roadmaptopandemicresilience_updated_4.20.20.pdf; and (3) American Enterprise Institute, "National coronavirus response: A road map to reopening," March 29, 2020, https://www.aei.org/research-products/report/national-coronavirus-response-a-road-map-to-reopening/.

[39] See, for example, LabPulse.com, "The case for a national COVID-19 testing strategy: A Q&A with Dr. Gary Procop," June 26, 2020, https://www.labpulse.com/index.aspx?sec=sup&sub=pth&pag=dis&ItemID=801411.

government. Recently, HHS announced the launch of the National COVID-19 Testing Implementation Forum, described as "a new program to capture feedback between federal officials and the private sector."[40] Information about the initiative is limited, but stated goals include gathering private sector input on end-to-end supply chain issues and implementation of a national surveillance strategy. In addition, seven states—Louisiana, Maryland, Massachusetts, Michigan, Ohio, North Carolina and Virginia—recently announced the formation of a bipartisan purchasing compact to procure large volumes of rapid antigen tests directly from the tests' manufacturers, bypassing the federal government and using their combined leverage in an effort to secure needed tests and ensure manufacturers of demand for their product.[41]

PPPHCEA required HHS to develop and submit to Congress a COVID-19 strategic testing plan.[42] The plan was required to help states understand the types of testing available for COVID-19, provide guidelines for testing and estimates of testing production, and outline how the HHS Secretary will increase testing capacity and testing supplies. This testing plan was submitted in report form to statutorily designated congressional committees on May 24, 2020, and was not required to be released publicly. The report provides detailed background on the types of COVID- 19 tests, as well as an overview of the types of laboratories carrying out testing (the testing "ecosystem"), among other things, but it did not provide an overarching federal level strategy. Instead, the report notes that the responsibility for implementing testing rests with the states.[43] The PPPHCEA also required

---

[40] HHS, "HHS Announces National COVID-19 Testing Implementation Forum," July 21 2020, https://www.hhs.gov/about/news/2020/07/21/hhs-announces-national-covid-19-testing-implementation-forum.html.

[41] Washington Post, "There's no national testing strategy for coronavirus. These states banded together to make one.," August 4, 2020, https://www.washingtonpost.com/coronavirus/coronavirus-state-testing-compact/2020/08/04/8b73bed8-d66f-11ea-9c3b-dfc394c03988_story.html.

[42] P.L. 116-139, Division B, "Additional Emergency Appropriations for Coronavirus Response," Title I, Department of Health and Human Services.

[43] HHS, "Report to Congress: COVID Strategic Testing Plan," May 24, 2020, "The role of the Federal government is to enable innovation, help scale supplies, and provide strategic guidance. States, territories, and tribes are responsible for formulating and implementing testing plans; and the private sector will continue to develop and produce technologies,

states and other jurisdictions receiving funding pursuant to the act to submit testing plans that include the following information: the number of tests needed; estimates of laboratory and testing capacity, including related to workforce, equipment and supplies, and available tests; and a description of how the state, locality, territory, tribe, or tribal organization will use its resources for testing, including how such use relates to easing any COVID-19 community mitigation policies.[44] According to the national report submitted by HHS to Congress, "States are requested to detail how a minimum of two percent of the State's population will be tested each month beginning immediately; as well as plans to increase that number by the fall of 2020."[45] The state plans were initially required to be submitted to HHS 30 days post-enactment, but states were given an extension to May 30 for plans covering May and June, and until June 15 for plans covering the remainder of 2020. Although these state plans were not required to be released publicly, HHS made them publicly available on July 10, 2020.[46] In late June, Representative Frank Pallone sent a letter to HHS requesting the public release of the state testing plans.[47]

What Supply Chain-Related Issues Are Affecting COVID-19 Testing?

It has been widely reported that supply chain issues related to COVID-19 diagnostic testing have affected access to testing nationally.[48] The supply

supplies, and services to meet the needs of the States," pp. 7, https://delauro.house.gov/sites/delauro.house.gov/files/ HHS_COVID_Testing_Report.pdf.

[44] P.L. 116-139, Division B, "Additional Emergency Appropriations for Coronavirus Response," Title I, Department of Health and Human Services.

[45] HHS, "Report to Congress: COVID-19 Strategic Testing Plan," May 24, 2020, pp. 71-81, https://delauro.house.gov/ sites/delauro.house.gov/files/HHS_COVID_Testing_Report.pdf (hereinafter, HHS, "COVID-19 Strategic Testing Plan").

[46] HHS, "Coronavirus (COVID-19) Testing Plans by State and Jurisdiction," July 10, 2020, https://www.hhs.gov/ coronavirus/testing-plans/index.html.

[47] 360dx.com, "US Congressman Requests State COVID-19 Testing Plans From HHS," June 26, 2020, https://www.360dx.com/infectious-disease/us-congressman-requests-state-covid-19-testing-plans-hhs#.XxY7EJ5Kg4k.

[48] See for example McKinsey & Company, "COVID-19: Overcoming supply shortages for diagnostic testing," July 15, 2020, https://www.mckinsey.com/industries/pharmaceuticals-

chain for molecular diagnostics—the type of testing most in demand and, as a result, the one putting the most stress on its supply chain—is not streamlined and has not been developed to support the high-volume capacity, rapid sample-to- answer testing required during the pandemic. The testing industry has been described as "bespoke,"[49] meaning it has generally focused on developing tailor- or custom-made products, rather than mass production of a uniform product. It is not centrally coordinated, is composed of multiple providers, facilities, and laboratories, and relies on a wide variety of platforms and instruments that are not interoperable. As a result, most laboratories' supply chains rely on a unique combination of inputs from various manufacturers, which can be difficult to characterize and optimize.

As the FDA has granted EUAs for more laboratory-developed tests (LDTs) and test kits— including POC tests—and testing volume has increased, laboratories across the country have reported shortages of virtually all necessary supplies for testing.[50] PCR-based molecular diagnostic testing involves sample collection, nucleic acid extraction, and testing to identify the presence of the SARS-CoV-2 virus. Since testing began, there have been shortages of the supplies needed for each of these steps: swabs needed for sample collection; viral transport media needed to stabilize and store the samples after collection and during transport; ribonucleic acid (RNA)[51] extraction kits and reagents needed to extract viral RNA from the samples prior to testing; test kits and testing reagents needed to amplify and detect viral nucleic acid; and instruments needed to run tests.

and-medical-products/our-insights/covid-19-overcoming- supply-shortages-for-diagnostic-testing#.

[49] Andrew Slavitt, "Here's How The US Can Start Testing More People for Covid-19," May 5, 2020. https://coronavirus.medium.com/heres-how-the-us-can-start-testing-more-people-for-covid-19-ed3f10bb9952.

[50] Association of Molecular Pathology, "SARS-CoV-2 Molecular Testing, Summary of Recent SARS-CoV-2 Molecular Testing Survey," survey conducted from late April to early May, 20202, https://www.amp.org/AMP/assets/AMP_SARS-CoV-2_Survey_Report_FINAL.pdf?pass=28.

[51] RNA (ribonucleic acid) is defined as a "complex compound of high molecular weight that functions in cellular protein synthesis and replaces DNA (deoxyribonucleic acid) as a carrier of genetic codes in some viruses." https://www.britannica.com/science/RNA.

PPE needed during sample collection has similarly been in short supply, as has laboratory space and trained personnel needed to physically run the tests, as well as common laboratory consumables (e.g., pipette tips).

These testing shortages have been anecdotally reported by laboratories and were documented in an April 3 report by the HHS Office of the Inspector General (OIG) addressing hospitals experience responding to COVID-19. The report notes that "severe shortages of testing supplies and extended waits for test results limited hospitals' ability to monitor the health of patients and staff."[52] In an April-May survey of clinical laboratories on a number of issues relevant to that community, the Association for Molecular Pathology (AMP) found that 85% of clinical laboratories reported that supply interruptions have delayed testing or decreased their testing capacity, and that "the types of supply chain interruptions that laboratories experienced were vast and include testing platforms, testing kits, reagents, swabs, viral transport media (VTM), laboratory consumables, and PPE."[53] Overall, AMP received 118 completed responses from U.S.- based labs, including community hospital or health system laboratories, academic medical centers, and commercial reference laboratories. In addition, states have reported significant and ongoing difficulty in obtaining needed supplies and, in some cases, have noted that competition for limited supplies has been intense.[54]

---

[52] HHS Office of Inspector General (OIG), "Hospital Experiences Responding to the COVID-19 Pandemic: Results of a National Pulse Survey March 23–27, 2020," April 2020, OEI-06-20-00300, https://www.oig.hhs.gov/oei/reports/oei- 06-20-00300.pdf.

[53] Association of Molecular Pathology, "SARS-CoV-2 Molecular Testing, Summary of Recent SARS-CoV-2 Molecular Testing Survey," https://www.amp.org/AMP/assets/AMP_SARS-CoV-2_Survey_Report_FINAL.pdf?pass= 28.

[54] See, for example, Forbes, "States Are Being Forced Into Bidding Wars To Get Medical Equipment To Combat Coronavirus," March 28, 2020, https://www.forbes.com/sites/claryestes/2020/03/28/states-have-are-being-forced-into-bidding-wars-to-get-medical-equipment-to-combat-coronavirus/#6f27fb571cde.

**Selected Approaches to Increasing Testing Capacity:
Sample Pooling and Point-of-Care (POC) and At-Home Tests**

As the country faces increasing demand for all types of COVID-19 testing—especially as cases increased in the Sun Belt states and consideration is being given to reopening schools and nonessential workplaces—several approaches have been touted as possible partial solutions to easing testing capacity and supply chain concerns.

One of these is using sample pooling to screen asymptomatic individuals in low-prevalence areas. Sample pooling combines multiple individual samples (the number varies depending on disease prevalence and test sensitivity) to create a single sample to be tested, using only a single test for the pooled sample. If this returns a positive result, then the individual samples are each tested. In this way, test reagents and other supplies may be conserved. The FDA has provided guidance to test manufacturers and laboratories that would like to use sample pooling in their test EUA to help manage concerns about decreased sensitivity due to sample dilution resulting from combining multiple samples, and the agency has authorized Quest to use pooled sampling with its COVID-19 PCR diagnostic test.

In addition, POC tests, and specifically antigen tests, have been identified as key to a rapid and cost-effective scale- up of testing. The FDA has approved two rapid antigen tests, and millions are expected to be made available over the coming months. However, as currently authorized, these tests must be carried out under the auspices of CLIA and require a physician or other health care professional to order them. As a result, their use in decentralized non-health care or community settings is limited. An at-home test that does not require a physician order—similar to a home pregnancy test—would improve access, capacity, and turnaround time, and would facilitate testing in any setting at any frequency (e.g., homes, workplaces, schools). These types of tests are currently under development by several researchers using a paper-based and CRISPR-based (gene editing) method.

Sources: (1) FDA, "Molecular Diagnostic Template for Commercial Manufacturers," https://www.fda.gov/medical-devices/coronavirus-disease-2019-covid-19-emergency-use-authorizations-medical-devices/vitro-diagnostics-euas; (2) FDA, "Coronavirus (COVID-19) Update: FDA Issues First Emergency Authorization for Sample Pooling in Diagnostic Testing," July 18, 2020, https://www.fda.gov/news-events/press-announcements/coronavirus-covid-19-update-fda-issues-first-emergency-authorization-sample-pooling-diagnostic; (3) 360dx.com, "HHS to Purchase BD Rapid Antigen Tests, Instruments for Coronavirus Detection," July 15, 2020, https://www.360dx.com/immunoassays/hhs-purchase-bd-rapid-antigen-tests-instruments-coronavirus-detection#.Xw-MAShKg4k; and (4) 360dx.com, "SARS-CoV-2 Pandemic May Promote Progress in Paper MDx," July 10, 2020, https://www.360dx.com/molecular-diagnostics/sars-cov-2-pandemic-may-promote-progress-paper-mdx#.Xw-MSihKg4k.

Which Federal Agencies Are Involved in the Testing Supply Chain?

The FDA has worked with industry to identify and mitigate shortages by modifying test EUAs to allow for the use of alternate supplies when carrying out a test and by providing information for manufacturers and laboratories relating to testing supply substitution strategies.[55] However, as noted above, shortages reportedly persist due to global demand and the unprecedented level of testing, as well as a lack of coordinated ascertainment, production, and allocation of supplies. The FDA does not have the authority to allocate or distribute supplies.

By virtue of the national emergency, Federal Emergency Management Agency (FEMA) has played a key federal role in procuring and distributing testing supplies (see the "What Is FEMA's Role in Distributing Testing Materials to Providers?" section of this chapter), and the Defense Production Act (DPA) is an available mechanism for compelling production of testing supplies.[56] For example, the President invoked the DPA for the production of nasal swabs, and the Department of Defense announced $75 million in DPA investments to increase nasal swab production.[57] The Assistant Secretary of Preparedness and Response (ASPR) at HHS also has a significant role in supply chain issues for medical countermeasures in public health emergencies, including, for example, through the management of the Strategic National Stockpile.[58]

[55] FDA, "FAQs on Testing for SARS-CoV-2," https://www.fda.gov/medical-devices/coronavirus-covid-19-and- medical-devices/faqs-testing-sars-cov-2.

[56] For more information about the Defense Production Act, see CRS Insight IN11387, *COVID-19: Defense Production Act (DPA) Developments and Issues for Congress*.

[57] Department of Defense (DOD), "DOD Details $75 Million Defense Production Act Title 3 Puritan Contract," April 29, 2020, https://www.defense.gov/Newsroom/Releases/Release/Article/2170355/dod-details-75-million-defense-production-act-title-3-puritan-contract/.

[58] See "HHS Office of the Assistant Secretary for Preparedness and Response," https://www.phe.gov/about/aspr/Pages/ default.aspx.

What Is FEMA's Role in Distributing Testing Materials to Providers?

FEMA procures and distributes testing materials directly to states, tribes, territories, local governments, and nonprofit medical facilities to expand testing capacity.[59] In addition, FEMA and HHS lead the Laboratory Diagnostics Task Force, which supports testing efforts undertaken by state and local governments, health care providers, and public health labs.[60]

FEMA and the White House have advised that the COVID-19 response, like other emergency and disaster response, is locally executed, state-managed, and federally supported.[61] However, FEMA may provide assistance directly when states, tribes, territories, local governments, and eligible private nonprofit organizations (public assistance applicants) are overwhelmed; this is referred to as direct federal assistance.[62] In these cases, FEMA tasks its own personnel or other federal agencies, such as HHS and CDC, to perform work eligible for public assistance on behalf of the requesting applicants. According to FEMA, the agency exercised this authority to procure and distribute testing supplies and services directly to states, tribes, territories, local governments, and eligible nonprofits.[63]

FEMA entered into a memorandum of understanding (MOU) with ASPR of HHS in April 2020 that enabled FEMA to acquire and distribute critical medical supplies through the Strategic National Stockpile.[64] The

---

[59] Federal Emergency Management Agency (FEMA), "FEMA, "Federal Support to Expand National Testing Capabilities," May 5, 2020, https://www.fema.gov/fact-sheet/federal-support-expand-national-testing-capabilities.

[60] Ibid.

[61] The White House, *Testing Blueprint*, April 5, 2020, p. 2, https://www.whitehouse.gov/wp-content/uploads/2020/04/ Testing-Blueprint.pdf; submitted testimony of FEMA Administrator Peter Gaynor and DOD representative John Polowczyk, in U.S. Congress, Senate Homeland Security and Governmental Affairs Committee (HSGAC), *Evaluating the Federal Government's Procurement and Distribution Strategies in Response to the COVID-19 Pandemic,* hearings, 116th Cong., 2nd sess., June 6, 2020, p. 7, https://www.hsgac.senate.gov/imo/media/doc/Testimony-Gaynor%20&%20Polowczyk-2020-06-09.pdf (hereinafter, Gaynor and Polowsczyk, HSGAC hearing).

[62] Authorized in Stafford Act Sections 402, 403, 418, 419, and 502; 42 U.S.C. §§5170a-b, 5185, 5186, and 5192. See also 44 C.F.R. §206.208.

[63] Email from FEMA Office of Congressional and Legislative Affairs to CRS, June 19, 2020.

[64] FEMA and HHS, "Memorandum of Understanding between the Federal Emergency Management Agency and the Department of Health and Human Services, Office of

MOU specifically included "testing supplies." The MOU called for ASPR to reimburse FEMA for the cost of acquired materials, as specified in subsequent interagency agreements.[65] According to FEMA, this MOU and subsequent interagency agreements enabled FEMA to procure and distribute testing supplies directly to states, tribes, territories, local governments, and nonprofits free of charge.[66]

Beginning in early May 2020, FEMA announced that the agency would begin delivering a limited amount of testing materials to states, tribes, and territories to support each government's own testing plan, in accordance with the Administration's *Testing Blueprint*.[67] FEMA Administrator Peter Gaynor explained that each government would begin receiving testing swabs and transport media from FEMA on May 15, 2020, and would continue to receive weekly distributions through the end of June 2020.[68] States, tribes, and territories are responsible for determining a distribution strategy to meet the needs of their own populations.[69]

DELIVERY OF TESTING FOR COVID-19

This set of questions addresses issues related to individuals accessing testing, including (1) who can receive testing, (2) the settings where testing is available, and (3) the settings where testing is available for individuals who are unable to pay for the full costs of testing.

Assistance Secretary of Preparedness Response," executed April 5, 2020, provided to CRS by FEMA Office of Congressional and Legislative Affairs.

[65] Ibid.

[66] Ibid and email from FEMA Office of Congressional and Legislative Affairs to CRS, June 19, 2020.

[67] FEMA, "Federal Support to Expand National Testing Capabilities;"; HHS, "Report to Congress: COVID-19 Strategic Testing Plan," May 24, 2020, pp. 20-21, https://www.democrats.senate.gov/imo/media/doc/COVID%20National%20Diagnostics%20Strategy%2005%2024%202020%20v%20FINAL.pdf (hereinafter, HHS, "COVID-19 Strategic Testing Plan").

[68] Gaynor and Polowsczyk, HSGAC hearing.

[69] FEMA, "Federal Support to Expand National Testing Capabilities," May 5, 2020, https://www.fema.gov/fact-sheet/ federal-support-expand-national-testing-capabilities.

How Is Diagnostic Testing Prioritized?

States and other jurisdictions are primarily responsible for setting prioritization criteria for COVID-19 testing. At an individual level, testing recommendations may rely on clinician judgement.[70] State approaches may differ depending on their respective testing capacities and the level of COVID-19 transmission in their communities.[71] The federal government, particularly through CDC, can inform these criteria by issuing guidance. In the early stages of the epidemic, CDC guidance recommended limiting COVID-19 testing mostly to individuals with relevant travel or exposure history.[72] As of July 17, 2020, CDC guidance includes considerations for the uses of diagnostic and serologic testing, and for testing symptomatic and asymptomatic individuals. CDC recommends that diagnostic tests be prioritized for the following five populations:

- individuals with signs or symptoms consistent with COVID-19;
- asymptomatic individuals with recent known or suspected exposure to SARS- CoV-2 to control transmission;
- asymptomatic individuals without known or suspected exposure to SARS-CoV-2 for early identification in special settings (e.g., congregate living settings); and
- individuals being tested for purposes of public health surveillance for SARS- CoV-2.[73]

---

[70] Centers for Disease Control and Prevention (CDC), "Testing for COVID-19," last updated June 24, 2020, https://www.cdc.gov/coronavirus/2019-ncov/symptoms-testing/testing.html.

[71] Bill McBride, *Memorandum: Capacity for COVID-19 Testing- Current Status*, National Governors Association, May 14, 2020, https://www.nga.org/wp-content/uploads/2020/04/Testing-Memo-Update-5-13-20.pdf.

[72] CRS Report R46219, *Overview of U.S. Domestic Response to Coronavirus Disease 2019 (COVID-19).*

[73] CDC, "Coronavirus Disease 2019 (COVID-19): Testing Overview," Updated July 2, 2020, https://www.cdc.gov/coronavirus/2019-ncov/hcp/testing-overview.html?CDC_AA_refVal=https%3A%2F%2Fwww.cdc.gov%2Fcoronavirus%2F2019-ncov%2Fhcp%2Fclinical-criteria.html.

CDC has also developed more specific guidance related to testing certain populations or testing programs in specific settings.[74]

Targeted screening testing of certain populations may be a key component of broader state or other jurisdictional plans to control the spread and impact of COVID-19. The National Governors Association (NGA) encourages states to consider public health criteria for testing recommendations, including considering prioritizing certain communities of color (such as American Indian/Native American populations) and lower-income populations. According to NGA, "Communities of color and lower-income Americans are more often essential workers, often live and work in densely populated areas, are more likely to have underlying conditions putting them at higher risk, and have chronic access to healthcare challenges."[75]

Where Can Individuals Get a COVID-19 Test?

Testing availability may vary by state and by the type of test sought. Generally, a range of both ambulatory and inpatient *health care settings* and providers (e.g., hospitals, doctors' offices, urgent care centers) provide testing, and some congregate living sites (e.g., nursing homes) may provide testing to their residents. In addition, many jurisdictions have established testing programs in *community-based settings*, such as walk-up or drive-through testing sites, public health departments, and those at retail pharmacies. A number of settings provide free or reduced- cost tests to the general population using another source of payment (see the "Where Are Free or Reduced Cost Tests Available?" section of this chapter).

---

[74] For example, CDC has issued testing guidelines for nursing homes: https://www.cdc.gov/coronavirus/2019-ncov/ hcp/nursing-homes-testing.html, and for high-density critical infrastructure workplaces: https://www.cdc.gov/ coronavirus/2019-ncov/community/worker-safety-support/hd-testing.html.

[75] Bill McBride, *Memorandum: Capacity for COVID-19 Testing- Current Status*, National Governors Association, May 14, 2020, https://www.nga.org/wp-content/uploads/2020/ 04/Testing-Memo-Update-5-13-20.pdf.

Generally, state law governs who may order a test, which in turn may affect the settings where testing is available. For example, not all states permit nurse practitioners to order tests, so in those states a person would need to see a physician to have a test ordered.[76] Two factors inform whether a complete test is available directly from a provider or if a central laboratory must be involved in its processing: (1) the settings that are able to provide tests (e.g., whether testing is available at a pharmacy), which may be affected by both state law and CLIA (Clinical Laboratory Improvement Amendments of 1988) requirements and (2) where a test is FDA-authorized to be provided (e.g., a waived or point-of-care setting). Test availability may also differ based on the locations where a given payor may pay for testing. For example, some payors may require the provider to be recognized as meeting federal (and sometimes state) conditions of participation requirements (e.g., Medicaid participating provider) in order to pay for a test that a program enrollee receives from that provider.

Where Are Free or Reduced Cost Tests Available?

A number of types of health care and other settings may administer COVID-19 tests; however, only a few types of facilities have requirements to provide care to all individuals regardless of their ability to pay. As such, not all testing sites provide free testing nor do all types of facilities test uninsured individuals.

Public Health Department Testing Programs

State, local, territorial, and tribal health departments may operate testing programs, though activities can vary by jurisdiction. For example, some local health departments operate temporary testing sites (e.g., drive-through

---

[76] National Alliance of State Pharmacy Associations, "COVID-19 Testing," https://naspa.us/resource/covid-19-testing/. On April 8, 2020, HHS released guidance authorizing pharmacists to order testing and providing immunity to do so.
See HHS, "Guidance for Licensed Pharmacists, COVID-19 Testing, and Immunity under the PREP Act," https://www.hhs.gov/sites/default/files/authorizing-licensed-pharmacists-to-order-and-administer-covid-19-tests.pdf.

testing sites), or so-called "mobile strike teams," to provide targeted testing in outbreak areas or for certain populations, such as uninsured or high-risk individuals.[77] Some of the community-based testing sites have been operated jointly by FEMA and/or HHS with health departments, while others have been operated in partnership with health care provider organizations or commercial partners such as retail pharmacies (e.g., CVS).[78] In the early stages of the pandemic, many of the health department testing programs were focused on target populations, such as health care workers and first responders.[79] Some health department testing programs have expanded to become more broadly available in some jurisdictions, though the availability of testing and the populations that can access such testing can vary by jurisdiction.

Testing provided by or in partnership with health departments is often available free of charge to individuals, though testing is often limited to residents of a certain jurisdiction and some programs may seek to bill private health insurance plans or public payors (e.g., Medicaid) for individuals with applicable coverage or to charge certain individuals for testing.[80] CDC grant funding provided through several coronavirus supplemental appropriations measures can support testing programs run by health departments.[81] In particular, the $10.25 billion in funding awards made to states and other jurisdictions pursuant to the PPPHCEA can be used in part to support health

---

[77] National Association of City and County Health Officials (NACCHO), *Local Health Departments Standing Strong on the Frontlines of COVID-19 Response*, April 9, 2020, https://www.naccho.org/uploads/downloadable-resources/Press-Release-NPHW-2020-Role-of-LHDs-in-COVID-19-Response_4.9.20.pdf.

[78] Bill McBride, *Memorandum: Capacity for COVID-19 Testing-Current Status*, National Governors Association, May 14, 2020, https://www.nga.org/wp-content/uploads/2020/04/Testing-Memo-Update-5-13-20.pdf.

[79] Association of State and Territorial Health Officials, *16 Key Considerations for Drive-Through or Mobile Testing*, March 19, 2020, https://astho.org/StatePublicHealth/16-Key-Considerations-for-Drive-Through-or-Mobile-Testing/03- 19-20/.

[80] For example, the District of Columbia (DC) operates free testing sites for D.C. residents experiencing any COVID- 19 symptoms or with known exposures and does not bill insurance providers, see https://coronavirus.dc.gov/testing. The Texas Department of State Health Services states "unless otherwise stated, deductible, co-pay, or co-insurance may apply." Public health testing programs vary by local jurisdiction in Texas. See https://dshs.texas.gov/coronavirus/ testing.aspx.

[81] For a list of CDC grant amounts to jurisdictions as of June 2, 2020, see "CDC COVID-19 State, Tribal, Local, and Territorial Funding Update," https://www.cdc.gov/ coronavirus/2019-ncov/downloads/php/funding-update.pdf.

department testing programs, especially those aimed at high-risk populations and institutional settings.[82]

Emergency Departments

Hospitals with emergency departments are required to provide an appropriate medical screening examination and stabilization care regardless of a patient's eligibility to participate in Medicare. This obligation is required under the Emergency Medical Treatment and Active Labor Act (EMTALA),[83] and it generally extends to individuals who come to the emergency department and are suspected to have COVID-19.[84] EMTALA does permit hospitals to bill individuals for services provided pursuant to their EMTALA obligation. Although some individuals may pay for these services, hospitals that provide care pursuant to their EMTALA obligation may seek payment from the uninsured testing fund discussed below. As mentioned above, some community-based and facility-specific testing may be available to individuals who do not have a source of payment. In addition, the federal government has created an uninsured fund to reimburse facilities for testing provided to uninsured individuals. Congress has enacted legislation that has expanded Medicaid eligibility under limited circumstances so that Medicaid funds may be available for testing for some individuals who are otherwise ineligible for Medicaid (see the "How Can Facilities That Provide Testing for Uninsured Individuals Be Reimbursed?" section of this chapter).

Health Centers

Federal health centers (also called federally qualified health centers or FQHCs) are outpatient facilities that receive federal grants to provide

---

[82] HHS, "Report to Congress: COVID-19 Strategic Testing Plan," May 24, 2020, pp. 71-81, https://www.democrats.senate.gov/imo/media/doc/COVID%20National%20Diagnostics%20Strategy%2005%2024%202020%20v%20FINAL.pdf (hereinafter, HHS, "COVID-19 Strategic Testing Plan).

[83] 42 U.S.C. §1395dd.

[84] HHS, Center for Medicare and Medicaid Services (CMS), "Emergency Medical Treatment and Labor Act (EMTALA) Requirements and Implications Related to Coronavirus Disease 2019 (COVID-19)," memorandum, March 9, 2020, at https://www.cms.gov/files/document/qso-20-15-emtala-requirements-and-coronavirus-0311-updated- 003pdf.pdf-1.

primary care and other services. They must be located in medically underserved areas and provide care to all individuals regardless of their ability to pay. They may bill patients with public or private insurance coverage for the services provided, and they are required to use a sliding scale fee schedule for individuals who do not have coverage.[85] Health centers have received more than $2 billion in supplemental funding to provide COVID-19 testing and related care. Of that amount, $600 million was explicitly appropriated for testing; however, all of the funds appropriated to health centers were to prevent, prepare for, and respond to COVID-19, which includes testing.[86] The Health Resources and Services Administration (HRSA), which administers the health center program, surveyed health centers on the impact of COVID-19 on their operations. The survey found that more than 90% of responding health centers were offering testing, with 70% offering drive-up or walk-up testing.[87]

Federally Qualified Health Center Look-Alikes

Federally Qualified Health Center Look-Alikes (called Look-Alikes) are outpatient centers similar to the health centers described above, but Look-Alikes do not receive a health center grant. Like health centers, these entities serve an underserved population, must be located in medically underserved areas, and are required to provide care to all individuals regardless of their ability to pay. As such, Look-Alikes are a setting where uninsured individuals may receive COVID-19 testing. The majority (87.8%) of Look-Alikes reported to HRSA that they have COVID-19 testing capacity, with approximately half providing walk-up or drive-up testing.[88]

---

[85] CRS Report R43937, *Federal Health Centers: An Overview*.

[86] CRS Insight IN11367, *Federal Health Centers and COVID-19*.

[87] HHS, Health Resources and Services Administration (HRSA), "Health Center Covid-19 Survey: National Summary Report," https://bphc.hrsa.gov/emergency-response/coronavirus-health-center-data.

[88] HHS, HRSA, "Health Center Program Look-Alike COVID-19 Survey National Summary Report," latest data from June 26, 2020.

Federal Community-Based Testing Sites

FEMA collaborated with HHS to establish community-based testing sites (CBTS) in partnership with state and local governments. Since late March 2020, FEMA and HHS helped establish 41 CBTS throughout the country.[89] Initially, local staff at each site were supplemented by one federal physician and by U.S. Public Health Service personnel. The federal government also provided assistance with contracts, logistics, lab processing, and patient notification.[90] The sites initially focused on testing for health care professionals and first responders, though later they tested a broader population.[91] For example, a number of New Jersey's community-based testing sites offered testing only to symptomatic health care workers, first responders, and law enforcement on Saturdays beginning in early April, but those sites are now open to the public during the rest of the week.[92]

On April 10, 2020, FEMA announced the option for CBTS to transition to full state management, with states assuming responsibilities such as staffing, procurement, and testing.[93] FEMA's guidance explains that states and local governments managing these sites may seek reimbursement for eligible expenses associated with running CBTS (e.g., eligible staff costs, testing supplies) through FEMA's Public Assistance (PA) program, subject to a federal 75% cost share.[94] Alternatively, states, tribes, and territories may

---

[89] FEMA, "Weekly Update: Coronavirus Pandemic Whole-of-America Response," June 18, 2020, p. 2, provided by FEMA Congressional and Legislative Affairs. FEMA, "Coronavirus (COVID-19) Pandemic Whole-of-Government Response," Wednesday, March 25, 2020, p. 3; FEMA, "Option to Transition Federal Community-Based Testing Sites to State Management," April 9, 2020, https://www.fema.gov/news-release/20200726/option-transition-federal-community-based-testing-sites-state-management, hereinafter, FEMA, "Community-Based Testing Sites").

[90] HHS, "Report to Congress: COVID-19 Strategic Testing Plan," May 24, 2020, pp. 24-25, https://www.democrats.senate.gov/imo/media/doc/COVID%20National%20Diagnostics%20Strategy%2005%2024%202020%20v%20FINAL.pdf (hereinafter, HHS, "COVID-19 Strategic Testing Plan").

[91] FEMA, "Community-Based Testing Sites."

[92] New Jersey.gov, "What's the difference between community-based testing, local testing, pharmacy testing sites, and private testing sites?," https://covid19.nj.gov/faqs/nj-information/symptoms-tests-and-treatment/whats-the-difference- between-community-based-testing-local-testing-pharmacy-testing-sites-and-private-testing-sites.

[93] FEMA, "Community-Based Testing Sites," May 24, 2020, https://www.fema.gov/news-release/20200726/option-transition-federal-community-based-testing-sites-state-management.

[94] Ibid.

request testing supplies for CBTS directly from FEMA for a limited time after transition.[95]

As of June 24, 2020, FEMA reported that 13 sites continued to operate under federal control, 20 have transitioned to state management, and 8 have closed in consultation with states.[96] At that point, FEMA reported that these sites had processed 287,312 samples while under full federal control.[97] HHS reported that CBTS remain operational in Colorado, Illinois, New Jersey, Pennsylvania, and Texas, as of June 9, 2020.[98] According to FEMA, all remaining community- based testing sites were due to close or transition to full state management on June 30, 2020, though the status of federal financial support is unclear.[99] Numerous news outlets reported that federal support for all sites would end on June 30,[100] though FEMA indicated that financial support for state-managed testing sites will continue through the PA program.[101]

In late June, dozens of Members of Congress appealed to FEMA and HHS to extend federal support for sites given record new COVID-19 cases across the country.[102] Several news outlets reported that HHS had extended

---

[95] FEMA, "Community-Based Testing Sites." HHS explains that sites were provided with materials for 7-14 days after the transition to state management (HHS, "COVID-19 Strategic Testing Plan," p. 24).

[96] FEMA, "Weekly Update: Coronavirus Pandemic Whole-of-America Response," June 25, 2020, p. 2, provided by FEMA Office of Congressional and Legislative Affairs.

[97] Ibid.

[98] Submitted testimony of HHS Assistant Secretary for Health Brett Giroir, *Evaluating the Federal Government's Procurement and Distribution Strategies in Response to the COVID-19 Pandemic,* hearings, 116th Cong., 2nd sess., June 6, 2020, p. 6.

[99] FEMA Office of Congressional and Legislative Affairs, email to CRS, June 24, 2020, noted that all sites were due to close or transition by June 30, 2020. FEMA guidance indicates community-based testing sites under state management remain eligible for Public Assistance. FEMA, "Community-Based Testing Sites."

[100] See, for example, David Lim, "Trump administration ending support for drive-thru testing sites," *Politico*, June 24, 2020, https://www.politico.com/news/2020/06/24/trump-administration-drive-through-coronavirus-testing-338217.

[101] FEMA, "Community Based Testing Sites"; FEMA, email to CRS, June 26, 2020.

[102] See, for example, Representative James E. Clyburn et al. Letter to Alex Azar, Secretary, HHS, June 26, 2020, https://coronavirus.house.gov/sites/democrats.coronavirus.house.gov/files/2020-06-25.Clyburn%20Foster%20Kim%20et%20al.%20to%20Azar%20II-HHS%20re%20Federal%20Testing.pdf; Senators John Cornyn and Ted Cruz, Letter to Peter Gaynor, Administrator, FEMA, and Alex Azar, Secretary, HHS, June 25, 2020, https://www.cruz.senate.gov/files/documents/Letters/06.25.20%20-%20Letter%20HHS%20FEMA%20CBTS%20Testing%20Sites%20-%20FV.pdf.

support for five of seven sites in Texas in response to congressional urging and an appeal by Texas Governor Greg Abbott.[103] Governor Abbott confirmed the extension, noting, "I thank our federal partners for extending these operations in Texas, and for their flexibility in allocating their resources to the communities of Dallas and Houston that are experiencing a high number of COVID-19 cases right now."[104]

In May, 2020, FEMA announced that the federal government, led by HHS, would build upon the first CBTS model to expand testing nationwide. Under this public-private partnership, the federal government provides a flat fee for each test administered to pharmacy and retail companies to offer testing at hundreds of sites throughout the country.[105] According to HHS, the private sector partners are responsible for coordinating the full testing process, including registration, scheduling, provider order, patient notifications, medical supplies, equipment, and lab testing.[106] FEMA reported that 623 sites established through the public-private partnership were operating in 48 states, Washington, DC, and Puerto Rico, as of June 24, 2020, and had processed 712,849 samples since the program initiation.[107] HHS has asserted that the majority of the sites are located in areas with moderate to high social vulnerability.[108] The HHS-operated Community

---

[103] Reese Oxner, "Federal government postpones plans to close five coronavirus testing sites in Texas," *Texas Tribune,* June 26, 2020, https://www.texastribune.org/2020/06/26/texas-federal-coronavirus-testing-sites/; David Lim, "Trump administration restores federal funding for Texas testing sites," *Politico*, June 26, 2020, https://www.politico.com/news/2020/06/26/trump-texas-coronavirus-testing-sites-341795.

[104] Office of the Texas Governor, "Governor Abbott Secures Extension Of Federally-Supported COVID-19 Testing Sites In Texas," June 26, 2020, https://gov.texas.gov/news/post/governor-abbott-secures-extension-of-federally-supported-covid-19-testing-sites-in-texas.

[105] FEMA, "Federal Support to Expand National Testing Capabilities," May 5, 2020, https://www.fema.gov/fact-sheet/ federal-support-expand-national-testing-capabilities (hereinafter FEMA, "FEMA, "Federal Support to Expand National Testing Capabilities"). HHS, "COVID-19 Strategic Testing Plan, pp. 24-25; HHS, "HHS Extends COVID-19 Testing Public-Private Partnership," June 30, 2020, https://www.hhs.gov/about/news/2020/06/30/hhs-extends-covid-19-testing- public-private-partnership.html.

[106] HHS, "HHS Extends COVID-19 Testing Public-Private Partnership," June 30, 2020, https://www.hhs.gov/about/ news/2020/06/30/hhs-extends-covid-19-testing-public-private-partnership.html.

[107] FEMA, "Weekly Update: Coronavirus Pandemic Whole-of-America Response," June 25, 2020, provided by FEMA Congressional and Legislative Affairs, p. 2.

[108] HHS, "COVID-19 Strategic Testing Plan, p. 25. Submitted testimony of HHS Assistant Secretary for Health Brett Giroir, *Evaluating the Federal Government's Procurement and*

Based Testing Sites website lists retail partners by state.[109] On June 30, HHS announced that the partnerships will be extended through August 2020.[110] Significant aspects of the community- based sites public-private partnership remain unclear, and official documentation of the effort by FEMA and HHS remains limited. Outstanding questions include, but are not limited to the following:

- What are the terms of the partnership between HHS (or, if applicable, other federal agencies) and private retailers, including questions of eligibility for testing?
- When will the partnership(s) expire?
- What is the source of federal funding supporting payments to private retail partners?
- What is the amount and frequency of bundled federal payments to retailers?
- Do private retailers and pharmacies in the partnership attempt to bill client insurance companies for all or part of the costs associated with testing?

Can COVID-19 Testing Be Done at Home?

There has been significant interest in, and some confusion around, at-home testing for coronavirus. Although testing at home would have benefits—including increased access to testing, decreased use of PPE, decreased risk of illness transmission—this type of testing requires more rigorous FDA oversight to ensure that the lay user conducting the test can do so safely and with accurate results. Although this type of testing has

---

Distribution Strategies in Response to the COVID-19 Pandemic, hearings, 116th Cong., 2nd sess., June 6, 2020, p. 7.

[109] HHS, "Community-Based Testing Sites for COVID-19: Public-Private Partnership," https://www.hhs.gov/ coronavirus/community-based-testing-sites/index.html.

[110] HHS, "HHS Extends COVID-19 Testing Public-Private Partnership," June 30, 2020, https://www.hhs.gov/about/ news/2020/06/30/hhs-extends-covid-19-testing-public-private-partnership.html.

traditionally been termed "at-home" by the FDA, this type of test may actually be carried out in any non-laboratory setting, including and especially relevant for COVID-19, schools, daycares, workplaces, or high-risk settings. The "at- home" designation means that the test may be conducted outside of a CLIA-regulated environment.

Testing for COVID-19 in a home environment can involve either: (1) a sample being self- collected at home using a kit and sent to a central laboratory for processing, or (2) a complete test, including sampling, testing, and interpretation, being conducted in the home. Complete home testing may involve telehealth visits with a health care provider to supervise the sample collection and help interpret the test result and develop a treatment plan, if indicated. Complete at-home testing generally requires a prescription or order from a health care provider, although the FDA does allow certain at-home tests to be offered over-the-counter (OTC), or without a prescription. Although test developers may pursue this option, it requires additional data and studies to determine that its use would be simple and safe, and would not result in harm to the lay user.[111] Advantages to OTC at-home tests would be increased access and the ability to access a test and results entirely outside of the health care setting (with no prescription or interaction with a health care provider necessary).

The FDA must approve or authorize for marketing all at-home COVID-19 tests, at-home sample self-collection kits, or modifications to existing EUAs for tests to specifically allow for at-home sample collection methods. To date, no complete at-home test has been approved or authorized for marketing by the agency, so none of these tests are currently available. However, at-home sample collection kits have been approved and EUAs have been modified to allow for use of at- home sample collection.[112] The agency has noted that it is open to this type of testing and encourages submission of EUAs, as long as the submission contains accompanying data

[111] See for example, FDA, "Over-the-Counter Diagnostic Tests for the Detection of Pathogens Causing Infectious Diseases," August 2016, https://www.fda.gov/media/99903/download.

[112] See for example, FDA, "Coronavirus (COVID-19) Update: FDA Authorizes First Test for Patient At-Home Sample Collection," April 21, 2020, https://www.fda.gov/news-events/press-announcements/coronavirus-covid-19-update-fda- authorizes-first-test-patient-home-sample-collection.

"demonstrating the ability of a lay user to collect their specimen, run the test, and interpret their results accurately."[113] Flexibilities in the EUA process granted for many commercial and laboratory-developed COVID-19 tests do not apply to at-home testing or sample collection, and a EUA is required prior to clinical use or commercial distribution of these tests in any case.[114]

Private Health Insurance Coverage of Testing

Private health insurance is the predominant source of health insurance coverage in the United States. Private health insurance includes both the group market (largely made up of employer- sponsored insurance) and the nongroup market (commonly referred to as the individual market, which includes plans directly purchased from an insurer both on and off health insurance exchanges).[115] The federal government may regulate private health insurance plans, including by requiring plans to cover certain benefits. The questions below address federal requirements related to private health insurance coverage of COVID-19 testing, including types of tests that must be covered, coverage of related items and services, coverage of testing for public health surveillance and employment purposes, and coverage of testing conducted by out-of-network providers. The questions address the types of plans subject to federal COVID-19 testing coverage requirements, and whether states may impose their own coverage requirements.

---

[113] FDA, "FAQs on Testing for SARS-CoV-2," https://www.fda.gov/medical-devices/emergency-situations-medical- devices/faqs-testing-sars-cov-2.

[114] FDA, "Policy for Coronavirus Disease-2019 Tests During the Public Health Emergency (Revised)," May 11, 2020, https://www.fda.gov/regulatory-information/search-fda-guidance-documents/policy-coronavirus-disease-2019-tests-during-public-health-emergency-revised.

[115] The CRS Report R46359, *COVID-19 and Private Health Insurance Coverage: Frequently Asked Questions* has additional background information on private health insurance and types of plans. Also see "What Types of Plans Are Subject to the FFCRA and CARES Act Requirements?" in this chapter.

Are Private Health Insurance Plans Required to Cover Testing, and Does That Differ by Type of Test?

Prior to the enactment of the Families First Coronavirus Response Act (FFCRA, P.L. 116-127), no federal requirements specifically mandated that private health insurance cover items or services related to COVID-19 testing.

Section 6001 of the FFCRA, as amended, requires most private health insurance plans to cover COVID-19 testing, including administration of the test and related items and services, as defined in the act. The coverage must be provided without consumer cost-sharing, including deductibles, copayments, or coinsurance.[116] Prior authorization or other medical management requirements are prohibited. These coverage requirements are discussed in more detail below.

FFCRA Section 6001(a)(1), as amended by the Coronavirus Aid, Relief, and Economic Security act (CARES, P.L. 116-136) Section 3201, describes the types of tests that must be covered, along with the administration of such tests. In addition, the Department of Labor (DOL), HHS, and the Treasury issued FAQ documents on April 11, 2020,[117] and June 23, 2020[118] (hereinafter, "Tri- Agency April 11 FAQ" and "Tri-Agency June 23 FAQ," respectively), on the private health insurance coverage requirements in FFCRA and the CARES Act.[119]

---

[116] A *deductible* is the amount an insured consumer pays for covered health care services before coverage begins (with exceptions). *Coinsurance* is the share of costs, figured in percentage form, an insured consumer pays for a covered health service. A *copayment* is the fixed dollar amount an insured consumer pays for a covered health service.

[117] Department of Labor (DOL), HHS, and the Treasury, "FAQS ABOUT FAMILIES FIRST CORONAVIRUS RESPONSE ACT AND CORONAVIRUS AID, RELIEF, AND ECONOMIC SECURITY ACT IMPLEMENTATION PART 42," April 11, 2020, at https://www.cms.gov/files/document/FFCRA-Part-42-FAQs.pdf. Hereinafter referred to as "Tri-Agency April 11 FAQ."

[118] DOL, HHS, and the Treasury, "FAQS ABOUT FAMILIES FIRST CORONAVIRUS RESPONSE ACT AND CORONAVIRUS AID, RELIEF, AND ECONOMIC SECURITY ACT IMPLEMENTATION PART 43," June 23, 2020, at https://www.cms.gov/files/document/FFCRA-Part-43-FAQs.pdf. Hereinafter referred to as "Tri-Agency June 23 FAQ."

[119] For a discussion of the agencies' implementation authority and the force of law of these documents, see the "Are Plans Required to Cover Testing for Public Health Surveillance or Employment Purposes?" section of this chapter.

The acts together require coverage of IVDs, as defined in FDA regulation,[120] that detect SARS- CoV-2 or diagnose the virus that causes COVID-19 and that are approved, cleared, or authorized for marketing by the agency or being marketed or clinically used pursuant to an allowed flexibility in FDA guidance. The acts didn't explicitly state whether this included serology testing.[121] The Tri-Agency April 11 FAQ interpreted the coverage requirement as applying to diagnostic (i.e., molecular and antigen) and serological (i.e., antibody) tests.

Together, the acts, as interpreted by the agencies through guidance, also require coverage without cost-sharing of "items and services furnished to an individual during [specified types of visits; discussed below] that result in an order for or administration of [an applicable COVID-19 test; see above], but only to the extent such items and services relate to the furnishing or administration of such product or to the evaluation of such individual for purposes of determining the need of such individual for such product."[122] Per an example provided in guidance, "if the individual's attending provider determines that other tests (e.g., influenza tests, blood tests, etc.) should be performed during a visit…to determine the need of such individual for COVID-19 diagnostic testing, and the visit results in an order for, or administration of, COVID-19 diagnostic testing, the plan or issuer must provide coverage for the related tests under section 6001(a) of the FFCRA."[123] In addition, consumers must not face cost-sharing for "facility fees" or other fees, to the extent they are related to COVID-19 testing or related items and services that are required to be covered under FFCRA Section 6001.[124]

---

[120] 21 C.F.R. §809.3(a).

[121] Although both serology tests and molecular and antigen diagnostic tests meet the regulatory definition of "in vitro diagnostic," applicability to serology testing was not clear based only on the statutory language, as it refers to detection and identification of the virus. Serology testing does not detect or identify the virus; rather, it detects antibodies. (See the "What Are the Different Types of COVID-19 Tests?" section of this chapter for more information).

[122] FFCRA §6001(a)(2). Also see the Tri-Agency April 11 FAQ, including questions five, six, and eight.

[123] Tri-Agency April 11 FAQ, question five.

[124] For more information, see the Tri-Agency June 23 FAQ, question seven, including its footnote 16.

However, the coverage requirements do not encompass treatment for illnesses associated with COVID-19.[125] They also do not apply to any services or items furnished at a testing visit that are not related to COVID-19 (e.g., if someone received testing or treatment for an unrelated condition at the same visit). In addition, the law and guidance do not explicitly address coverage and cost- sharing for the "related" items and services discussed above, if the individual does not ultimately receive the test.[126]

Per FFCRA Section 6001(a)(2), the coverage requirements apply to the specified items and services, discussed above, when furnished at visits including to health care provider offices (including in-person and telehealth visits), urgent care centers, and emergency rooms. Per the Tri- Agency April 11 FAQ, the requirements also apply at "nontraditional" settings, "including drive- through screening and testing sites where licensed healthcare providers are administering COVID-19 diagnostic testing."[127] Also see, in this section, "Are Plans Required to Cover Testing for Public Health Surveillance or Employment Purposes?"

In addition, guidance indicates that the coverage requirements apply to at-home COVID-19 tests, including at-home swab kits that may be sent to a lab for processing, when such tests are "ordered by an attending health care provider who has determined that the test is medically appropriate for the individual," as specified in guidance.[128]

These coverage requirements apply only to the specified items and services furnished during the COVID-19 public health emergency period

---

[125] For more information on private health insurance coverage of COVID-19 treatment, see CRS Report R46359, *COVID-19 and Private Health Insurance Coverage: Frequently Asked Questions*.

[126] Per the Tri-Agency April 11 FAQ, question five, the coverage of related items and services is required when "the visit results in an order for, or administration of, COVID-19 diagnostic testing." This language also appears in FFCRA Section 6001(a)(2). The statute and guidance do not explicitly address whether the coverage requirements apply if an individual receives the related items and services, even for purposes of determining the need for COVID-19 testing, but does not actually receive a COVID-19 test. Other federal and/or state requirements could be applicable.

[127] See Tri-Agency April 11 FAQ, question eight regarding "nontraditional" visits. Also see question 13 for more information about telehealth visits.

[128] Tri-Agency June 23 FAQ, question four. Also see question three regarding "attending providers."

described in FFCRA, as of the date the FFCRA was enacted (March 18, 2020).[129]

What Types of Plans Are Subject to the FFCRA and CARES Act Requirements?

These requirements apply to individual health insurance coverage and to small- and large-group plans, whether fully insured or self-insured.[130] The individual and small-group markets include plans sold on and off the individual and small-group health insurance exchanges, respectively. This includes grandfathered individual or group plans, which are exempt from certain other federal private health insurance requirements. Per the definition of individual health insurance coverage cited in FFCRA, the coverage requirements do not apply to short-term, limited duration insurance (STLDI). The Tri-Agency April 11 FAQ specifies other types of private health insurance coverage that are, or are not, subject to the COVID-19 testing coverage requirements.

This section of this chapter focuses mainly on coverage requirements for private sector plans stemming from Section 6001 of the FFCRA and other federal provisions. Section 6006 of the FFCRA separately addresses the Federal Employees Health Benefits Program (FEHB), which provides health insurance to federal employees, retirees, and their dependents. That section requires that no federal civil servants enrolled in a health benefits plan or

---

[129] Some coverage requirements in FFCRA and the CARES Act refer to the "emergency period" or similar construction. This emergency period refers to the public health emergency declared with respect to the COVID-19 outbreak by HHS Secretary Alex Azar on January 31, 2020, effective as of January 27, pursuant to Section 319 of the Public Health Service Act (PHSA). Hence, the emergency period began on January 27, 2020, and remains in effect as long as the declaration, or any renewal of it, is in effect. See "Duration of Emergency Period" in CRS Report R46316, *Health Care Provisions in the Families First Coronavirus Response Act, P.L. 116-127*, for more information.

[130] The requirements are technically applicable to group health plans and health insurers offering individual and group health insurance coverage. In this section, references to "plans" include applicable plans and insurers. More information on the types of plans discussed in this paragraph, and the applicability of FFCRA and CARES Act requirements to them, is available in CRS Report R46359, *COVID-19 and Private Health Insurance Coverage: Frequently Asked Questions*.

FEHB enrollees may be required to pay a copayment or other cost-sharing related to COVID-19 testing, administration of the test, or related items and services for visits during the emergency period.

Are Plans Required to Cover Testing for Public Health Surveillance or Employment Purposes?

As discussed above, Section 6001 of the FFCRA, as amended by the CARES Act, generally requires plans to cover specified testing for the detection or diagnosis of COVID-19 and administration of such tests, without cost-sharing, during the COVID-19 emergency period.[131] Following enactment of this provision, questions arose about the parameters of covered testing, including whether plans must pay for testing that is not mainly intended for the clinical or treatment needs of individual patients.[132] These questions centered on whether Section 6001 compels plans to cover testing for other reasons, such as public health surveillance or return-to- work purposes.[133]

Although the statutory language of Section 6001 does not articulate the precise circumstances under which testing must be covered, it generally restricts the ability of plans to limit coverage of COVID-19 testing. More specifically, Section 6001 indicates that plans cannot "impose prior authorization or other medical management requirements" with respect to required COVID-19 testing coverage.[134] Although not defined in the federal statute, medical management requirements commonly refer to standards or processes that plans follow to determine medically appropriate coverage

---

[131] See Families First Coronavirus Response Act, P.L. 116-127, §6001, 134 Stat. 201 (2020); Coronavirus Aid, Relief, and Economic Security Act, P.L. 116-136, §3201, 134 Stat. 366 (2020) codified at 42 U.S.C. §1320b-5 note. For more information on the definition of "emergency period" see "Duration of Emergency Period" in CRS Report R46316, *Health Care Provisions in the Families First Coronavirus Response Act, P.L. 116-127*.

[132] See, for example, Letter from National Association of Insurance Commissioners and the Center for Insurance Policy and Research, to Alex Azar, Secretary of Health and Human Services, and Seema Verma, Administrator, Centers for Medicare and Medicaid Services, at https://www.naic.org/documents/NAIC_Letter_to_Azar_May_2020.pdf.

[133] See, for example, id.

[134] 42 U.S.C. §1320b-5 note.

limitations (e.g., limits on the frequency of covered treatments, or the health care setting for a specific item or service).[135] While Section 6001 makes clear that plans cannot use such techniques to restrict coverage of COVID-19 testing, the scope of covered testing, and whether the provision compels plans to cover testing in all instances, have been the subject of debate.[136]

Section 6001 authorizes the Secretaries of HHS, Labor, and the Treasury to implement the provision "through sub-regulatory guidance, program instruction or otherwise."[137] As part of implementation, the agencies issued the aforementioned Tri-Agency April 11 FAQ.[138] According to the agencies, this document constituted a policy statement under the Administrative Procedure Act.[139] Policy statements do not carry the force of law, but they may inform regulated parties about the agencies' enforcement priorities.[140] Under the guidance, the agencies interpreted Section 6001 to compel plans to provide testing coverage only "when medically appropriate for the individual, as determined by the individual's attending healthcare provider in accordance with accepted standards of current medical practice." The guidance did not further outline the circumstances in which COVID-19 tests were "medically appropriate"; however, under the agencies' interpretation, the availability of covered testing appeared contingent upon a medical decision by a health care provider responsible for providing care to a specific patient.

In June 2020, the agencies issued a second guidance document, the Tri-Agency June 23 FAQ, that squarely addresses coverage of COVID-19

---

[135] See, for example, Amy B. Monahan, T*he Regulatory Failure to Define Essential Health Benefits*, 44 AM. J. L. & MED. 529, 544 (2018).

[136] See, for example, the letter cited in footnote 132. See also generally, Katie Thomas, *Testing Nursing Home Workers Can Help Stop Coronavirus. But Who Should Pay?*, N.Y. TIMES (June 9, 2020), https://www.nytimes.com/2020/06/09/ health/testing-coronavirus-nursing-homes-workers.html. Also see Blake Farmer, *Insurers May Only Pay For Coronavirus Tests When They're 'Medically Necessary'*, NATIONAL PUBLIC RADIO (June 19, 2020), https://www.npr.org/sections/health-shots/2020/06/19/880543755/insurers-may-only-pay-for-coronavirus-tests-when- theyre-medically-necessary.

[137] 42 U.S.C. §1320b-5 note.

[138] See Tri-Agency April 11 FAQ.

[139] See Tri-Agency April 11 FAQ at 1.

[140] For information on agency use and judicial review of general statements of policy, see CRS Report R44468, *General Policy Statements: Legal Overview*.

testing for surveillance or employment purposes.[141] In this guidance, the agencies specified that testing "conducted to screen for general workplace health and safety (such as employee 'return-to-work' programs), for public health surveillance for SARS-CoV-2, or for any other purpose not primarily intended for individualized diagnosis or treatment of COVID-19 or another health condition is beyond the scope of section 6001 of the FFCRA."[142] Some Members of Congress have called on the Trump Administration to reexamine and revise its guidance, as "[t]his interpretation of [FFCRA] is not supported by the statute, which makes clear that health plans are required to cover, without any conditions or limitations, the specified items and services related to diagnostic tests for the detection of COVID-19."[143] As of the date of this chapter, it appears that the statutory text of Section 6001 has not been examined by a court.

Are Plans Required to Cover Multiple Tests or Tests for Asymptomatic Individuals?

Per the Tri-Agency June 23 FAQ, if individuals receive multiple diagnostic tests for COVID-19, the FFCRA coverage requirements apply each time, "provided that the tests are diagnostic and medically appropriate for the individual, as determined by an attending health care provider in accordance with current accepted standards of medical practice."[144] The guidance suggests that providers "consult guidance issued by the CDC, as well as state, tribal, territorial, and local health departments or professional

---

[141] See Tri-Agency April 11 FAQ.

[142] Id., question five.

[143] Letter from Frank Pallone, Jr., Chairman, Committee on Energy and Commerce, Robert C. "Bobby" Scott, Chairman, Committee on Education and Labor, Richard Neal, Chairman, Committee on Ways and Means, Patty Murray, Ranking Member, Committee on Health, Education, Labor, and Pensions, Ron Wyden, Ranking Member, Committee on Finance, to Alex Azar, Secretary of Health and Human Services, Eugene Scalia, Secretary of Labor, and Steven T. Mnuchin, Secretary of Treasury (July 7, 2020), https://edlabor.house.gov/imo/media/doc/Democratic%20Health%20Leaders%20Demand%20Trump%20Administration%20Immediately%20Revisit%20Guidance%20Limiting%20COVID-19%20Testing%20Coverage.pdf.

[144] Tri-Agency June 23 FAQ, question six. Also see question three regarding "attending providers."

societies, when determining whether diagnostic testing is appropriate for a particular individual."[145]

That guidance also states that "clinical decisions about testing are made by the individual's attending health care provider and may include testing of individuals with signs or symptoms compatible with COVID-19, as well as asymptomatic individuals with known or suspected recent exposure to SARS-CoV-2, that is determined to be medically appropriate by the individual's health care provider, consulting CDC guidelines as appropriate."[146]

What Coverage and Provider Reimbursement Requirements Apply to Out-of-Network Testing?

While Section 6001 of FFCRA establishes requirements for private health insurance plans to cover COVID-19 testing, administration of the test, and related items and services, it does so without regard to whether a provider is in a health plan's network. See the text box below for background on provider networks and private health insurance coverage. Section 3202 of the CARES Act establishes a methodology for determining insurer payments to in-network and out-of-network providers for COVID-19 testing, and the Tri-Agency April 11 FAQ clarifies that the FFCRA coverage requirements apply both in-network and out-of- network.[147] Per guidance, Section 3202 of the CARES Act does not address the amount that a health plan must reimburse a provider for any other item or service beyond COVID-19 testing.[148] Under the CARES Act, if a health plan had a negotiated rate with a provider of diagnostic testing prior to the declaration of the COVID-19 public health emergency declared under PHSA Section 319, then the health plan must apply that negotiated rate throughout the period of the COVID-19 public health emergency.[149]

---

[145] Ibid.

[146] Tri-Agency June 23 FAQ, question five.

[147] Tri-Agency April 11 FAQ, question seven.

[148] Tri-Agency June 23 FAQ, question eight.

[149] Some coverage requirements in FFCRA and the CARES Act refer to the "emergency period" or similar construction. This emergency period refers to the public health emergency declared

In-Network and Out-of-Network Coverage in Private Health Insurance

In private health insurance, the amount paid for covered items and services is generally contingent upon whether a consumer's health plan has negotiated with a provider to enter into a contract. The contract between the health plan and the provider generally specifies the total amount that a provider may receive for furnishing particular items or services to that health plan's enrollees. A provider that enters into a contract with a health plan is considered to be part of the health plan's network, otherwise referred to as being *in-network.*

A provider that does not enter into a contract with a health plan is considered *out-of-network*, and as such there is no negotiated rate between the provider and the health plan. In situations involving services provided by an out- of-network provider, the amount that a provider will receive from a health plan depends on whether the health plan covers out-of-network services. In situations where health plans *do not cover* out-of-network services, the health plan will not pay any amount to a provider for services provided to an enrollee of the health plan. In situations where plans *do cover* out-of-network services, as there is no negotiated rate between health plans and out-of-network providers, health plans will use their own methodologies for calculating how much they will pay out-of-network providers for services. If an out-of-network provider's total charge for a service exceeds the amount reimbursed by the health plan, the provider may directly bill (i.e., balance bill) a consumer for the amount of the difference, except when prohibited by applicable state law or other contractual agreements.

If a health plan did not have a negotiated rate with a provider of diagnostic testing prior to the emergency declaration, then the health plan must either reimburse the provider an amount that equals the cash price for the COVID-19 testing, as listed on the provider's public website, or the health plan and provider may negotiate a rate that is less than the cash price. If there is no cash price listed on the provider's website and the two parties cannot negotiate a rate, then the methodology for determining reimbursement depends on whether there is an applicable state law.[150]

---

with respect to the COVID-19 outbreak by HHS Secretary Alex Azar on January 31, 2020, effective as of January 27, pursuant to Section 319 of the Public Health Service Act (PHSA). Hence, the emergency period began on January 27, 2020, and remains in effect as long as the declaration, or any renewal of it, is in effect. See "Duration of Emergency Period" in CRS Report R46316, *Health Care Provisions in the Families First Coronavirus Response Act, P.L. 116-127*, for more information.

[150] Tri-Agency June 23 FAQ, question 11.

During the period of the COVID-19 public health emergency, providers of COVID-19 diagnostic testing must make public the cash price for the COVID-19 test on the provider's public website. Section 3202 of the CARES Act does not include any further requirements for providers regarding the cash price, including any limitation on the amount that a provider may post as the cash price. The HHS Secretary may impose a civil monetary penalty on a provider of COVID-19 diagnostic testing that is not in compliance with the above requirement to post the cash price and has not completed a corrective action plan to comply with the requirement. The amount of the civil monetary penalty may not exceed $300 per day that the violation is ongoing.

Are Out-of-Network Providers Allowed to Balance Bill Patients for COVID-19 Testing and Other Related Items and Services?

The Tri-Agency June 23 FAQ clarifies that the combination of the Families First Coronavirus Response Act (FFRCA, P.L. 116-127) requirement to provide coverage for COVID-19 testing without cost-sharing, and the CARES Act methodology for determining reimbursement for COVID-19 testing, means that an out-of-network provider is generally precluded from directly billing a patient for the difference between provider's charge for COVID-19 testing and the amount reimbursed by the health plan (i.e., balance bill).[151] However, a provider is not prevented from balance billing for other items and services unless there is an applicable state law or other prohibition (e.g., pursuant to the terms of the Provider Relief Fund).[152]

---

[151] Question nine in the Tri-Agency June 23 FAQ points out that out-of-network providers who accept funds from the Provider Relief Fund may not seek to collect from patients out-of-pocket expenses that would be "greater than what the patient would have otherwise been required to pay if the care had been provided by an in network provider." For background on this funding, see CRS Insight IN11438, *The COVID-19 Health Care Provider Relief Fund.*

[152] Ibid.

May States Require Plans to Cover Additional Types or Purposes of Testing?

States are the primary regulators of private health insurance, and each state may impose coverage requirements on insurers and the plans they sell in that state.

With regard to COVID-19 testing, states may require coverage that exceeds applicable federal requirements, as long as states do not prevent the implementation of any federal requirements.[153] Some states have done so.[154] For example, although the Tri-Agencies have stated that FFCRA Section 6001 does not require insurance coverage of COVID-19 testing for public health purposes (see above), New York requires insurers to cover testing for individuals who meet one or more criteria listed in the state's guidance, including "an individual is employed as a health care worker, first responder, or other essential worker who directly interacts with the public while working."[155]

State requirements may apply to individual health insurance coverage, fully insured group coverage, or both, but states cannot regulate self-insured group plans.[156] States may impose requirements on STLDI. (See "What Types of Plans Are Subject to the FFCRA and CARES Act Requirements?" for information on plan types.)

---

[153] See, for example, the introduction of the Tri-Agency April 11 FAQ.

[154] The National Association of Insurance Commissioners (NAIC) is tracking certain state actions related to insurance and COVID-19 at https://content.naic.org/naic_coronavirus_info.htm. To confirm whether a given state has enacted any requirements related to coverage of COVID-19 testing (or related to other topics) that may not be reflected in that tracking document, check with that state's department of insurance: https://content.naic.org/state_web_map.htm.

[155] New York State Department of Financial Services, "Insurance Circular Letter No. 11 (2020)," May 19, 2020, at https://www.dfs.ny.gov/industry_guidance/circular_letters/cl2020_11.

[156] Some coverage requirements in FFCRA and the CARES Act refer to the "emergency period" or similar construction. This emergency period refers to the public health emergency declared with respect to the COVID-19 outbreak by HHS Secretary Alex Azar on January 31, 2020, effective as of January 27, pursuant to Section 319 of the Public Health Service Act (PHSA). Hence, the emergency period began on January 27, 2020, and remains in effect as long as the declaration, or any renewal of it, is in effect. See "Duration of Emergency Period" in CRS Report R46316, *Health Care Provisions in the Families First Coronavirus Response Act, P.L. 116-127*, for more information.

Note that a state or local department of health or other administrative agency may announce requirements or guidelines regarding testing certain populations or testing for certain public health purposes. However, this does not necessarily mean that insurers in that state are required to cover such testing, although that would be the case if the state department of insurance or other relevant agency also requires such coverage, or if federal requirements are applicable.

PAYMENT FOR TESTING BY FEDERAL PROGRAMS: MEDICARE, MEDICAID, AND CHIP

The Social Security Act (SSA) defines a federal health care program as any plan or program that provides health benefits—whether directly, through insurance, or otherwise—and that is funded directly, in whole, or in part by the U.S. government or a state health care program (with the exception of the Federal Employees Health Benefits Program).[157] Key federal health programs include (1) Medicare, the national health insurance program that pays for covered services furnished to beneficiaries (generally the elderly and disabled); (2) Medicaid, the federal-state program for certain low-income individuals; and (3) the State Children's Health Insurance program (CHIP), which provides coverage for low-income, uninsured children. The questions below discuss how these federal health care programs provide, establish coverage, or pay for testing for their beneficiaries. FFRCA required each of these programs to cover COVID-19 testing for their enrollees without beneficiary cost-sharing, under certain circumstances. The specific testing-related requirements associated with each program are discussed below. In general, these federal health care programs provide coverage for testing of beneficiaries when ordered by an enrollee's physician or practitioner.[158]

---

[157] Section 1128B(f) of the Social Security Act (SSA).

[158] For adults under the Medicaid program, states are permitted to limit the extent to which a covered benefit is available under the state plan by defining medical necessity criteria, and the amount, duration, and scope of covered services (see SSA Section(s) 1901;

How Does Medicare Pay for Testing, and Does That Differ by Type or Use of Test?

In general, Medicare covers health care services furnished to diagnose or rule out a possible illness or condition.[159] Medicare pays for clinical laboratory tests that are medically necessary and ordered by a beneficiary's physician or practitioner for such purposes.[160] There is no cost-sharing required under Part B, nor for beneficiaries enrolled in Medicare Advantage (MA) plans, as MA plans must cover all benefits under Medicare Parts A and B.[161] Clinical tests to diagnose or aid in the diagnosis of the coronavirus disease, as well as some tests for related respiratory conditions given with the COVID-19 test, are covered under Medicare Part B.[162] FDA-authorized antibody (serology) tests for those beneficiaries diagnosed with a known current or prior COVID-19 infection or suspected current or past COVID-19 infection are also covered with no cost- sharing.[163] There is no limit on the number of tests, so long as each test satisfies the coverage requirement. The FFCRA eliminated the Medicare Part B beneficiary cost-sharing for provider visits during which a coronavirus diagnostic test is administered or ordered during the emergency period. Beneficiaries are not responsible for any coinsurance payments or deductibles for any specified COVID-19 testing-related service, defined as a medical visit that falls within the evaluation and management service codes for the following categories:

1902(a)(30)(A); and 1903(m)(2)(A)(vii)). For children under Medicaid and CHIP Medicaid expansion programs, medical necessity requirements are established under Early and Periodic Screening, Diagnostic, and Treatment (EPSDT) (see SSA Section 1905(r)(5)). For separate CHIP programs, medical necessity requirements are established under SSA Section 2110(a)(24).

159 SSA Section 1862(a)(1)(A) specifies that Medicare covered health care services must be "reasonable and necessary for the diagnosis or treatment of illness or injury or to improve the functioning of a malformed body member."

160 Some preventive or screening tests may also be covered, but these are explicitly addressed in SSA Section 1862(a)(1)(B)-(P) (e.g., screening tests for mammography, prostate cancer, and colorectal cancer).

161 See CRS Report R40425, *Medicare Primer* for information about Medicare.

162 CMS, "Coronavirus disease 2019 (COVID-19) tests" at https://www.medicare.gov/coverage/coronavirus-disease- 2019-covid-19-tests.

163 CMS "Coronavirus disease 2019 (COVID-19) antibody test" at https://www.medicare.gov/coverage/coronavirus- disease-2019-covid-19-antibody-test. For information about molecular pathogen tests versus screening antibody serology tests, see CRS In Focus IF11516, *COVID-19 Testing: Key Issues*.

office and other outpatient services; hospital observation services; emergency department services; nursing facility services; domiciliary, rest home, or custodial care services; home services; or online digital evaluation and management services.

Medicare Coverage of Nursing Home Testing

As of July 2020, under Original Medicare and Medicare Advantage, Medicare covers COVID-19 diagnostic testing of Medicare beneficiaries who are residents of nursing homes. Diagnostic testing includes

- testing residents with signs or symptoms of COVID-19;
- testing asymptomatic residents with known or suspected exposure to an individual infected with SARS-CoV- 2, including close and expanded contacts (e.g., if there is an outbreak in the facility);
- initial (baseline) testing of asymptomatic residents without known or suspected exposure to an individual infected with SARS-CoV-2 as part of the recommended reopening process; and
- testing to determine resolution of infection.

Sources: CMS, "Medicare Coverage of COVID-19 Testing for Nursing Home Residents and Patients," June 19, 2020, available at https://www.cms.gov/newsroom/press-releases/cms-news-alert-june-19-2020, and CMS, "Medicare Fee-For-Service (FFS) Response to the Public Health Emergency on the Coronavirus (COVID-19." Medicare Learning Network Matters Document SE20011, July 17, 2020, at https://www.cms.gov/files/document/ se20011.pdf.

Surveillance testing, whether it be for the novel coronavirus or other purposes, does not meet the Medicare coverage criteria that the care be "reasonable and necessary for the diagnosis or treatment of illness or injury or to improve the functioning of a malformed body member." Similarly, COVID-19 testing for "return-to-work" would not be covered under Medicare.

How Does Medicaid Pay for Testing, and Does That Differ by Type or Use of Test?

Medicaid is a joint federal-state program that finances the delivery of primary and acute medical services, as well as long-term services and supports (LTSS), to a diverse low-income population, including eligible children, pregnant women, adults, individuals with disabilities, and people aged 65 and older. States have flexibility to design their own versions of Medicaid within the federal statute's basic framework. This flexibility results in variability across state Medicaid programs regarding factors such as eligibility and covered benefits.

Section 6004 of the FFCRA, as amended by Section 3717 of the CARES Act, requires state Medicaid programs to cover testing and testing-related services[164] without beneficiary cost- sharing, beginning on or after March 18, 2020, through the public health emergency period, as defined.[165] Testing services are defined as in vitro diagnostic products as defined in FDA regulation[166] including the administration of such products, for the detection of SARS-CoV-2 or the diagnosis of COVID-19. According to guidance from the Centers for Medicare and & Medicaid Services (CMS), the FDA has advised that serological tests for COVID-19 meet the FDA definition of an in vitro diagnostic product for the detection of SARS-CoV-2 or the diagnosis of COVID-19, and thus must be covered under Medicaid.[167] To date, the

---

[164] CMS interpreted COVID-19 testing-related services to include items and services for which payment is available under the Medicaid state plan that are directly related to the administration of COVID-19 testing, or for the evaluation of an individual to determine the need for COVID-19 testing (e.g., an X-ray). For more information, see Centers for Medicare and Medicaid Services (CMS), *Families First Coronavirus Response Act (FFCRA),* P.L. 116-127*; Coronavirus Aid, Relief, and Economic Security (CARES) Act,* P.L. 116-136*; Frequently Asked Questions (FAQ)*, April 13, 2020.

[165] FFCRA, as amended by the CARES Act, also added a new optional Medicaid "COVID-19 testing" eligibility group to provide testing and diagnosis of COVID-19 for certain specified uninsured individuals during the COVID-19 public health emergency. For more information on this optional eligibility group and the limited benefit coverage enrollees in this group are entitled to, see the "Under What Circumstances Will Medicaid Pay for Uninsured Testing?" section of this chapter.

[166] 21 C.F.R. 809.3(a) defines in vitro diagnostic products as "reagents, instruments, and systems intended for use in the diagnosis of disease or other conditions, including a determination of the state of health, in order to cure, mitigate, treat, or prevent disease or its sequelae. Such products are intended for use in the collection, preparation, and examination of specimens taken from the human body." To date, FDA has authorized one emergency use authorization for a serological test that is intended for use by clinical laboratories. See U.S. Food and Drug Administration, Letter to Cellex Inc. Regarding qSARS-CoV-2 IgG/IgM Rapid Test (April 1, 2020), available at https://www.fda.gov/media/ 136622/download.

[167] CMS, "Families First Coronavirus Response Act (FFCRA), P.L. 116-127; Coronavirus Aid, Relief, and Economic Security (CARES) Act, P.L. 116-136; Frequently Asked Questions (FAQs)," April 13, 2020, https://www.medicaid.gov/state-resource-center/downloads/ covid-19-section-6008-CARES-faqs.pdf (hereinafter, *CMS Medicaid FAQs*).

Medicaid specific CMS guidance has not explicitly addressed the question of whether states can use Medicaid as a payer of public health surveillance testing for SARS-CoV-2 (to screen for general workplace health and safety, as in the case of employee "return to work" programs).

How Does CHIP Pay for Testing, and Does That Differ by Type or Use of Test?

CHIP provides health insurance coverage to low-income, uninsured children in families with incomes above applicable Medicaid income standards, and to certain pregnant women. States have the flexibility to design their own versions of CHIP within the federal statute's basic framework. This flexibility results in variability across state CHIP programs regarding factors such as eligibility and covered benefits.

FFCRA, as amended by the CARES Act, also requires CHIP programs to cover COVID-19 testing and testing-related services[168] for CHIP enrollees for the period beginning March 18, 2020, through the duration of the public health emergency period, as specified. States are prohibited from charging beneficiary cost-sharing for such testing, or for testing-related visits furnished to CHIP enrollees during this period. CMS guidance clarifies that, as under Medicaid, such testing must include diagnostic and serological tests for symptomatic and asymptomatic CHIP program enrollees when testing is driven by medical necessity.[169] To date, the CHIP specific CMS guidance has not explicitly addressed the question of whether states can use Medicaid as a payer of public health surveillance testing for SARS-CoV-2 (to screen for general workplace health and safety, as in the case of "return to school" programs).

---

[168] CMS interpreted COVID-19 testing-related services to include items and services for which payment is available under the Medicaid state plan that are directly related to the administration of COVID-19 testing, or for the evaluation of an individual to determine the need for COVID-19 testing (e.g., an X-ray). When defining testing-related services available under CHIP, the CMS guidance points to Medicaid specific responses in the Q&A. For more information, see CMS Medicaid FAQs.

[169] CMS Medicaid FAQs.

Provision of and Payment for COVID-19 Testing by Federal Systems: IHS, VA, DOD, and FEMA

In general, the federal government pays for care provided by nonfederal providers. In the cases of the Indian Health Service, the Veterans Health Administration (VHA), and the DOD through the Defense Health System, the federal government may provide care directly to a limited set of beneficiaries enrolled in these programs. Other federal programs, that that do not have as their primary purpose the delivery of health care, may also, in some cases, directly provide services to individuals who reside in their facilities (for example, the Bureau of Prisons may provide care to federal inmates). The questions below focus on federal health systems that have as their main purpose the provision of health care, and how these systems provide and pay for testing for their beneficiaries. FFRCA requires each of these agencies to cover testing for their beneficiaries; the specific requirements for each agency are discussed in the questions below. In addition, federally operated health systems generally do not provide care to non-beneficiaries except under limited circumstances, some of which have arisen as part of the COVID-19 pandemic. The provision of testing services to non-beneficiaries is also discussed in the questions below.

How Does the Indian Health Service Provide or Pay for Testing?

The Indian Health Service (IHS) within HHS is the lead federal agency charged with improving the health of American Indians and Alaska Natives. In FY2019, IHS provided health care to approximately 2.6 million eligible American Indians/Alaska Natives.[170] IHS has 12 areas, and the Navajo area

---

[170] HHS, Indian Health Service (IHS), FY2021, "Justification of Estimates for Appropriations Committees," https://www.ihs.gov/sites/budgetformulation/themes/responsive2017/display_objects/documents/FY_2021_Final_CJ- IHS.pdf. IHS provides health care directly through facilities it operates, or through facilities that are operated by Indian Tribes/Tribal Organizations or Urban Indian organizations.

represents one of the highest COVID-19 death rates nationally.[171] IHS provides care free of charge to its beneficiaries, who are generally members of federally recognized tribes.[172] These services include COVID-19 testing. IHS reports that most of its facilities have testing capacity, and it has been making data on testing at the area level available on its website.[173] To expand testing, IHS received and provided 250 rapid test analyzers to facilities in its system, prioritizing sites near hot spots and those that were not near centralized lab capacity.[174]

IHS has received approximately $1.850 billion in supplemental funding for COVID-19-related testing and care.[175] FFRCA provided an additional $64 million, to remain available until September 30, 2022 (i.e., through FY2021), for specified COVID-19 testing and related health services and administration.[176] The act also requires IHS to pay the cost of providing any COVID- 19-related items and services without imposing any cost-sharing requirements for the period of the COVID-19 emergency. This requirement applies to any American Indian[177] receiving services through the IHS,[178] including through Urban Indian Organizations. Generally, IHS facilities operated by the Indian Health Service do not charge cost-sharing; however, facilities that are operated by Indian tribes or by Urban Indian Organizations

---

[171] Kenzi Abou-Sabe, Cynthia McFadden and Didi Martinez, "'Hit us at our core': Vulnerable Navajo Nation fears a second COVID-19 wave," August 3, 2020, https://www.nbcnews.com/specials/navajo-nation-fears-second-covid-19- wave/index.html.

[172] For definition of Indian Tribe see Section 4 of the Indian Health Care Improvement Act (25 U.S.C. §1603(14)).

[173] See HHS, IHS, "Coronavirus (COVID-19)," https://www.ihs.gov/coronavirus/.

[174] HHS, IHS "Coronavirus (COVID-19), FAQs—Federal Response in Indian Country," https://www.ihs.gov/ coronavirus/faqs-federal-response-in-indian-country/.

[175] For a discussion of funding provided to the Indian Health Service and Indian Tribes to prepare for and respond to the coronavirus, see CRS Insight IN11333, *COVID-19 and the Indian Health Service*.

[176] CRS Report R46316, *Health Care Provisions in the Families First Coronavirus Response Act, P.L. 116-127*.

[177] FFRCA defines *Indian* with a reference to Section 4 of the Indian Health Care Improvement Act (25 U.S.C. §1603(13)).

[178] The phrase "receiving services through the IHS" is not defined, but it has been used in prior federal guidance to refer to non-IHS facilities that have care coordination agreements with IHS facilities to treat American Indians and Alaska Natives. See Letter to State Health Official: Re: Federal Funding for Services "Received Through" an IHS/Tribal Facility and Furnished to Medicaid-Eligible American Indians and Alaska Natives (SHO #16-002), February 26, 2016, https://www.medicaid.gov/sites/default/files/Federal-Policy-Guidance/Downloads/sho022616.pdf.

may do so. The CARES Act provided an additional $1.032 billion to IHS to prevent, prepare for, and respond to the coronavirus. This funding was not explicitly for testing, but it may be used for testing. PPPHCEA also appropriated $750 million the Public Health and Social Services Emergency Fund (PHSSEF) to be allocated by IHS for testing capacity (see the "What Funds Have Been Appropriated for Testing Capacity and Infrastructure?" section of this chapter).

Does the Department of Veteran Affairs Offer or Pay for Testing?

The Veterans Health Administration (VHA) of the Department of Veterans Affairs (VA) operates one of the nation's largest integrated direct health care delivery systems.[179] The VHA estimates that in FY2020 it will provide care to about 6.33 million unique veteran patients.[180] In the same year, the VHA estimates that it will employ a staff of about 347,000 full-time equivalent employees[181] at approximately 1,456 VA sites of care,[182] with an appropriation of approximately $80.6 billion.[183] The VHA provides a standard medical benefits package to enrolled veterans for services both related to and unrelated to their military service.[184] These services include

---

179 The Veterans Health Administration (VHA) operates under a different model from the predominant health care financing and delivery model in the United States, in which there is a payer for health care services (e.g., Medicare or private health insurance plan), a provider (e.g., hospital, physician), and a recipient of care (the patient). The VHA is not a health insurance financing program that provides reimbursement to providers for all or a portion of a patient's health care costs. The VHA is primarily a direct provider of care; it owns the hospitals and employs the clinicians.

180 Department of Veterans Affairs (VA), *FY2021 Congressional Submission, Medical Programs and Information Technology Programs*, vol. 2 of 4, February 2020, p. VHA-19.

181 VA, *FY2021 Congressional Submission, Budget in Brief*, February 2020, p. BiB-4.

182 Ibid., p. BiB-11. (Sites of care used in this calculation are VA hospitals, community living centers, health care centers, community-based outpatient clinics [CBOCs], other outpatient service sites, and dialysis centers.)

183 VA, *FY2021 Congressional Submission, Supplemental Information &Appendices*, vol. 1 of 4, February 2020, p. Supplemental Information-1.

184 For more information on the VHA health system in general, including who can enroll and the services that provided, see CRS Report R42747, *Health Care for Veterans: Answers to Frequently Asked Questions*.

COVID- 19 testing. The VA reports that it is capable of administering approximately 60,000 tests per week, with the ability to test asymptomatic individuals who request a test.[185] The VA has been making some data regarding testing publicly available on its website.[186]

Diagnostic testing is generally a covered service under the standard medical benefits package.[187] Some veterans are required to pay copayments for care that is not related to a service-connected disability. However, routine lab tests are exempt from copayment requirements.[188] Furthermore, the FFCRA prohibited the VA from charging any copayment or other cost-sharing payments for COVID-19 testing or medical visits during any period of this public health emergency.[189]

The VA has received supplemental funding for COVID-19-related testing and care.[190] The FFRCA provided an additional $30 million to the VHA medical services account, to remain available until September 30, 2022 (i.e., through FY2021) to fund health services and related items pertaining to COVID-19.[191] The CARES Act provides supplemental appropriations for FY2020 for certain VA accounts totaling $19.6 billion, designated as emergency spending. The VHA medical services account received $14.4 billion of that total, which is partially intended for testing.[192]

---

[185] VHA Daily COVID-19 Update, June 18, 2020. Testing capacity is accurate as of June 18, 2020. VA indicates that it is continuing to increase testing capacity.

[186] See VHA, VA, "Novel Coronavirus Disease (COVID-19)," https://www.publichealth.va.gov/n-coronavirus/.

[187] 38 C.F.R. §17.38.

[188] 38 C.F.R. §17.108(e)(14).

[189] Generally, diagnostic testing is a covered service under VA's standard medical benefits package, which is available to all veterans enrolled in the VA health care system (38 C.F.R. §17.38). Some veterans are required to pay copayments for care that is not related to a service-connected disability. However, routine lab tests are exempt from copayments. (38 C.F.R. §17.108(e)(14)). Prior to enactment of FFRCA, it was unclear whether VA was including COVID-19 testing under this exemption.

[190] For a discussion of funding provided to VA to prepare for and respond to the public health emergency, see CRS Report R46340, *Federal Response to COVID-19: Department of Veterans Affairs*.

[191] VHA's annual appropriations consist of five accounts: medical services, medical community care, medical support and compliance, medical facilities, and medical and prosthetic research accounts. The first four accounts cover the provision of health care and related services.

[192] Based on Senate Appropriations Committee, Coronavirus Supplemental Appropriations Summary, available at https://www.appropriations.senate.gov/download/coronavirus-emergency-supplemental-appropriations-summary.

Can the IHS and the VA Provide Testing for Individuals Who Are Not Otherwise Eligible for Services?

Generally, health services at facilities operated by the IHS are limited to IHS beneficiaries who are generally members of Indian tribes. Facilities operated by Indian tribes, tribal organizations, or Urban Indian Organizations may serve non-IHS beneficiaries, but they may not use IHS funds to do so. The Indian Health Care Improvement Act (IHCIA, P.L. 94-437), which provides general authority for much of IHS's activities, permits IHS facilities to serve non-beneficiaries under limited circumstances, as specified in Section 813 (25 U.S.C. §1680). These circumstances include preventing the spread of a communicable disease or to address a health hazard. IHS provided guidance to tribal facilities stating that tribes may choose to provide care to non- beneficiaries to reduce COVID-19 spread, including, but not limited to, members of Indian households who are not otherwise eligible for IHS services. In this guidance, IHS noted that the decision to provide services to non-beneficiaries would be made at the local level.[193] IHCIA generally requires that services provided to non-beneficiaries be reimbursed. As such, individuals who have another source of coverage would be tested at an IHS-facility billed to the relevant payer. HRSA has stated in its Frequently Asked Questions about the uninsured fund that COVID- 19 testing that IHS facilities provide to non-IHS beneficiaries may be reimbursed by the uninsured fund if the individual tested does not have another source of payment.[194]

Similarly, VA health services provided through the VHA are generally limited to veteran enrollees who are subject to specified eligibility and enrollment criteria.[195] The VHA's primary function is to "provide a complete medical and hospital service for the medical care and treatment of veterans"

[193] HHS, IHS, "IHS COVID-19 Interim Guidance for Care Services to Non-Beneficiaries," March 20, 2020, https://www.ihs.gov/sites/coronavirus/themes/responsive2017/display_objects/documents/IHS_COVID-19_InterimGuidanceCareServices_Non-Beneficiaries.pdf.

[194] HHS, HRSA, "Frequently Asked Questions," https://www.hrsa.gov/coviduninsuredclaim/frequently-asked- questions?field_faq_category_tid=All&combine=indian.

[195] For a detailed discussion of eligibility for VA health care and qualification for enrollment, see CRS Report R42747, *Health Care for Veterans: Answers to Frequently Asked Questions*.

(38 U.S.C. §7301). However, the VA may provide hospital care and medical services through a number of legal authorities to other individuals during periods of war, national disasters, emergencies, or humanitarian crisis.

The Veterans Administration and Department of Defense Health Resources Sharing and Emergency Operations Act (P.L. 97-174) was enacted to serve as the primary health care backup to the military health care system during and immediately following an outbreak of war or a national emergency.[196] Since then, Congress has provided additional authorities to the VA to "use its vast infrastructure and resources, geographic reach, deployable assets, and health care expertise, to make significant contributions to the Federal emergency response effort in times of emergencies and disasters."[197]

The VHA may care for nonveterans and veterans not enrolled in the VA health care system.[198] The VA also has authority to provide certain health services such as medical counter measures[199] to VA employees.[200] The authority to care for nonveterans applies in situations where the President has declared a major disaster or emergency under the Robert T. Stafford Disaster Relief and Emergency Assistance Act (Stafford Act), or where the

---

[196] 38 U.S.C. §811A.

[197] VA, *Department of Veterans Affairs FY 2018—2024 Strategic Plan*, Refreshed May 31, 2019, May 31, 2019, p. 35.

[198] 38 U.S.C. §1785 and 38 C.F.R. §17.86 establish VA authority to provide hospital care and medical services to nonveterans responding to, involved in, or otherwise affected by a disaster or emergency. These individuals may include active duty servicemembers, as well as National Guard and Reserve component members activated by state or federal authority. This authority also allows the VA to treat veterans not enrolled in the VA health care system. Unless another federal agency reimburses the VA, individuals could be charged for this care. "[I]ndividuals who receive hospital care or medical services under this section [38 C.F.R. §17.86] are responsible for the cost of the hospital care or medical services when charges are mandated by Federal law (including applicable appropriation acts) or when the cost of care or services is not reimbursed by other-than-VA Federal departments or agencies." 38 C.F.R. §17.86.

[199] Medical counter measures are "are life-saving medicines and medical supplies regulated by the U.S. Food and Drug Administration (FDA) that can be used to diagnose, prevent, protect from, or treat conditions associated with chemical, biological, radiological, or nuclear (CBRN) threats, emerging infectious diseases, or a natural disaster" (https://www.cdc.gov/cpr/readiness/mcm.html); see CRS Report R46427, *Development and Regulation of Medical Countermeasures for COVID-19 (Vaccines, Diagnostics, and Treatments): Frequently Asked Questions*.

[200] 5 U.S.C. §7901; also see Appendix A of Department of Veterans Affairs, Veterans Health Administration, *All- Hazards Emergency Cache Program*, VHA Directive 1047, Washington, DC, April 21, 2020, pp. A-1-A-2.

HHS Secretary has declared a disaster or emergency activating the National Disaster Medical System established pursuant to Section 2811(b) of the Public Health Service Act (42 U.S.C. §300hh-11(b)). The President's March 13, 2020, declaration of a national emergency under Section 501(b) of the Stafford Act allows the VA to use this authority.

Does the Department of Defense Offer or Pay for Testing?

Under Chapter 55 of Title 10, *U.S. Code*, the DOD administers statutory health entitlements to approximately 9.5 million beneficiaries (i.e., servicemembers, military retirees, and family members).[201] Collectively, these entitlements are organized under a program called TRICARE that is administered by the Military Health System (MHS). The MHS offers health care services in military hospitals and clinics—known as military treatment facilities (MTFs)—and through civilian health care providers participating in TRICARE.[202] With the exception of active duty servicemembers, MHS beneficiaries may have a choice of TRICARE plan options depending on their status and geographic location. Each plan option has different beneficiary cost-sharing features, including annual enrollment fees, deductibles, copayments, and an annual catastrophic cap.[203]

COVID-19 diagnostic and serologic testing is a TRICARE-covered benefit when deemed medically necessary by a health care provider.[204] Beneficiaries may receive COVID-19 testing at certain MTFs or through TRICARE-authorized civilian heath care providers or laboratories. DOD

---

[201] Defense Health Agency, "Patients by Beneficiary Category," accessed June 10, 2020, https://www.health.mil/I-Am-A/Media/Media-Center/Patient-Population-Statistics/Patients-by-Beneficiary-Category.

[202] For more on the Military Health System, see CRS In Focus IF10530, *Defense Primer: Military Health System*.

[203] For more on TRICARE cost-sharing features, see Defense Health Agency, TRICARE Fact Sheet, *TRICARE Costs and Fees 2020*, May 2020, https://tricare.mil/-/media/Files/TRICARE/Publications/Misc/Costs_Sheet_2020.pdf.

[204] DOD generally follows CDC guidance on COVID-19 screening, testing, diagnosis, and treatment. For more on DOD-specific clinical guidance, see DOD, "DoD COVID-19 Practice Management Guide," May 14, 2020, https://www.health.mil/Reference-Center/Technical-Documents/2020/05/14/DoD-COVID-19-Practice-Management- Guide-Version-2.

has approximately 100 clinical laboratories (stand-alone or embedded at MTFs) worldwide with COVID-19 diagnostic capabilities and can support up to 16,000 tests per day.[205]

There are no out-of-pocket costs for MHS beneficiaries obtaining medically necessary COVID- 19 tests. Pursuant to FFRCA Section 6006(a), DOD is required to waive all TRICARE cost- sharing requirements related to COVID-19 testing, administration of the test, and related items and services provided during an associated health care office, urgent care, or emergency department visit for the duration of the declared public health emergency.[206] In addition to COVID-19 diagnostic and serologic testing, DOD conducts asymptomatic screening and ongoing surveillance testing of certain active duty servicemembers to mitigate potential impacts to national security or ongoing military operations. Servicemembers subjected to mandatory surveillance testing include those assigned to strategic and nuclear deterrence positions, initial recruitment or accession training, and forward-deployed forces.[207]

Does FEMA Pay for COVID-19 Testing?

FEMA may provide direct and financial assistance for certain costs incurred for COVID-19 testing. The presidential declarations of emergency

---

[205] Email from the Defense Health Agency (DHA), Armed Forces Health Surveillance Branch, Integrated Biosurveillance Section, June 4, 2020; and CRS discussion with other DHA officials, June 10, 2020.

[206] For more on DOD-specific requirements and appropriations included in the FFCRA, see CRS Report R46316, *Health Care Provisions in the Families First Coronavirus Response Act, P.L. 116-127*; and Defense Health Agency, *Decision Memorandum on TRICARE Implementation of the "Families First Coronavirus Response Act*, April 7, 2020, https://www.health.mil/Reference-Center/Publications/2020/04/07/TRICARE-Implementation-of-the-Families-First- Coronavirus-Response-Act.

[207] See Jim Garamone, "DOD Starts Tiered COVID-19 Testing Process to Ensure Safety," *DOD News*, April 22, 2020, https://www.defense.gov/Explore/News/Article/Article/2160008/dod-starts-tiered-covid-19-testing-process-to-ensure- safety/; and DOD, "Force Health Protection Guidance (Supplement 9) – Department of Defense Guidance for Deployment and Redeployment of Individuals and Units during the Novel Coronavirus Disease 2019 Pandemic," May 26, 2020, https://media.defense.gov/2020/May/26/2002305748/-1/-1/1/FORCE-HEALTH-PROTECTION- GUIDANCE-SUPPLEMENT-9.PDF.

and major disaster for COVID-19[208] under the Robert T. Stafford Disaster Relief and Emergency Assistance Act (hereinafter the Stafford Act) specifically authorized Public Assistance (PA) Category B: Emergency Protective Measures, defined as work undertaken to save lives and protect property or public health and safety, or to avert the threat of a catastrophe.[209] This work includes the provision of specific medical care costs directly related to the COVID-19 pandemic, including "triage and medically necessary tests and diagnosis related to COVID-19 patients."[210] Related eligible costs include, but are not limited to

- the costs of consumable and durable medical supplies;
- the costs of temporary and expanded medical facilities;
- overtime for budgeted medical staff treating COVID-19 patients;
- regular time and overtime for temporary and contracted medical staff treating COVID-19 patients; and
- the purchase and delivery of specialized medical equipment, PPE, and durable and consumable medical supplies.[211]

---

[208] The President issued an emergency declaration, and subsequently issued major disaster declarations for all 50 states, five territories, the District of Columbia, and one tribe, authorizing Public Assistance (PA) for COVID-19 response efforts (Federal Emergency Management Agency (FEMA), "COVID-19 Disaster Declarations," https://www.fema.gov/coronavirus/disaster-declarations (Stafford Act Declarations as of June 16, 2020).

[209] Public Assistance (PA) provides grant assistance to state, tribal, territorial, and local governments, as well as eligible private nonprofit organizations, for the costs of urgent response and long-term recovery work following an emergency or major disaster declared under the Robert T. Stafford Disaster Relief and Emergency Assistance Act (Stafford Act; P.L. 93-288, as amended; 42 U.S.C. §§5121 et seq.). Assistance for emergency protective measures is authorized under Stafford Act Sections 402, 403, 407, 418, and 419 for major disasters, and Section 502 for emergencies; 42 U.S.C. §§5170a, 5170b, 5173, 5185, 5186, and 5192. See 44 C.F.R. §206.220 for general eligibility for public assistance. FEMA released guidance specific to COVID-19, including a nonexclusive list of emergency protective measures. FEMA, "Coronavirus (COVID-19) Pandemic: Eligible Emergency Protective Measures," fact sheet, March 19, 2020, https://www.fema.gov/fact-sheet/eligible-emergency-protective-measures.

[210] FEMA, "Coronavirus (COVID-19) Pandemic: Medical Care Costs Eligible for Public Assistance," FP 104-010-04, May 9, 2020, p. 3, https://www.fema.gov/media-library-data/1589208038530-19c77b9558076c303b4ebec5f0631697/PA_Medical_Care_Policy_for_COVID-19_508.pdf (hereinafter, FEMA, "COVID-19: Eligible Medicare Care Costs").

[211] Eligibility for the costs of PPE and medical supplies are subject to disposition requirements. For a nonexclusive list of eligible medical care costs and requirements, see FEMA, "COVID-19: Eligible Medicare Care Costs."

For COVID-19, FEMA will reimburse PA Applicants, which can include state, tribal, territorial, and local governments, as well as eligible private nonprofit organizations[212] (including nonprofit medical facilities), for 75% of eligible costs incurred while performing eligible work, including medically necessary tests.[213] For example, news sources have reported that FEMA reimbursed the State of Iowa for contract testing services provided by TestIowa, a public-private partnership to provide COVID-19 testing.[214]

There is no predetermined limit on the amount of funding available through the PA program.[215] However, FEMA will not reimburse costs covered by another source, which may include private or publicly funded insurance, funding provided through the CARES Act (P.L. 116-136), the COVID-19 Uninsured Program for uninsured patients, or programs overseen by HHS, among others.[216] In addition, to be eligible for reimbursement, FEMA must confirm that costs are reasonable.[217] FEMA has advised it will use Medicare rates as the basis to determine cost reasonability for eligible medical care.[218]

---

[212] FEMA describes eligible private nonprofit organizations in FEMA, *Public Assistance Program and Policy Guide (PAPPG)*, FP 104-009-2, effective June 1, 2020, pp. 43-48, https://www.fema.gov/media-library-data/1594239534694-ea876c73c2135c4273e49145867879f/PAPPG_V4_Final_6-1-2020_508.pdf.

[213] FEMA, "COVID-19 Emergency Protective Measures." For information on eligibility of PA applicants, work, and costs, see 44 C.F.R. §206.220 and FEMA, *PAPPG*, pp. 42-47, 51-59, 65-96. To receive reimbursement, work must be the legal responsibility of the applicant (44 C.F.R. §206.223(a)(3)). Emergency protective measures are "generally" the responsibility of state, local, tribal, and territorial governments, but may be the responsibility of certain private nonprofit organizations including medical care providers (FEMA, Coronavirus [COVID-19] Pandemic: Private Nonprofit Organizations," April 2, 2020, https://www.fema.gov/fact-sheet/coronavirus-covid-19-pandemic-private-nonprofit-organizations).

[214] News 7 KWWL.com, "FEMA Awards Iowa with $78 million for COVID-19 Response," May 7, 2020, https://kwwl.com/2020/05/07/fema-awards-iowa-with-78-million-for-covid-19-response/. The TestIowa website is available at https://www.testiowa.com/en.

[215] Stafford Act assistance is subject to the availability of funds in the Disaster Relief Fund, as discussed below.

[216] FEMA, "COVID-19: Eligible Medicare Care Costs," p. 7-8; Stafford Act Section 312 (42 U.S.C. §5155). The HHS Uninsured Program fund is discussed in the "How Can Facilities That Provide Testing for Uninsured Individuals Be Reimbursed?" section of this chapter.

[217] 2 C.F.R. §200.404; FEMA, *PAPPG*, 65-96; and FEMA, "Public Assistance: Reasonable Cost Evaluation," Job Aid, https://www.fema.gov/media-library-data/1539879525279-d00ae1c43f9765c5a4b415e1a31202c5/PA_Reasonable_Cost_Evaluation_Job_Aid_508_FINAL_10-16-2018.pdf.

[218] FEMA will use standard Medicare rates that do not include the 20% increase in COVID-19 Medicare DRG rates implemented by the CARES Act. FEMA, "COVID-19: Eligible Medicare Care Costs," p. 5.

PA is funded through the Disaster Relief Fund (DRF), the primary source of funding for the federal government's domestic general disaster relief programs. DRF appropriations are not allocated for specific emergencies, disasters, or forms of assistance, including PA. Division B of the CARES Act (P.L. 116-136) included $45 billion for the DRF in March 2020, bringing its available balance for the costs of major disasters to more than $87 billion at the end of that month.[219] This is the first time FEMA has exercised Stafford Act authorities as a primary response to a pandemic, so FEMA has not provided projections for future spending from the DRF—including PA—on the COVID-19 response.[220]

Payment for Testing for Individuals with No Source of Coverage

As mentioned above, some community-based testing and testing at some types of facilities may be available to individuals who do not have a source of payment. The federal government has created an uninsured fund that may reimburse facilities for testing provided to uninsured individuals. In addition, Congress has enacted legislation that has expanded Medicaid eligibility under limited circumstances so that Medicaid funds may be available for testing for some uninsured individuals who are otherwise ineligible for Medicaid.

How Can Facilities That Provide Testing for Uninsured Individuals Be Reimbursed?

Various laws enacted in response to the COVID-19 pandemic may provide reimbursement to providers who offer testing to uninsured

---

[219] FEMA, "Disaster Relief Fund: Monthly Report, as of March 31, 2020," April 8, 2020, p. 7, https://www.fema.gov/media-library-data/1586553202915-6ad14cfec022590b2485cba9039190b0/Apr2020DisasterReliefFundReport.pdf.

[220] For more information, see CRS Report R45484, *The Disaster Relief Fund: Overview and Issues*; and CRS Report R46326, *Stafford Act Declarations for COVID-19 FAQ*.

individuals. FFRCA provides $1 billion for testing of individuals who are uninsured as defined in FFRCA.[221] The CARES Act appropriated $100 billion for provider relief, termed the Provider Relief Fund (PRF), which was established "to reimburse, through grants or other mechanisms, eligible health care providers for health care related expenses or lost revenues that are attributable to coronavirus."[222] An unspecified portion of this fund will be used to treat the uninsured.[223] PPPHCEA provided an additional $75 billion for the PRF, as well as an additional $1 billion for testing for the uninsured.[224]

These funding streams are being administered by HRSA. Entities that seek reimbursement for testing and related services under the FFRCA/PPPHCEA allocation must comply with certain terms and conditions.[225] For example, entities must register with the fund, provide required information about the services provided and the patient the services were provided to, agree to accept the Medicare rate as full payment, and may not seek cost-sharing from individuals. For patients who were tested prior to the funds' establishment, and for whom a facility may have already sought reimbursement, the facility must agree to return the already collected cost-sharing to individuals.[226] Facilities are not required to seek reimbursement from this fund, and they may provide care to individuals who are uninsured and seek payment from the patient who received testing or treatment directly.

---

[221] For more information, see CRS Report R46316, *Health Care Provisions in the Families First Coronavirus Response Act, P.L. 116-127*, and HHS, HRSA, "COVID-19 Claims Reimbursements to Health Care Providers and Facilities for the Testing and Treatment of the Uninsured," https://coviduninsuredclaim.linkhealth.com/.

[222] P.L. 116-136.

[223] CRS Report R46353, *COVID-19: Overview of FY2020 LHHS Supplemental Appropriations*.

[224] For information on the HHS Provider Relief Fund, see CRS Insight IN11438, *The COVID-19 Health Care Provider Relief Fund*.

[225] HHS, HRSA, "FFCRA Relief Fund Payment Terms and Conditions," https://www.hhs.gov/sites/default/files/terms-and-conditions-ffcra-relief-fund.pdf.

[226] HHS, HRSA, "COVID-19 Claims Reimbursements to Health Care Providers and Facilities for the Testing and Treatment of the Uninsured," https://coviduninsuredclaim.linkhealth.com/.

Under What Circumstances Will Medicaid Pay for Uninsured Testing?

Section 6004 of the FFCRA, as amended by the CARES Act, added, at state option, a new Medicaid eligibility group to provide testing and diagnosis of COVID-19, including testing- related services (as specified under that law's new Medicaid mandatory service category), testing- related visit and the administration of the testing, without beneficiary cost-sharing for certain specified uninsured individuals during the public health emergency period. FFCRA provides a 100% federal medical assistance percentage (FMAP or federal matching rate) for medical assistance and administrative costs associated with Medicaid enrollees under this group.

Medicaid coverage under what is being referred to as the "COVID-19 testing" eligibility group is limited to in vitro diagnostic products for the detection of SARS-CoV-2 or the diagnosis of COVID-19.[227] Coverage under this optional eligibility group is tied to the COVID-19 public health emergency, beginning no earlier than March 18, 2020, through the end of the COVID-19 public health emergency period, as specified. The law defines "uninsured individuals" as

- individuals who are not enrolled in another health care program funded by the federal government, including CHIP, Basic Health Program (BHP), Medicare, TRICARE and the VA, and federal employee health plans;
- individuals who are not enrolled in a group health plan or health insurance coverage offered by a health insurance issuer (as defined in PHSA Section 2791), including a qualified health plan through an exchange, employer-sponsored health insurance, retiree health

[227] As with the new Medicaid mandatory coverage of in vitro diagnostic testing added under FFCRA, as amended by the CARES Act, diagnostic and serological testing may be covered for symptomatic and asymptomatic Medicaid enrollees determined eligible via the "COVID-19 testing" pathway, as long as such tests are driven by medical necessity. To date, the Medicaid specific CMS guidance has not explicitly addressed the question of whether states can use Medicaid as a payer of public health surveillance testing for SARS-CoV-2 (to screen for general health and safety).

plans and Consolidated Omnibus Budget Reconciliation Act (COBRA) continuation coverage;[228]

- individuals who are not eligible to receive coverage under one of Medicaid's existing mandatory eligibility groups (e.g., poverty-related children);
- individuals who would be eligible for Medicaid via the Affordable Care Act (ACA, P.L. 111-148) Medicaid expansion pathway in states that have not adopted this eligibility pathway (i.e., non-ACA Medicaid expansion states); and
- certain specified Medicaid enrollees who, by virtue of their Medicaid eligibility pathway, are entitled to limited Medicaid benefits, including
    - low-income tuberculosis-infected individuals who are entitled to services related to the tuberculosis infection,
    - individuals eligible only for family planning services and supplies,
    - individuals eligible through the Medically Needy pathway[229] whose coverage does not meet minimum essential health coverage,[230] and
    - certain low-income pregnant woman who are entitled to limited pregnancy- related services.

While there is no income or resource test associated with the "COVID-19 testing" eligibility pathway, applicants must be otherwise eligible for

[228] CMS Medicaid FAQs. For questions about these types of private health insurance plans, congressional clients may contact Vanessa Forsberg.

[229] Medically needy individuals (e.g., children, pregnant women, aged, blind, or disabled) are those who are otherwise eligible for Medicaid but who have incomes too high to qualify and spend down their income on medical care. For this medically needy subgroup, states may offer a more restrictive benefit package than is available to other enrollees.

[230] For more information on the CMS criteria used to evaluate whether a given state's medically needy coverage meets the minimum essential health coverage standard, see CMS, Dear State Health Official, Dear State Medicaid Director, SHO# 14-002, Re: Minimum Essential Coverage, November 7, 2014, https://www.medicaid.gov/sites/default/files/ Federal-Policy-Guidance/downloads/SHO-14-002.pdf. For more general information on minimum essential coverage under Medicaid, see https://www.medicaid.gov/medicaid/eligibility/minimum-essential-coverage/index.html.

Medicaid (e.g., they must meet federal and state requirements regarding residency, immigration status, and documentation of U.S. citizenship). Like all other Medicaid eligibility pathways, applicants for the optional "COVID-19 testing" pathway are required to provide a Social Security number.[231]

Can the Uninsured Fund Reimburse Testing Provided to the Optional Medicaid COVID-19 Testing Group?

Medicaid enrollees eligible through the optional "COVID-19 testing" group are not eligible for coverage of COVID-19 testing and testing-related services through the HRSA-administered COVID-19 Claims Reimbursement Program. In instances where an HRSA-administered COVID- 19 Claims Reimbursement Program pays a claim for COVID-19 testing or testing-related services to a provider, but later determines that such services were delivered to a Medicaid enrollee (regardless of that person's Medicaid eligibility pathway), HRSA is required to recover payment(s) made to the provider and to advise the provider to bill Medicaid as the primary payer.[232]

How Can Individuals Who Are Unauthorized Immigrants Obtain Testing?

Unauthorized (sometimes referred to as *undocumented*) immigrants are eligible to obtain testing anywhere that COVID-19 testing is offered; for example, doctors' offices, public health sites, hospitals' emergency departments, and community health centers.

---

[231] 42 C.F.R. §435.910.

[232] Centers for Medicare & Medicaid Services, *NEW FAQs- Released June 30, 2020*, COVID-19 Frequently Asked Questions (FAQs) for State Medicaid and Children's Health Insurance Program (CHIP) Agencies, June 30, 2020, https://www.medicaid.gov/state-resource-center/downloads/covid-19-new-faqs.pdf.

Over half (55%) of the nonelderly[233] unauthorized population in the United States has health insurance.[234] Nonelderly unauthorized immigrants who are uninsured can receive free or reduced- cost testing at some of the aforementioned locations. Health care providers can seek reimbursement through the HRSA-administered COVID-19 Claims Reimbursement Program.

HRSA has stated that "health care providers are not required to confirm immigration status prior to submitting claims for reimbursement."[235]

Under What Circumstances Will Medicaid Pay for Testing for Unauthorized Immigrants?

With a few exceptions,[236] state Medicaid programs are prohibited from covering unauthorized immigrants.[237] Under one such exception, emergency Medicaid, unauthorized immigrants who are otherwise eligible for Medicaid except for their immigration status may receive "medical assistance under Title XIX of the Social Security Act … for care and emergency services that are necessary for the treatment of an emergency medical condition (as defined in Section 1903(v)(3) of such Act) of the alien involved and are not related to an organ transplant procedure."[238]

In response to the COVID-19 public health emergency, some states have extended coverage for certain specified COVID-19-related health care

---

233 Individuals under the age of 65.

234 Samantha Artiga and Maria Diaz, "Healthcare Coverage and Care of Undocumented Immigrants," Kaiser Family Foundation, July 15, 2019, at https://www.kff.org/disparities-policy/issue-brief/health-coverage-and-care-of- undocumented-immigrants/.

235 HRSA, "Frequently Asked Questions for the COVID-19 Claims Reimbursement to Health Care Providers and Facilities for Testing and Treatment of the Uninsured Program," at https://www.hrsa.gov/coviduninsuredclaim/ frequently-asked-questions.

236 These exceptions are (1) emergency Medicaid; (2) State Children's Health Insurance Coverage (CHIP) coverage for fetuses as permitted through federal regulation (often referred to as the CHIP unborn child pathway); and (3) the CHIPRA option that allows states to provide Medicaid coverage to certain lawfully residing children and/or pregnant women within the five-year waiting period when certain conditions are met.

237 For more information, see CRS Report RL33809, *Noncitizen Eligibility for Federal Public Assistance: Policy Overview*.

238 See Personal Responsibility and Work Opportunity Reconciliation Act of 1996 (PRWORA; P.L. 104-193), §401(a)(1)(A).

expenses (e.g., testing) to otherwise eligible unauthorized immigrants under emergency Medicaid.[239] The duration and scope of COVID-19- related emergency Medicaid coverage vary depending on the state.[240]

Also, on May 20, 2020, CMS approved a temporary Emergency Medicaid State Plan Amendment (SPA) that permits the Commonwealth of Northern Mariana Islands (CNMI) to adopt the FFCRA "COVID-19 testing" eligibility pathway to extend COVID-19 testing without cost-sharing to uninsured individuals (as defined in FFCRA and as amended by CARES).[241] Through this temporary emergency SPA, CMNI is extending the COVID testing for uninsured pathway to individuals regardless of their immigration status. This is done by using the presumptive eligibility Medicaid enrollment facility tool to relax requirements regarding citizenship documentation. This SPA temporarily extends Medicaid to unauthorized immigrants outside of emergency Medicaid and is in place from April 1, 2020, through the end of the public health emergency period, including any extensions.

EMERGENCY SUPPLEMENTAL FUNDING FOR TESTING

Testing includes the direct provision of diagnostic tests in traditional health care settings, the provision of testing in community-based and other less traditional settings, and the provision of public health testing outside of the clinical context. As described above, the testing supply chain has been under stress, as has the capacity of clinical laboratories to carry out necessary testing. To help address these issues, Congress and the President have appropriated emergency supplemental FY2020 funding to be used for the clinical provision of tests, as well as for support of developing testing infrastructure and capacity.

---

239 For more information about states that are covering COVID-19 testing and treatment under emergency Medicaid, see Jane Shubel, *States are Leveraging Medicaid to Respond to COVID-19*, Center on Budget and Policy Priorities, June 18, 2020, https://www.cbpp.org/sites/default/files/atoms/files/5-7-20health.pdf#page=7.

240 For more information, see CRS Report R46339, *Unauthorized Immigrants' Eligibility for COVID-19 Relief Benefits: In Brief.*

241 The Commonwealth of the Northern Mariana Islands (CNMI) emergency Medicaid state plan amendment is available at https://www.medicaid.gov/sites/default/files/State-resource-center/Medicaid-State-Plan-Amendments/ Downloads/CNMI/MP-20-0001.pdf.

What Funds Have Been Appropriated for Testing Capacity and Infrastructure?

Recently enacted supplemental appropriations have included funding for several accounts that can be used to support COVID-19 testing capacity and infrastructure. Testing capacity and infrastructure are defined here as activities and functions intended to help provide COVID-19 testing at scale to help control the spread of the virus. Such activities and functions can include increasing laboratory capacity (facilities, equipment, and workforce); procuring testing supplies and improving supply chains; establishing and supporting community-based testing sites; and supporting public health testing programs.

Many of the accounts in the table include funding that can be used for many purposes—testing infrastructure and capacity related activities are among the *possible* uses of the funds. Although this table is inclusive of all budgetary resources in relevant accounts that, among their purposes, could support testing, the dollar amounts in the table should not be interpreted as representing the amount of funding that will eventually go to support testing. It is expected that these funds will also go toward supporting a variety of non-testing-related purposes.

Though funding testing capacity and infrastructure differ from funding for testing individuals (covered in the next question), this distinction is not always clear cut. For example, CDC and FEMA funds can be used for testing capacity and infrastructure, as well as to pay for testing of individuals. In Table 2, CDC and FEMA amounts are included because the accounts support testing capacity and infrastructure activities. In addition, CDC- and FEMA-supported testing programs are aimed at providing testing to individuals as a part of multifaceted disease control and emergency response effort rather than to specifically fund COVID-19 testing in health care settings for clinical purposes.

Table 2 shows accounts from which funding can be used in part for testing and infrastructure activities as provided in the following coronavirus-related supplemental appropriations acts:[242]

- Division A, Coronavirus Preparedness and Response Supplemental Appropriations Act, 2020 (P.L. 116-123), enacted on March 6, 2020.
- Division B, Coronavirus Aid, Relief, and Economic Security Act (P.L. 116-136), enacted on March 27, 2020.
- Division B, Paycheck Protection Program and Health Care Enhancement Act (P.L. 116-139), enacted on April 24, 2020.

Table 2. Funding available for testing infrastructure and capacity in coronavirus supplemental appropriations
Accounts with funding available for testing capacity and infrastructure. Budget authority in millions or billions of dollars as specified

Account	Amount	Purpose	Availability
Coronavirus Preparedness and Response Supplemental Appropriations Act, 2020 (P.L. 116-123)[a]			
Department of Health and Human Services (HHS)—Centers for Disease Control and Prevention (CDC)— CDC-Wide Activities and Program Support	$2.2 billion including relevant set- asides or transfers below (less specified set-aside of not less than $300 million)[b]	"to prevent, prepare for, and respond to coronavirus, domestically or internationally." CDC may direct this funding for testing- related activities, such as for public health laboratories and testing programs.	September 30, 2022
Grants/cooperative agreements with states, localities, territories, tribes, tribal organizations, urban Indian health organizations, or health service providers to tribes (non-add)	*Not less than $950 million, including $40 million allocated to tribes, tribal organizations, urban Indian health organizations, or health service providers to tribes*	*As above "including to carry out surveillance, epidemiology, laboratory capacity, infection control, mitigation, communications, and other preparedness and response activities."*	*As above*

[242] The second supplemental appropriations measure, the Families First Coronavirus Response Act (P.L. 116-127) did not include available funding for MCM research and development.

Account	Amount	Purpose	Availability
Coronavirus Preparedness and Response Supplemental Appropriations Act, 2020 (P.L. 116-123)[a]			
Transfer to the Infectious Disease Rapid Response Reserve Fund (IDRRRF; non-add)	*$300 million*	*As specified by 42 U.S.C. §247d-4a IDRRRF funds may be used "for carrying out titles II, III, and XVII of the Public Health Service Act to prevent, prepare for, or respond to an infectious disease emergency"* *CDC may direct this funding for testing-related activities, such as for public health laboratories and testing programs.*	*As above*
HHS Office of the Secretary (OS)—Public Health and Social Services Emergency Fund (PHSSEF)	$3.1 billion and $300 million in contingent appropriations (less specified transfers of not more than $102 million)[c]	"to prevent, prepare for, and respond to coronavirus, domestically or internationally, including the development of necessary countermeasures and vaccines, prioritizing platform-based technologies with U.S.-based manufacturing capabilities, and the purchase of vaccines, therapeutics, diagnostics, necessary medical supplies, medical surge capacity, and related administrative activities." The HHS Secretary may use funding in this account to pay for procurement of tests or testing-related equipment and supplies.	September 30, 2024
Coronavirus Aid, Relief, and Economic Security Act (CARES Act; P.L. 116-136)[d]			
Department of Defense (DOD)—National Guard Personnel, Army[e]	$746.6 million	"to prevent, prepare for, and respond to coronavirus, domestically or internationally." In some states, National Guard personnel aid in testing programs. DOD personnel accounts fund basic and specialty pays and certain fringe benefits	September 30, 2020
DOD—National Guard Personnel, Air Force	$482.1 million	As above	September 30, 2020

Table 2. (Continued)

Account	Amount	Purpose	Availability
DOD—Operation and Maintenance, Army	$160.3 million	"to prevent, prepare for, and respond to coronavirus, domestically or internationally." DOD Operation and Maintenance accounts fund general mission-related operations, including supporting testing infrastructure and programs.	September 30, 2020
DOD—Operation and Maintenance, Navy	$360.3 million	As above	September 30, 2020
DOD—Operation and Maintenance, Marine Corps	$90.0 million	As above	September 30, 2020
Coronavirus Aid, Relief, and Economic Security Act (CARES Act; P.L. 116-136)[d]			
DOD—Operation and Maintenance, Air Force	$155.0 million	As above	September 30, 2020
DOD—Operation and Maintenance, Army Reserve	$48.0 million	As above	September 30, 2020
DOD—Operation and Maintenance. Army National Guard	$186.7 million	As above	September 30, 2020
DOD—Operation and Maintenance, Air National Guard	$75.8 million	As above	September 30, 2020
DOD—Operation and Maintenance, Defense-Wide	$827.8 million	As above	September 30, 2020
DOD—Defense Production Act Purchases	$1 billion	"to prevent, prepare for, and respond to coronavirus, domestically or internationally."[f]	Until expended[g]
Department of Veterans Affairs (VA)—Veterans Health Administration (VHA)—Medical Services	$14.4 billion	"to prevent, prepare for, and respond to coronavirus, domestically or internationally, including related impacts on health care delivery ... " Per the Senate Appropriations Committee summary, funding can be used for purchase of testing kits and related supplies for the VHA system.[h]	September 30, 2022

Account	**Amount**	**Purpose**	**Availability**
Department of Homeland Security— Federal Emergency Management Agency (FEMA)- Disaster Relief Fund[i]	$45 billion	The Disaster Relief Fund (DRF) is the primary source of funding for the federal government's domestic general disaster relief programs. While diagnostic testing and testing sites may get funded from the DRF through the FEMA Public Assistance Program, only a portion of DRF resources will go to COVID-19-related activities.	Until expended
HHS—CDC—CDC-Wide Activities and Program Support	$4.3 billion (less specified set-asides of not less than $1 billion)[j]	"to prevent, prepare for, and respond to coronavirus, domestically or internationally."	September 30, 2024
Coronavirus Aid, Relief, and Economic Security Act (CARES Act; P.L. 116-136)[d]			
		CDC may direct this funding for testing- related activities, such as for public health laboratories and testing programs.	
Grants/cooperative agreements with states, localities, territories, tribes, tribal organizations, urban Indian health organizations, or health service providers to tribes (non-add)	*$1.5 billion, including $125 million to tribes, tribal organizations, urban Indian health organizations, or health service providers to tribes*	*As above including "to carry out surveillance, epidemiology, laboratory capacity, infection control, mitigation, communications, and other preparedness and response activities."*	*As above*
Transfer to the IDRRRF (non-add)	*$300 million*	*As specified by 42 U.S.C. §247d-4a IDRRRF funds may be used "for carrying out titles II, III, and XVII of the Public Health Service Act to prevent, prepare for, or respond to an infectious disease emergency," CDC may direct this funding for testing-related activities, such as for public health laboratories and testing programs.*	*As above*

Table 2. (Continued)

Account	Amount	Purpose	Availability
HHS—OS—PHSSEF[k]	$27 billion including the set-asides below of not more than $16 billion (less other specified set-asides and transfers of roughly $4 billion)[l]	"to prevent, prepare for, and respond to coronavirus, domestically or internationally, including the development of necessary countermeasures and vaccines, prioritizing platform-based technologies with U.S.-based manufacturing capabilities, the purchase of vaccines, therapeutics, diagnostics, necessary medical supplies, as well as medical surge capacity, addressing blood supply chain, workforce modernization, telehealth access and infrastructure, initial advanced manufacturing, novel dispensing, enhancements to the U.S.	September 30, 2024
Coronavirus Aid, Relief, and Economic Security Act (CARES Act; P.L. 116-136)[d]			
		Commissioned Corps, and other preparedness and response activities."	
		The HHS Secretary may use funding in this account to pay for procurement of tests or testing-related equipment and supplies.	
Strategic National Stockpile (SNS)	*Not more than $16 billion*	*As above. The HHS Secretary may procure testing-related supplies for SNS and use it as a distribution mechanism.*	*As above*
Paycheck Protection Program and Health Care Enhancement Act (P.L. 116-139)[m]			
HHS—OS—PHSSEF[n]	$25 billion including set-asides and transfers below (less other specified set-asides or transfers of roughly $4.4 billion)[o]	"to prevent, prepare for, and respond to coronavirus, domestically or internationally, for necessary expenses to research, develop, validate, manufacture, purchase, administer, and expand capacity for COVID–19 tests to effectively monitor and suppress COVID–19, including tests for both active infection and prior exposure, including molecular, antigen, and	Until expended

Account	Amount	Purpose	Availability
		serological tests, the manufacturing, procurement and distribution of tests, testing equipment and testing supplies, including personal protective equipment needed for administering tests, the development and validation of rapid, molecular point-of-care tests, and other tests, support for workforce, epidemiology, to scale up academic, commercial, public health, and hospital laboratories, to conduct surveillance and contact tracing, support development of COVID–19 testing plans, and other related activities related to COVID–19 testing."	
Paycheck Protection Program and Health Care Enhancement Act (P.L. 116-139)[m]			
Grants/cooperative agreements with states, localities, territories, tribes, tribal organizations, urban Indian health organizations, or health service providers to tribes (non-add).	*Not less than $11 billion, of that amount, not less than $750,000,000 shall be allocated in coordination with the Director of the Indian Health Service, to tribes, tribal organizations, urban Indian health organizations, or health service providers to tribes.*	*"to develop, purchase, administer, process, and analyze COVID–19 tests, including support for workforce, epidemiology, use by employers or in other settings, scale up of testing by public health, academic, commercial, and hospital laboratories, and community-based testing sites, health care facilities, and other entities engaged in COVID–19 testing, conduct surveillance, trace contacts, and other related activities related to COVID–19 testing."*	*As above*
CDC-Wide Activities and Program Support	*Not less than $1 billion*	*"for surveillance, epidemiology, laboratory capacity expansion, contact tracing, public health data surveillance and analytics infrastructure modernization, disseminating information about testing, and workforce support necessary to expand and improve COVID–19 testing."*	*As above*

Table 2. (Continued)

Account	Amount	Purpose	Availability
Rural health clinics	*$225 million*	*"additional funding for COVID–19 testing and related expenses, through grants or other mechanisms, to rural health clinics as defined in section 1861(aa)(2) of the Social Security Act, with such funds also available to such entities for building or construction of temporary structures, leasing of properties, and retrofitting facilities as necessary to support COVID–19 testing."*	*As above*

Source: CRS analysis of COVID-19 response legislation.

[a] HHS may transfer nearly all the funds appropriated to it in Title III, Division A, of P.L. 116-123, among accounts at CDC, NIH, or PHSSEF, provided the transfers are made to prevent, prepare for, and respond to the COVID-19 pandemic, domestically or internationally (see §304). HHS is to notify the House and the Senate appropriations committees 10 days in advance of such a transfer.

[b] Not less than $300 million of the total $2.2 billion for CDC is for global disease detection and emergency response.

[c] Transfers specified are $100 million to the Health Resources and Services Administration (HRSA) for grants for health centers and up to $2 million to the HHS Office of Inspector General (OIG).

[d] HHS may transfer nearly all the funds appropriated to it in Title VIII, Division B, of P.L. 116-136 among accounts at CDC, PHSSEF, NIH, Administration for Children and Families, and the Administration for Community Living, provided the transfers are made to prevent, prepare for, and respond to the COVID-19 pandemic, domestically or internationally (see §18111). HHS is to notify the House and the Senate appropriations committees 10 days in advance of such a transfer.

[e] Funds in DOD accounts: "Funds appropriated by this title may be transferred to, and merged with, other applicable appropriations of the Department of Defense, except for 'Drug Interdiction and Counter-Drug Activities, Defense,' for expenses incurred in preventing, preparing for, or responding to coronavirus, including expenses of the Department of Defense incurred in support of other Federal Departments and agencies, and State, local, and Indian tribal governments, to be merged with and to be available for the same purposes, and for the same time period, as the appropriation or fund to which transferred."

[f] Thus far, the only public announcement of a testing-related allocation of the DPA funding was on April 29 with $75 million for nasal swab production. See CRS Insight IN11387, COVID-19: Defense Production Act (DPA) Developments and Issues for Congress.

[g] The CARES Act suspended the year-to-year funding cap of $750 million for DPA for two years.

[h] Based on Senate Appropriations Committee, Coronavirus Supplemental Appropriations Summary, available at https://www.appropriations.senate.gov/download/coronavirus-emergency-supple-mental-appropriations-summary.

[i] Public Assistance is funded through the Disaster Relief Fund (DRF), the primary source of funding for the federal government's domestic general disaster relief programs. DRF appropriations are not allocated to specific emergencies, disasters, or specific forms of assistance, including food assistance. Division B of the CARES Act (P.L. 116-136) included $45 billion for the DRF in March 2020, bringing its available balance for the costs of major disasters to more than $87 billion. As of June 30, 2020, almost $7.3 billion had been obligated for COVID-19 costs—and the unobligated balance of the fund was approximately $76 billion.

[j] Specified set-asides for purposes that are not primarily related to domestic testing include not less than $500 billion for global disease detection and emergency response and not less than $500 million for "public health data

surveillance and analytics modernization." The public health data funds are not included in the table as they are primarily for "modernization" of data systems (including testing-related data among others) rather than to support testing-related data collection specifically.

[k] Not more than $4 million per Title VIII, Division B, Section 8113, is to be transferred to the HHS OIG from the $127.29 billion total appropriated to PHSSEF for oversight of all activities supported with funds appropriated to HHS to prevent, prepare for, and respond to the COVID-19 pandemic.

[l] Other specified set-asides for purposes that are not primarily related to domestic testing include not less than $250 million for Hospital Preparedness Program grantees or subgrantees; not less than $3.5 billion for the Biomedical Advanced Research and Development Authority; not more than $289 million for other federal agencies for the care of persons under federal quarantine; and $1.5 million for a National Academies of Science, Medicine, and Engineering study on the medical supply chain.

[m] HHS may transfer certain funds appropriated to it in Title I, Division B, of P.L. 116-139 among accounts at CDC, NIH, PHSSEF, and FDA, provided the transfers are made to prevent, prepare for, and respond to the COVID-19 pandemic (see §102). HHS is to notify the House and the Senate appropriations committees 10 days in advance of such a transfer.

[n] Not more than $6 million per Title I, Division B, Section 103, of P.L. 116-139, is to be transferred to the HHS OIG from the $100 billion total appropriated to PHSSEF for oversight of all activities supported with funds appropriated to HHS to prevent, prepare for, and respond to the COVID-19 pandemic.

[o] Other specified set-asides or transfers include not less than $306 million transfer for the National Cancer Institute, not less than $500 million transfer for the National Institute of Biomedical Imaging and Bioengineering, not less than $1 billion transfer for the NIH Office of Director, not less than $1 billion for BARDA, $22 million transfer to the FDA, $600 million transfer to the HRSA, Community Health Centers program, not more than $1 billion for testing for the uninsured.

In some cases, funds are appropriated to relevant accounts; in others, transfers or set-asides to relevant agencies or accounts are either directed or allowed. (This transfer authority in several instances is either "not more than" or "not less than" a specified amount.) Funds to be transferred are shown in the account to which they were appropriated, not in the account to which they may be transferred.

The purpose of the funds indicates their allowed uses as specified in the respective appropriations acts. Additional contextual information is included where appropriate. The period of availability is either the date after which funds are no longer available for obligation or "until expended." To identify accounts in this table, CRS exercised professional judgement based on knowledge of agency activities. The goal was to be comprehensive; however, CRS cannot ensure that the below table is comprehensive of all accounts that can be used for testing capacity and infrastructure.

The table does not include funding for research and development for, or FDA approval of, new COVID-19 tests.

Paycheck Protection Program and Health Care Enhancement Act Testing Funding

As noted in Table 2, the PPPHCEA appropriated funds specifically to increase testing capacity. Specifically, PPPHCEA appropriated $25 billion to the PHSSEF—an account that may be used in appropriations acts to provide the HHS Secretary with one-time or emergency funding—to support the expansion of testing infrastructure and capacity broadly. These funds were in some cases transferred to specific agencies (e.g., HRSA, CDC) for certain purposes. For example, NIH received $1.5 billion for research and development of rapid point-of-care and other diagnostics, and FDA received a $22 million transfer to support in vitro diagnostic review activities at the agency. In addition, the act appropriated $11 billion to the states, localities, territories, and tribes to support broad public health activities related primarily to testing and contact tracing. The remaining funds were authorized to be used for notably broad activities to boost testing infrastructure, production, capacity, and administration, including for the purchase of testing supplies; for "construction, alteration, renovation, or equipping of non-federally owned facilities for the production of diagnostic, serologic, or other COVID–19 tests"; and "for grants for the rent, lease, purchase, acquisition, construction, alteration, renovation, or equipping of non- federally owned facilities to improve preparedness and response capability at the State and local level for diagnostic, serologic, or other COVID–19 tests."[243] The law also included a number of reporting and other requirements, including the development of a national testing strategy; that each state develop and submit to HHS its own state testing plan; and several on identifying racial and ethnic disparities related to COVID-19 testing, hospitalizations, and outcomes, including mortality.

PPPHCEA appropriated $225 million for testing at rural health clinics (RHCs), outpatient facilities located in rural areas. Each facility received approximately $50,000 for testing infrastructure, including expenses related to implementing a testing program, procuring supplies, and training providers and staff on issues related to testing. HRSA awarded these funds

---

[243] PPPHCEA (P.L. 116-139), Division B—Additional Emergency Appropriations for Coronavirus Response, Title I— Department of Health and Human Services.

and awarded $500,000 of the amount appropriated for technical assistance to support RHCs in implementing testing programs.[244] IHS also received $750 million in PPHCEA for testing capacity. IHS announced its plan to allocate these funds in a letter to tribal leaders on May 21.

The letter stated that the funds may be used to

> analyze COVID-19 tests, including support for workforce, epidemiology, and use by employers or in other settings. In addition, these funds can be used to scale up testing by public health, academic, commercial, and hospital laboratories, and community-based testing sites, health care facilities, and other entities engaged in COVID-19 testing. Funds may also be used to conduct surveillance, trace contacts, and perform other related activities related to COVID-19 testing.[245]

In terms of amounts, IHS announced that it will provide $50 million to urban Indian organizations for testing and $550 million for programs operated by the Indian Health Service or by tribes. IHS retains $150 million for nationwide coordination, epidemiological research, and surveillance.[246] Tribes that received funding were, like states, required to submit a testing plan to HHS that includes testing goals for the remainder of 2020. The plan was required to include the number of tests monthly by type; monthly estimates of laboratory and testing capacity, including the workforce needed to process tests and the relevant supplies; and a description of how funds will be used for testing and to meet the goals laid out in the testing plan.[247]

---

[244] HHS, HRSA, "HHS Providers $225 Million for COVID-19 Testing in Rural Communities," https://www.hhs.gov/about/news/2020/05/20/hhs-provides-225-million-for-covid19-testing-in-rural-communities.html.

[245] Letter from Michael D. Weahkee, Director Indian Health Service, to Dear Tribal Leader and Urban Indian Organization Leader, May 20, 2020, https://www.ihs.gov/sites/newsroom/themes/responsive2017/display_objects/documents/2020_Letters/DTLL_DUIOLL_05192020.pdf, p. 1.

[246] Ibid., p. 2.

[247] HHS, "HHS Delivers Funding to Expand Testing Capacity for States, Territories, Tribes," press release, May 18, 2020, https://www.hhs.gov/about/news/2020/05/18/hhs-delivers-funding-to-expand-testing-capacity-for-states- territories-tribes.html.

What Funds Have Been Appropriated for the Clinical Provision of Tests?

Congress and the President have also provided supplemental funding in several accounts to help pay for COVID-19 testing for individuals for clinical purposes. Table 3 shows FY2020 supplemental *discretionary appropriations* for accounts that can primarily be used to pay for testing of individuals for primarily *clinical purposes.*[248] Relevant funding has been included in two coronavirus-related supplemental appropriations measures:

- Division A, Families First Coronavirus Response Act (P.L. 116-127), enacted on March 18, 2020.[249]
- Division B, Paycheck Protection Program and Health Care Enhancement Act (P.L. 116-139), enacted on April 24, 2020.

The below table does not include the mandatory spending budgetary effects of clinical testing- related provisions carried in COVID-19 response legislation. For example, FFCRA and the CARES Act included several provisions to expand coverage of testing paid by federal health programs, such as Medicare and Medicaid, as well as private insurance. (Note that these are covered earlier in this chapter and in other CRS reports.)[250] In addition, discretionary accounts that can be used for a broad set of health care purposes (including testing among others), such as the Provider Relief Fund and funding for the Health Centers program are not included in the below table, as these funds have not been provided specifically for testing.

With regard to the discretionary funding in the below table, in some cases, funds are appropriated to relevant accounts; in others, transfers or set-asides to relevant agencies or accounts are either directed or allowed.

---

[248] For more information on clinical testing, see "For What Purposes Is COVID-19 Testing Used?"

[249] Division G of the Families First Coronavirus Response act included requirements about the use of testing funds. See CRS Report R46316, *Health Care Provisions in the Families First Coronavirus Response Act, P.L. 116-127.*

[250] See also CRS Report R46334, *Selected Health Provisions in Title III of the CARES Act (P.L. 116-136)* and CRS Report R46316, *Health Care Provisions in the Families First Coronavirus Response Act, P.L. 116-127.*

Table 3. Discretionary funding for clinical provision of tests in coronavirus supplemental appropriations Accounts with specific funding available for testing of individuals for clinical purposes; Budget authority in millions or billions of dollars, as specified

Account	Amount	Purpose	Availability
Families First Coronavirus Response Act (P.L. 116-127)[a]			
Department of Defense (DOD)—Defense Health Programs	$82 million	COVID-19 testing, administration of the test, and related items and services for Defense Health Program beneficiaries.	September 30, 2022
Department of Health and Human Services (HHS)—Indian Health Service	$64 million	COVID-19 testing, administration of the test, and related items and services for Indian Health Service Beneficiaries.	September 30, 2022
Department of Veterans Affairs (VA)—Veterans Health Administration (VHA)—Medical Services	$30 million	COVID-19 testing, administration of the test, and related items and services for covered veterans at Veterans Health Administration facilities.	September 30, 2022
Veterans Health Administration (Medical Community Care)	$30 million	COVID-19 testing, administration of the test, and related items and services through the Veterans Health Administration Community Care program.	September 30, 2022
HHS—Office of the Secretary (OS)—Public Health and Social Services Emergency Fund (PHSSEF)—Testing for the Uninsured	$1 billion	COVID-19 testing, administration of the test, and related items and services for uninsured individuals as defined.	Until expended
HHS—OS—PHSSEF-Testing for the Uninsured	Not more than transfer of $1 Billion	COVID-19 testing, administration of the test, and related items and services for uninsured individuals as defined.	Until expended
HHS—OS—PHSSEF—Health Resources and Services Administration Transfer	$600 million	Transferred to the Health Resources and Services Administration for Health Center Grants[c]	Until expended

Source: CRS analysis of legislation.

Notes: Comprehensive information about HHS transfer authorities and relevant transfers to the HHS Office of the Inspector General for the respective appropriations acts is included in Table 2.

[a] Division A appropriated testing funds, while Division G specified how these funds would be used. See CRS Report R46316, *Health Care Provisions in the Families First Coronavirus Response Act, P.L. 116-127.*

[b] CRS Report R46325, *Fourth COVID-19 Relief Package (P.L. 116-139): In Brief.*

[c] Health center funds were to supplement grants and were awarded specifically to expand testing capacity. See HHS, HRSA, "HHS Awards More than Half Billion Dollars Across the Nation to Expand COVID-19 Testing," https://www.hhs.gov/about/news/2020/05/07/hhs-awards-more-than-half-billion-across-the-nation- to-expand-covid19-testing.html.

(This transfer authority in several instances is either “not more than” or “not less than” a specified amount.) Funds to be transferred are shown in the account to which they were appropriated, not in the account to which may be transferred.

The purpose of the funds summarizes their allowed uses as specified in the respective appropriations acts. Unlike for the previous table, exact bill text is not cited for several accounts because of references to other provisions in the respective bills. For example, several of the provisions in the FFRCA use the construction, “for health services consisting of SARS–CoV–2 or COVID–19 related items and services as described in section 6006(b) of division F of the Families First Coronavirus Response Act (or the administration of such products).” Additional contextual information is included where appropriate. The period of availability is either the date after which funds are no longer available for obligation, or “until expended.”

As noted previously, CRS exercised professional judgement to distinguish accounts that pay for testing infrastructure and capacity from those that pay for testing of individuals, however this distinction is not always clear cut. Several of the accounts covered in the previous question can also be used to pay for testing of individuals and are not repeated in the below table, as the clinical provision of tests is not the primary purpose of those accounts. In addition, a number of the accounts discussed below received additional appropriations in the CARES Act that was not specific to testing, as such, these funds are not included in the table below. The below table shows accounts that primarily fund testing of individuals for clinical (rather than public health or emergency response) purposes.

PUBLIC HEALTH REPORTING OF COVID-19 TEST DATA

What Types of Testing Data Are Collected?

CDC collects many types of data related to testing, some provided by states or other jurisdictions and some provided directly by laboratories to

CDC.[251] These data are used to monitor public health trends, understand the virus, and better understand disease trends and affected populations. Some testing data are being collected directly by HHS from hospital-based academic and clinical laboratories.[252] Existing testing-related surveillance (i.e., data collection) systems include the following:

- Case-based surveillance. Positive COVID-19 test results are reported by laboratories to jurisdictions that then link and collect detailed information on each case, including demographic and health information. Jurisdictions use a case reporting system to report to CDC.[253] Case reporting occurs through two CDC data systems: the National Notifiable Diseases Surveillance System (NNDSS) and the Data Collation and Integration for Public Health Event Response (DCIPHER) platform.[254]
- Virological surveillance. Overall test positivity rates are captured across all public health laboratories and a subset of clinical and commercial laboratories.[255]
- Virus characterization. Viral samples from laboratories are used to monitor genomic changes in virus in CDC's SARS-CoV-2 Sequencing for Public Health Emergency Response, Epidemiology, and Surveillance (SPHERES) consortium.[256]

---

[251] CDC, *CDC Activities and Initiatives Supporting the President's Plan for Opening Up America Again*, May 2020, https://www.cdc.gov/coronavirus/2019-ncov/downloads/php/CDC-Activities-Initiatives-for-COVID-19-Response.pdf.

[252] HHS, "COVID-19 Guidance for Hospital Reporting and FAQs For Hospitals, Hospital Laboratory, and Acute Care Facility Data Reporting" updated July 10, 2020," https://www.hhs.gov/sites/default/files/covid-19-faqs-hospitals-hospital-laboratory-acute-care-facility-data-reporting.pdf.

[253] CDC, "Coronavirus Disease 2019: Reporting a Confirmed Case," updated May 5, 2020, https://www.cdc.gov/coronavirus/2019-ncov/php/reporting-pui.html.

[254] CRS correspondence with CDC, May 6, 2020.

[255] CDC, "COVIDView: A Weekly Surveillance Summary of U.S. COVID-19 Activity: Purpose and Methods," updated July 15, 2020, https://www.cdc.gov/coronavirus/2019-ncov/covid-data/covidview/purpose- methods.html#virologic.

[256] CDC, "Coronavirus Disease 2019: SARS-CoV-2 Sequencing (SPHERES)," updated July 7, 2020, https://www.cdc.gov/coronavirus/2019-ncov/covid-data/spheres.html?CDC_AA_refVal=https%3A%2F%2Fwww.cdc.gov%2Fcoronavirus%2F2019-ncov%2Fcases-updates%2Fspheres.html.

Traditionally, most public health data reporting requirements have been based in state law. States or other jurisdictions can mandate that laboratories or health care providers report data related to certain diseases to jurisdictions' public health departments. States then voluntarily share de-identified data with CDC as a part of national surveillance.[257] CDC can also form partnerships with specific jurisdictions, other federal agencies, and academic and nonprofit research institutions for public health data, an approach taken with SPHERES.[258]

Where Do COVID-19 Results Get Reported, and What Data Are Collected?

COVID-19 cases are reported to 60 U.S.-affiliated jurisdictions that then report to CDC, including the 50 states; the District of Columbia; New York City, the U.S. territories of American Samoa, Guam, the Commonwealth of the Northern Mariana Islands, Puerto Rico, and the U.S Virgin Islands; and three freely-associated states (Federated States of Micronesia, Republic of the Marshall Islands, and Republic of Palau).[259] Case reporting and other surveillance allow jurisdiction-level public health officials to respond to positive cases, conduct contact tracing, and make decisions about state and local public health policy. The data can also be used by researchers to inform an understanding of the disease and affected populations.[260]

---

257 Lawrence O. Gostin and Lindsay F. Wiley, "Chapter Nine: Surveillance and Public Health Research: Privacy, Security, and Confidentiality of Personal Health Information," in *Public Health Law: Duty, Power, and Restraint*, 3rd ed. (University of California Press), pp. 303-344.

258 CDC, "Coronavirus Disease 2019: SARS-CoV-2 Sequencing (SPHERES)," Updated July 7, 2020, https://www.cdc.gov/coronavirus/2019-ncov/covid-data/spheres.html?CDC_AA_refVal=https%3A%2F%2Fwww.cdc.gov%2Fcoronavirus%2F2019-ncov%2Fcases-updates%2Fspheres.html.

259 CDC, "About CDC Data," last updated July 13, 2020, https://www.cdc.gov/coronavirus/2019-ncov/cases-updates/ about-us-cases-deaths.html.

260 CDC, *CDC Activities and Initiatives Supporting the President's Plan for Opening Up America Again*, May 2020, https://www.cdc.gov/coronavirus/2019-ncov/downloads/php/CDC-Activities-Initiatives-for-COVID-19-Response.pdf.

Throughout the COVID-19 pandemic, many jurisdictions have faced issues with incomplete data from laboratories. In many reported cases, testing data reported from laboratories were missing key patient information needed to contact the patient and conduct contact tracing. In addition, much of the early COVID-19 data lacked information about patient demographic characteristics, such as on race and ethnicity.[261] After a positive test result, public health departments usually have to follow up with patients and providers to obtain full details about the case—a difficult and time-consuming task, especially when cases rise rapidly. In addition, many public health departments rely on fax or paper records shared by health care providers, which can be error- prone and add to delays.[262] Though the situation has somewhat improved, such missing data issues have hindered the public health response and experts' ability to analyze and understand the situation. Though CDC implements standardized reporting systems, states and other jurisdictions are usually responsible for deciding what information to collect and share with CDC.[263] In the early stages of the pandemic, many states were not collecting and/or reporting patient demographic information, such as on patients' race and ethnicity.[264] Guidance issued pursuant to a provision in the CARES Act changed federal reporting requirements for jurisdictions (as described below).

According to July 22nd data, 47 states report COVID-19 cases by race/ethnicity, 45 states report COVID-19 deaths by race, and 5 states report testing data by race.[265]

---

261 Kelly Servick, ""Huge Hole" in Testing Data Blurs Racial, Ethnic Disparities," *Science*, July 17, 2020, https://science.sciencemag.org/content/369/6501/237.

262 Darius Tahir, "Virus Hunters Rely on Faxes, Paper Records as More States Reopen," *Politico*, May 10, 2020; and Council of State and Territorial Epidemiologists, *Driving Public Health in the Fast Lane: The Urgent Need for a 21st Century Data Superhighway*, September 2019, https://cdn.ymaws.com/www.cste.org/resource/resmgr/pdfs/pdfs2/Driving_PH_Display.pdf.

263 Lawrence O. Gostin and Lindsay F. Wiley, "Chapter Nine: Surveillance and Public Health Research: Privacy, Security, and Confidentiality of Personal Health Information," in *Public Health Law: Duty, Power, and Restraint*, 3rd ed. (University of California Press), pp. 303-344.

264 Kelly Servick, ""Huge Hole" in Testing Data Blurs Racial, Ethnic Disparities," *Science*, July 17, 2020, https://science.sciencemag.org/content/369/6501/237.

265 Johns Hopkins University (JHU) Coronavirus Resource Center, "Racial Data Transparency: States that have Released COVID-19 Data by Race," last viewed July 22, 2020, https://coronavirus.jhu.edu/data/racial-data- transparency.

The CARES Act added new authorities for the HHS Secretary related to COVID-19 testing data. Specifically, Section 18115 of the CARES Act requires that every laboratory that performs or analyzes a test intended to detect or diagnose a possible case of COVID-19 report the test results to the HHS Secretary in such form and manner, and at such timing and frequency, as the Secretary may prescribe until the end of the Secretary's Public Health Emergency declaration (PHSA §319) with respect to COVID-19 or any extension of such declaration. The provision allows the Secretary to decide which laboratories must submit reports pursuant to that section and does not require the data be made publicly available.

On June 4, 2020, HHS issued guidance to implement Section 18115 of the CARES Act. As a part of the guidance, the Secretary requires that all laboratories report data with a minimum set of required elements to state or local public health departments using existing reporting channels.

The minimum required data elements that must be reported for each test include, among other things, patient age, race, ethnicity, sex, zip code, and county. The guidance also states that state and local public health departments should collect information about a patient's address and phone number, but should not share this information with CDC.[266] The press release accompanying the guidance stated,

> "HHS and the entire Trump Administration are deeply concerned that COVID-19 is having a disproportionate impact on certain demographics, including racial minorities and older Americans," said HHS Secretary Alex Azar. "High quality data is at the core of any effective public health response, and standardized, comprehensive reporting of testing information will give our public health experts better data to guide decisions at all levels throughout the crisis."[267]

[266] HHS, "COVID-19 Pandemic Response, Laboratory Data Reporting: CARES Act Section 18115," June 4, 2020, https://www.hhs.gov/sites/default/files/covid-19-laboratory-data-reporting-guidance.pdf.

[267] HHS, "HHS Announces New Laboratory Data Reporting Guidance for COVID-19 Testing," press release, June 4, 2020, https://www.hhs.gov/about/news/2020/06/04/hhs-announces-new-laboratory-data-reporting-guidance-for-covid- 19-testing.html.

The guidance gives laboratories several options for submitting the data. Laboratories may use existing reporting systems, as required by state or local law or policy, or through a state or regional health information exchange systems. State governments then share data with CDC on a daily basis.[268] Laboratories also may submit through an automated platform that shares data automatically with both state and local authorities as well as with CDC—the Association of Public Health Laboratories' (APHL's) Informatics Messaging Services (AIMS) platform.[269] According to CDC, as of July 7, 2020, 57% of jurisdictions were using the AIMS platform, with additional jurisdictions converting their systems.[270] A map with compiled case counts from all three systems is available on CDC's website.[271]

Separately, Vice President Michael R. Pence and HHS have issued testing-related data requests from hospital-based academic and clinical laboratories, several of which requested hospital-based laboratories to submit aggregate testing data directly to HHS on a daily basis.[272] As specified in updated guidance for hospitals on July 29, hospitals that perform "in-house" laboratory testing are to follow the June 4 guidelines pursuant to the CARES Act. For hospitals that are not reporting all data to their state health department or are located in a jurisdiction that has not converted to COVID-19 electronic laboratory reporting to CDC, they are requested to submit aggregate daily data to HHS until they confirm that CDC is receiving their data through the state. Such hospitals can use one of three methods: (1) the HHS Protect data system; (2) their state reporting system, if the state is reporting to the APSR administrator; or (3) their health information technology vendor, as authorized by the hospital to submit daily data to HHS/CDC. Hospitals do not need to report testing results for tests sent to commercial laboratories or to public health laboratories.[273]

---

[268] Ibid.

[269] Association of Public Health Laboratories (APHL), "APHL AIMS Platform," https://www.aphl.org/programs/ informatics/pages/aims_platform.aspx.

[270] Correspondence with CDC, July 7, 2020.

[271] CDC, "Coronavirus Disease 2019: Cases in the United States," https://www.cdc.gov/ coronavirus/2019-ncov/cases- updates/cases-in-us.html.

[272] CRS Insight IN11361, *COVID-19: U.S. Public Health Data and Reporting*.

[273] HHS, *COVID-19 Guidance for Hospital Reporting and FAQs for Hospitals, Hospital Laboratory, and Acute Care Facility Data Reporting Updated July 29, 2020*, July 29, 2020,

Appendix A. Acronyms Used in This Chapter

Acronym	Definition
ACA	Patient Protection and Affordable Care Act
AIMS	APHL Informatics Messaging Services
APHL	Association of Public Health Laboratories
AMP	Association for Molecular Pathology
ASPR	Assistant Secretary of Preparedness Response
BHP	Basic Health Program
CARES Act	Coronavirus Aid, Relief, and Economic Security Act
CBTS	Community-Based Testing Sites
CDC	Centers for Disease Control and Prevention
CFR	Code of Federal Regulations
CHIP	Children's Health Insurance Program
CLIA	Clinical Laboratory Improvement Amendments
CMS	Centers for Medicare & Medicaid Services
CNMI	Commonwealth of Northern Mariana Islands
COBRA	Consolidated Omnibus Budget Reconciliation Act
DCIPHER	Data Collation and Integration for Public Health Event Response
DOD	Department of Defense
DOL	Department of Labor
DPA	Defense Production Act
DRF	Disaster Relief Fund
EMTALA	Emergency Medical Treatment and Active Labor Act
EPSDT	Early and Periodic Screening, Diagnostic, and Treatment
EUA	Emergency Use Authorization
FAQ	Frequently Asked Questions
FDA	Food and Drug Administration
FEHB	Federal Employees Health Benefits Program
FEMA	Federal Emergency Management Agency
FFRCA	Families First Coronavirus Response Act
FMAP	Federal Medical Assistance Percentage
FQHC	Federally Qualified Health Center
HHS	Department of Health and Human Services
HRSA	Health Resources and Services Administration
HSGAC	Homeland Security and Governmental Affairs Committee
IDRRRF	Infectious Disease Rapid Response Reserve Fund
IHCIA	Indian Health Care Improvement Act
IHS	Indian Health Service
IVD	In Vitro Diagnosis
LDT	Laboratory-Developed Test

https://www.hhs.gov/sites/default/files/covid-19-faqs-hospitals-hospital-laboratory-acute-care-facility-data-reporting.pdf%3C.

Acronym	Definition
LTCF	Long-Term Care Facility
LTSS	Long-Term Services and Support
MA	Medicare Advantage
MHS	Military Health Services
MOU	Memorandum of Understanding
MTF	Military Treatment Facility
NAIC	National Association of Insurance Commissioners
NCI	National Cancer Institute (of the National Institutes of Health)
NF	Nursing Facility
NGA	National Governors Association
NIH	National Institutes of Health
NNDS	National Notifiable Diseases Surveillance System
OIG	Office of Inspector General (HHS)
OS	Office of the Secretary (HHS)
OTC	Over-the-Counter
PA	Public Assistance (FEMA)
PAPPG	Public Assistance Program and Policy Guide (FEMA)
PCR	Polymerase Chain Reaction
PHSA	Public Health Service Act
PHSSEF	Public Health and Social Services Emergency Fund
POC	Point-of-Care
PPE	Personal Protection Equipment
PPPHCEA	Paycheck Protection Program and Health Care Enhancement Act
PRF	Provider Relief Fund
PRWORA	Personal Responsibility and Work Opportunity Reconciliation Act of 1996
RHC	Rural Health Clinic
RNA	Ribonucleic acid
SNF	Skilled Nursing Facility
SNS	Strategic National Stockpile
SPA	State Plan Amendment
SPHERES	Sequencing for Public Health Emergency Response, Epidemiology, and Surveillance
SSA	Social Security Act
STLDI	Short-term, limited duration insurance
TTSI	Testing, Tracing, and Supported Isolation
USC	United States Code
VA	Department of Veterans Affairs
VHA	Veterans Health Administration
VTM	Viral Transport Media

APPENDIX B. POLICY EXPERTS TABLE

Topic	Contact
Types of COVID-19 Testing and Their Uses	Amanda K. Sarata
Test Accuracy	Amanda K. Sarata
Testing Infrastructure, Capacity and Strategies	Amanda K. Sarata
Testing Supply Chain	Amanda K. Sarata Erica A. Lee
Priority for Testing Individuals	Kavya Sekar
Role of Federal Emergency Management Agency in Testing: Infrastructure, Delivery and Payment	Erica A. Lee
Role of Public Health Departments in Testing	Kavya Sekar Sarah Lister
Nursing Home Testing	Phoenix Voorhies
Testing for Uninsured Individuals	Elayne J. Heisler
Defense Health Care	Bryce H. P. Mendez Alan Ott
Veterans Health Care	Sidath Viranga Panangala Jared S. Sussman
Indian Health Service	Elayne J. Heisler
Medicaid and the State Children's Health Insurance Program (CHIP)	Evelyne P. Baumrucker
Medicare	Jim Hahn
Private Health Insurance	Vanessa C. Forsberg
Private Health Insurance (Out of Network)	Noah D. Isserman
Private Health Insurance (Legal Issues)	Jennifer A. Staman
Funding for Testing Infrastructure	Amanda K. Sarata Kavya Sekar
Funding for Testing Individuals	Elayne J. Heisler
Unauthorized Immigrants' Access to Testing	Abigail F. Kolker
Use of Uninsured Fund for Testing	Elayne J. Heisler
Medicaid Funding for Testing Uninsured Individuals	Evelyne P. Baumrucker
Testing Data Reporting	Kavya Sekar Sarah Lister
Resources on Testing	Kate M. Costin

APPENDIX C. ADDITIONAL RESOURCES

Below are frequently cited resources related to COVID-19 testing in the United States. This appendix includes selected federal, academic, and stakeholder resources available at the time of this chapter's publication. Federal agencies continue to update guidance to reflect the current situation. Please note, this is not a comprehensive list of resources.

Data Repositories

Preliminary data reported by U.S. Laboratories including Commercial and Reference, Public Health, and Hospital; totals may include antibody data from some states.

Centers for Disease Control and Prevention (CDC)

- CDC COVID Data Tracker: United States Laboratory Testing, updated regularly, https://www.cdc.gov/covid-data-tracker/#testing
- Previous U.S. Viral Testing Data, May 19, 2020, https://www.cdc.gov/coronavirus/2019-ncov/cases-updates/previous-testing-in-us.html.

Coronavirus Resource Center, John Hopkins University & Medicine

For a complete list of data contributors, visit https://github.com/CSSEGISandData/COVID-19/ blob/master/README.md

- COVID-19 Dashboard by the Center for Systems Science and Engineering (CSSE) at Johns Hopkins University, updated regularly, https://coronavirus.jhu.edu/map.html
- Johns Hopkins COVID-19 Testing Insights Initiative, updated regularly, https://coronavirus.jhu.edu/testing
- Testing Trends Tool, updated regularly, https://coronavirus.jhu.edu/testing/ tracker/overview
- All State Comparison of Testing Efforts, updated regularly, https://coronavirus.jhu.edu/testing/states-comparison
- Daily State-by-State Testing Trends, updated regularly, https://coronavirus.jhu.edu/testing/individual-states
- Testing Trends Tool, updated regularly, https://coronavirus.jhu.edu/testing/ tracker/overview

- Which U.S. States Meet WHO Recommended Testing Criteria?, updated regularly, https://coronavirus.jhu.edu/testing/testing-positivity
- International Comparison of Positivity Rates and Tests Per Capita, updated regularly, https://coronavirus.jhu.edu/testing/international-comparison
- Racial Data Transparency: States that have released breakdowns of Covid-19 data by race, updated regularly, https://coronavirus.jhu.edu/data/racial-data- transparency.

The COVID Tracking Project by the Atlantic

- Our Data, updated regularly, https://covidtracking.com/data

Department of Health and Human Services (HHS) Guidance

Department of Health and Human Services (HHS)

- COVID-19 Pandemic Response, Laboratory Data Reporting: CARES Act Section 18115, https://www.hhs.gov/sites/default/files/covid-19-laboratory-data- reporting-guidance.pdf
- COVID-19 Guidance for Hospital Reporting and FAQs For Hospitals, Hospital Laboratory, and Acute Care Facility Data Reporting, https://www.hhs.gov/sites/ default/files/covid-19-faqs-hospitals-hospital-laboratory-acute-care-facility-data-reporting.pdf%3C.

Centers for Disease Control and Prevention (CDC)

- Interim Guidelines for Collecting, Handling, and Testing Clinical Specimens for COVID-19, https://www.cdc.gov/coronavirus/2019-ncov/lab/guidelines-clinical- specimens.html

- Testing Guidelines for Nursing Homes, https://www.cdc.gov/coronavirus/2019- ncov/hcp/nursing-homes-testing.html
- Interim Guidance on Testing Healthcare Personnel for SARS-CoV-2, https://www.cdc.gov/coronavirus/2019-ncov/hcp/testing-health-care- personnel.html
- Interim SARS-CoV-2 Testing Guidelines for Nursing Home Residents, https://www.cdc.gov/coronavirus/2019-ncov/hcp/nursing-homes-testing.html
- Interim Considerations for Institutions of Higher Education Administrators for SARS-CoV-2 Testing, https://www.cdc.gov/coronavirus/2019-ncov/community/ colleges-universities/ihe-testing.html
- Interim Guidelines for COVID-19 Antibody Testing, https://www.cdc.gov/coronavirus/2019-ncov/lab/resources/antibody-tests-guidelines.html.

Centers for Medicare & Medicaid Services (CMS)

- Clinical Laboratory Improvement Amendments (CLIA) Laboratory Guidance During COVID-19 Public Health Emergency, https://www.cms.gov/files/ document/qso-20-21-clia.pdf-0
- Frequently Asked Questions: SARS-CoV-2 Surveillance Testing, https://www.cms.gov/files/document/06-19-2020-frequently-asked-questions- covid-surveillance-testing.pdf
- Medicare Administrative Contractor (MAC) COVID-19 Test Pricing, https://www.cms.gov/files/document/mac-covid-19-test-pricing.pdf
- COVID-19 Frequently Asked Questions (FAQs) for State Medicaid and Children's Health Insurance Program (CHIP) Agencies, https://www.medicaid.gov/state-resource-center/downloads/covid-19-faqs.pdf
- Current emergencies, Coronavirus Disease 2019, updated regularly, https://www.cms.gov/About-CMS/Agency-Information/

Emergency/EPRO/Current-Emergencies/Current-Emergencies-page

- Coronavirus Disease 2019 (COVID-19) Guidance, Updated as new Center for Consumer Information and Insurance Oversight guidance documents are published, https://www.cms.gov/CCIIO/Resources/Fact-Sheets-and- FAQs#COVID-19.

Food and Drug Administration (FDA)

- Policy for Coronavirus Disease-2019 Tests During the Public Health Emergency (Revised), May 2020, https://www.fda.gov/regulatory-information/search-fda-guidance-documents/policy-coronavirus-disease-2019-tests-during-public-health-emergency-revised
- FAQs on Testing for SARS-CoV-2, https://www.fda.gov/medical-devices/emergency-situations-medical-devices/faqs-testing-sars-cov-2.

HHS, Department of Labor, and the Treasury

- FAQS about Families First Coronavirus Response Act and Coronavirus Aid, Relief, and Economic Security Act Implementation Part 42, April 11, 2020, https://www.cms.gov/files/document/FFCRA-Part-42-FAQs.pdf
- FAQS about Families First Coronavirus Response Act and Coronavirus Aid, Relief, and Economic Security Act Implementation Part 43, June 23, 2020, https://www.cms.gov/files/document/FFCRA-Part-43-FAQs.pdf.

Federal COVID-19 Guidance (Non-HHS)

U.S. Equal Employment Opportunity Commission (EEOC)

- What You Should Know About COVID-19 and the ADA, the Rehabilitation Act, and Other EEO Laws, https://www.eeoc.gov/wysk/what-you-should-know-about-covid-19-and-ada-rehabilitation-act-and-other-eeo-laws.

White House

- Testing Blueprint: Opening Up America Again, April 2020, https://www.whitehouse.gov/wp-content/uploads/2020/04/Testing-Blueprint.pdf
- Testing Overview: Opening Up America Again, April 2020, https://www.whitehouse.gov/wp-content/uploads/2020/04/Testing-Overview- Final.pdf
- Guidance on Interpreting COVID-19 Test Results, May 6, 2020, https://www.whitehouse.gov/wp-content/uploads/2020/05/Testing-Guidance.pdf
- Addendum to the Testing Blueprint, June 2020, https://www.whitehouse.gov/wp-content/uploads/2020/06/Addendum-to-the-testing-blueprint-FINAL.pdf.

Test Strategies

Centers for Disease Control and Prevention (CDC)

- SARS-CoV-2 Testing Strategy: Considerations for Non-Healthcare Workplaces, https://www.cdc.gov/coronavirus/2019-ncov/community/organizations/testing-non-healthcare-workplaces.html

- Testing Strategy for Coronavirus (COVID-19) in High-Density Critical Infrastructure Workplaces after a COVID-19 Case is Identified, https://www.cdc.gov/coronavirus/2019-ncov/community/worker-safety-support/ hd-testing.html
- COVID-19 Serology Surveillance Strategy, https://www.cdc.gov/coronavirus/2019-ncov/covid-data/serology-surveillance/index.html.

Department of Health and Human Services (HHS)

- Report to Congress: COVID-19 Strategic Testing Plan, May 24, 2020, https://www.democrats.senate.gov/imo/media/doc/ COVID%20National%20Diagnostics%20Strategy%2005%2024%202020%20v%20FINAL.pdf
- Coronavirus (COVID-19) Testing Plans by State and Jurisdiction, updated regularly, https://www.hhs.gov/coronavirus/testing-plans/index.html.

The Johns Hopkins Center for Health Security

- Developing a National Strategy for SARS-CoV-2 Serosurveys in the United States, June 18, 2020, https://www.centerforhealthsecurity.org/our-work/publications/developing-a-national-strategy-for-sars-cov-2-serosurveys-in-the- united-states.

The John Hopkins Bloomberg School of Public Health

- A National Plan to Enable Comprehensive COVID-19 Case Finding and Contact Tracing in the US, April 2020, https://www.centerforhealthsecurity.org/our-work/pubs_archive/pubs-pdfs/2020/200410-national-plan-to-contact-tracing.pdf.

The Rockefeller Foundation

- National COVID-19 Testing and Tracing Action Plan, https://www.rockefellerfoundation.org/national-covid-19-testing-and-tracing- action-plan/.

Relevant Reports and Other Resources

Centers for Disease Control and Prevention (CDC)

- Overview of Testing for SARS-CoV-2, https://www.cdc.gov/coronavirus/2019-ncov/hcp/testing-overview.html
- Report to Congress on Paycheck Protection Program and Health Care Enhancement Act Disaggregated Data on U.S. Coronavirus Disease 2019 (COVID-19) Testing, May 2020, https://www.help.senate.gov/imo/media/doc/FY%202020%20CDC%20RTC%20on%20COVID-19%20Testing%20Data%20-%20CDCfinalclean.pdf
- CDC Activities and Initiatives Supporting the COVID-19 Response and the President's Plan for Opening America Up Again, May 2020, https://www.cdc.gov/coronavirus/2019-ncov/downloads/php/CDC-Activities-Initiatives-for-COVID-19-Response.pdf.

Centers for Medicare & Medicaid Services (CMS)

- Frequently Asked Questions: COVID-19 Testing at Skilled Nursing Facilities/ Nursing Homes, August 5, 2020, https://www.cms.gov/files/document/covid- faqs-snf-testing.pdf.

Department of Health and Human Services (HHS)

- Community-Based Testing Sites for COVID-19, updated regularly, https://www.hhs.gov/coronavirus/community-based-testing-sites/index.html.

Federal Emergency Management Agency (FEMA)

- Federal Support to Expand National Testing Capabilities, May 4, 2020, https://www.fema.gov/fact-sheet/federal-support-expand-national-testing- capabilities.

Food and Drug Administration (FDA)

- Independent Evaluations of COVID-19 Serological Tests, updated regularly, https://open.fda.gov/apis/device/covid19serology/.

Government Accountability Office (GAO)

- COVID-19: Opportunities to Improve Federal Response and Recovery Efforts, June 25, 2020, https://www.gao.gov/products/ GAO-20-625.

National Academy of Medicine (NAM)

- Evaluating Data Types: A Guide for Decision Makers using Data to Understand the Extent and Spread of COVID-19, 2020, https://www.nap.edu/catalog/25826/evaluating-data-types-a-guide-for-decision-makers-using-data
- Rapid Expert Consultation on SARS-CoV-2 Laboratory Testing for the COVID- 19 Pandemic, April 8, 2020, https://www.nap.edu/ catalog/25775/rapid-expert-consultation-on-sars-cov-2-laboratory-testing-for-the-covid-19-pandemic-april-8- 2020.

In: Testing and Contract Tracing … ISBN: 978-1-53618-857-8
Editor: Ernesto M. Batista © 2020 Nova Science Publishers, Inc.

Chapter 3

DEVELOPMENT AND REGULATION OF DOMESTIC DIAGNOSTIC TESTING FOR NOVEL CORONAVIRUS (COVID-19): FREQUENTLY ASKED QUESTIONS*

Amanda K. Sarata

ABSTRACT

On December 31, 2019, the World Health Organization (WHO) was informed of a cluster of pneumonia cases in Wuhan City, Hubei Province of China. Illnesses have since been linked to a disease caused by a previously unidentified strain of coronavirus, designated Coronavirus Disease 2019, or COVID-19. Despite containment efforts in China, the United States, and elsewhere, by late February there were indications that the COVID-19 outbreak may have entered a new phase, with community spread occurring or suspected in several countries other than China, including in the United States.

---

* This is an edited, reformatted and augmented version of Congressional Research Service, Publication No. R46261, dated March 9, 2020.

Diagnostic testing is a critical part of the public health response to and clinical management of COVID-19, caused by the SARS-CoV-2 virus. Efforts in the United States to develop and disseminate a test for COVID-19 have faced challenges. Manufacturing and quality issues with the nation's test—developed by the Centers for Disease Control and Prevention (CDC)—resulted in significant delay in access to testing throughout the country. In this context, on February 29, 2020, in an effort to facilitate the expansion of testing capacity as the first cases of community spread were confirmed in the United States, the Food and Drug Administration (FDA) announced a new policy, issued via agency guidance and effective immediately, that would allow certain laboratories—principally clinical and large commercial and reference laboratories—that have developed and validated their own COVID-19 diagnostic to begin to use the test prior to it receiving an Emergency Use Authorization (EUA) from the agency.

FDA's February 29 guidance aims to facilitate the expansion of diagnostic testing from the public health setting into the clinical health care and commercial settings. Doing so may help the country meet the increasing and substantial demand for testing generated by community spread of the disease and expanded clinical testing guidelines issued by the CDC. This chapter does not address financing or coverage of diagnostic testing for COVID-19.

INTRODUCTION

On December 31, 2019, the World Health Organization (WHO) was informed of a cluster of pneumonia cases in Wuhan City, Hubei Province of China. Illnesses have since been linked to a disease caused by a previously unidentified strain of coronavirus, designated Coronavirus Disease 2019, or COVID-19. Despite containment efforts in China, the United States, and elsewhere, by late February there were indications that the COVID-19 outbreak may have entered a new phase, with community spread occurring or suspected in several countries other than China, including in the United States.[1]

Diagnostic testing is a critical part of the public health response to and clinical management of the COVID-19 caused by the SARS-CoV-2 virus.

---

[1] For more information about the domestic response to the novel coronavirus, see CRS Report R46219, *Overview of U.S. Domestic Response to Coronavirus Disease 2019 (COVID-19)*.

Efforts in the United States to develop and disseminate a test for COVID-19 have faced challenges. Manufacturing and quality issues with the nation's test—developed by the Centers for Disease Control and Prevention (CDC)—resulted in essentially all testing going through CDC's laboratory facility in Atlanta through early March, despite distribution of test kits to state and local public health labs beginning in early February.

CDC's initial test kits had to be remanufactured and redistributed, which, along with other factors, has significantly delayed access to testing throughout the country. It has been reported that the CDC's Atlanta laboratory is currently under investigation by the Department of Health and Human Services (HHS) for possible quality issues related to its manufacture of the test kits, which may have led to the contamination of one reagent and thus to the quality issues with the test.[2]

In this context, on February 29, 2020, in an effort to facilitate the expansion of testing capacity as the first cases of community spread were confirmed in the United States, the Food and Drug Administration (FDA) announced a significant new policy. This policy, issued via agency guidance and effective immediately, allows certain laboratories—principally clinical and commercial laboratories—that have developed and validated their own COVID-19 diagnostics to begin to use the tests prior to the test receiving an Emergency Use Authorization (EUA) from the agency.[3]

Diagnostic testing for COVID-19, in part because it is caused by a novel pathogen, has been led and carried out to date through the country's public health infrastructure. This includes primarily the CDC and the country's network of state and local public health laboratories. In contrast, in most situations, diagnostic testing is carried out by a number of facilities, including private commercial laboratories (e.g., Quest, LabCorp), hospital

---

[2] "U.S. agency investigating production of faulty coronavirus test kits," March 1, 2020, https://www.reuters.com/article/us-china-health-test-kits/u-s-agency-investigating-production-of-faulty-coronavirus-test-kits-idUSKBN20P09Y.

[3] See generally FDA, "Policy for Diagnostics Testing in Laboratories Certified to Perform High Complexity Testing under CLIA prior to Emergency Use Authorization for Coronavirus Disease-2019 during the Public Health Emergency," February 29, 2020, https://www.fda.gov/media/135659/download.

and other clinical laboratories, and laboratories in academic medical centers, among others.

FDA's February 29 guidance aims to facilitate the expansion of diagnostic testing from the public health setting into the clinical health care and commercial settings, leveraging significant standing resources throughout the country, including facilities, trained personnel, expertise, materials, and equipment. It is FDA's intention that this expansion will help the country meet the increasing and substantial demand for testing generated by community spread of the disease and expanded clinical testing guidelines issued by the CDC. In addition, because many cases of COVID-19 are reportedly mild or asymptomatic, widespread access to testing—which informs development of important metrics such as the case fatality rate—is critical to understanding the scope and extent of the disease in the United States, and to efficiently directing resources to mitigate its impact in the broader community.

Diagnostic tests—formally called in vitro diagnostic (IVD) devices—may be commercially developed and distributed as "kits" or developed, validated, and carried out by a single laboratory. This second type of test—known as a laboratory-developed test, or an LDT—is the more commonly used type of test because of its flexibility and differing federal regulatory requirements, among other reasons. Although the CDC's test is being manufactured as a test kit and initially has been distributed to specific CDC-qualified labs, the FDA guidance targets LDTs that are generally carried out in clinical and academic settings or private commercial laboratories. All clinical laboratories in the United States, regardless of whether they are part of the country's public health infrastructure or part of the health care delivery system, are regulated by the Clinical Laboratory Improvement Amendments of 1988 (CLIA) program, administered by the Centers for Medicare & Medicaid Services (CMS).

Federal agencies involved in the regulation of IVDs include FDA and CMS. FDA derives its authority to regulate the sale and distribution of medical devices, such as IVDs, from the Federal Food, Drug, and Cosmetics Act (FFDCA) and the Public Health Service Act (PHSA). CMS's authority to regulate IVDs is through CLIA (P.L. 100-578). FDA regulates the safety and effectiveness of diagnostic tests, as well as the quality of the design and manufacture of the diagnostic test. CMS regulates the quality of clinical laboratories and the clinical testing process.

Diagnostic Tests

What Are IVD Tests?

In vitro diagnostic devices are defined in FDA regulation as a specific subset of medical devices that include "reagents, instruments, and systems intended for use in the diagnosis of disease or other conditions ... in order to cure, mitigate, treat, or prevent disease ... [s]uch products are intended for use in the collection, preparation, and examination of specimens taken from the human body." As indicated by this definition, an IVD may also include components of tests, which can include both non-diagnostic ingredients, called general purpose reagents (GPRs), and the active ingredient in a diagnostic test, referred to as the analyte specific reagent (ASR).

In general, an IVD device may be a "commercial test kit" (a product developed, produced, and sold by a manufacturer for distribution to multiple laboratories) or a "laboratory developed test" (a product developed by and used in a single laboratory). LDTs may use components (e.g., general purpose reagents like a buffer) that are either manufactured in-house by the laboratory or commercially developed and distributed.

What Is an LDT?

A laboratory-developed test is a class of IVD that is designed, manufactured, and used within a single laboratory. LDTs are often used to test for conditions or diseases that are either rapidly changing (e.g., new strains of known infectious diseases) or the subject of quickly advancing scientific research (e.g., genomic testing for cancer). The majority of genetic tests—a type of IVD that analyzes various aspects of an individual's genetic material (e.g., DNA, RNA)—are LDTs.

How Are IVD Tests Regulated?

In general, oversight of in vitro diagnostic devices focuses on ensuring their safety and effectiveness; their accuracy and reliability; the quality of clinical laboratories that carry out IVD testing; the utility of the information generated by IVDs in clinician and patient decision-making; and the truthfulness of claims made about IVDs that are marketed directly to consumers. As with other medical devices, the application of FDA regulatory requirements to IVDs depends on the IVD's risk classification according to its intended use. Classification is based, in turn, on the risk the device poses to the patient. For IVDs, which are informational tests, the risk to the patient is that of an incorrect test result, either a false positive or a false negative result, either of which may cause serious harm to the individual. In the case of infectious diseases—for example, COVID- 19—the risk of a false negative test extends beyond the individual patient into the community at large. The FDA has three classes of medical device: Class I (low risk), Class II (moderate risk), and Class III (high risk). Regulatory controls are dependent on the class of a given medical device. COVID-19 diagnostics would most likely fall in Class III, as they would be considered to be high-risk devices.

How Are LDTs Regulated?

The regulation of laboratory-developed tests has been the subject of ongoing debate over the past 20 years, driven in large part by an increase in the number and complexity of genetic tests over this time. In general, the FDA has maintained that it has clear regulatory authority over LDTs, as it does with all IVDs that meet the definition of medical device in the FFDCA.[4] However, the FDA traditionally exercised enforcement discretion over LDTs—choosing not to enforce applicable statutory and regulatory requirements with respect to such tests—meaning that most of these tests have neither undergone premarket review nor received FDA clearance or approval for marketing. To date, FDA has instead focused its enforcement efforts on commercial IVD kits, which are broadly commercially marketed. In recent years, despite the absence of specific agency guidance on the regulation of LDTs, FDA has nevertheless begun to assert authority over LDTs, and specifically over some direct-to-consumer (DTC) genetic tests, that it considers to be higher- risk tests.

What Is CLIA and How Is It Involved in LDT Regulation?

CLIA of 1988 provides CMS with authority to regulate clinical laboratories.[5] CLIA establishes quality standards for clinical laboratory testing and a certification program for clinical laboratories that perform testing using IVD devices. All laboratories that perform diagnostic testing for health-related reasons (i.e., with results returned to the patient or a health care practitioner) are regulated by CMS under the authority of CLIA. For CLIA to apply, testing must be carried out on a human specimen. CLIA certification is based on the level of complexity of testing that the laboratory performs, specifically (1) low (therefore, waived) complexity, (2) moderate complexity, and (3) high complexity. FDA is responsible for categorizing tests according to their level of complexity. CLIA requirements are used to evaluate a test's *analytical validity*, defined as the ability of a test to detect or measure the analyte it is intended to detect or measure. Laboratories that perform moderate- and high-complexity testing must meet specific standards and requirements as a condition of certification, including proficiency testing (PT), patient test management, quality control, personnel qualifications, and quality assurance. All LDTs, including genetic tests offered as LDTs, are considered high-complexity tests under CLIA. All

---

[4] The term *medical device* is defined in FFDCA §201(h) [21 U.S.C. §321(h)].

[5] PHSA §353; 42 U.S.C. §263a.

COVID-19 diagnostics would be considered to be high complexity tests under CLIA.

How Are IVDs Regulated by the FDA During an Emergency Such as the Outbreak of COVID-19?

In certain public health or other emergency situations, the HHS Secretary may declare that existing circumstances justify the use of unapproved medical products for certain uses, or approved medical products for unapproved uses.[6] This declaration facilitates access to not-yet- approved medical products in an expedited manner during certain emergency situations. In the case of the COVID-19 disease, HHS Secretary Azar determined that "there is a public health emergency and [declared] that circumstances exist justifying the authorization of emergency use of in vitro diagnostics for detection and/or diagnosis of the novel coronavirus."[7] On the basis of this declaration, FDA issued an Emergency Use Authorization authorizing the emergency use of the CDC-developed diagnostic test for COVID-19.[8] The FDA also issued an EUA to the state of New York for an LDT developed by the state public health labs. To date, these are the only two EUAs for coronavirus diagnostics that the FDA has issued.[9]

How Does the Emergency Use Authority Apply to LDTs if They Are Generally Exempted from Premarket Requirements?

During an emergency, all laboratory-developed tests testing for the relevant pathogen (in this case, SARS-CoV-2) must either be approved, cleared, or authorized under an EUA to be legally carried out. As noted

---

[6] FFDCA §564 [21 U.S.C. §360bbb–3].

[7] FDA, "Policy for Diagnostics Testing in Laboratories Certified to Perform High Complexity Testing under CLIA prior to Emergency Use Authorization for Coronavirus Disease-2019 during the Public Health Emergency," February 29, 2020, https://www.fda.gov/media/135659/download, page 1.

[8] Letter of authorization from FDA to CDC, advising of the authorization for emergency use of the CDC-developed diagnostic test, available at "Novel coronavirus (COVID-2019) EUA Information" on the FDA web page "Emergency Use Authorization," https://www.fda.gov/emergency-preparedness-and-response/mcm-legal-regulatory-and-policy-framework/emergency-use-authorization.

[9] FDA, Emergency Use Authorization, https://www.fda.gov/emergency-preparedness-and-response/mcm-legal- regulatory-and-policy-framework/emergency-use-authorization.

above, FDA generally waives most regulatory requirements (e.g., premarket review) for LDTs in normal situations; nevertheless, LDTs may only be used with authorization (e.g., an EUA) during an emergency declaration pursuant to FFDCA Section 564.[10] That is, statutory requirements under FFDCA Section 564 apply to LDTs as they do to other medical products, and they apply to both commercial test kits—which are normally subject to FDA regulatory requirements—and to LDTs.

The EUA process is usually used to expedite access to medical products that would otherwise need premarket approval or clearance in emergency situations. However, because premarket approval requirements for LDTs are generally waived through enforcement discretion by the agency, the EUA represents additional regulatory requirements for the use of an LDT in emergency situations. This is because, among other things, in the case of a communicable disease, the test result has implications beyond the individual being tested, and so a false negative result could have serious consequences for the community.[11] Therefore, FDA states that these tests need an EUA in an emergency prior to clinical use as do other medical products. In contrast, for commercial test kits, the EUA represents an abbreviated mechanism that allows the unapproved product to be used without undergoing the FDA premarket review typically required (for a complex molecular test for a novel pathogen, that review would generally be a Premarket Approval, or PMA, for high-risk medical devices).

Despite a request from the Association of Public Health Laboratories (APHL) to FDA, the agency declined to exercise enforcement discretion with respect to LDTs that detect SARC-CoV-2 and diagnose COVID-19 and the requirement that they receive an EUA prior to use. APHL maintains that these labs are regulated by CLIA, and that this regulatory oversight is sufficient.[12] However, on February 29, 2020, FDA announced a new policy

[10] 21 U.S.C. §360bbb–3.

[11] FDA, "Information for Laboratories Implementing IVD Tests Under an EUA," https://www.fda.gov/emergency- preparedness-and-response/mcm-legal-regulatory-and-policy-framework/information-laboratories-implementing-ivd- tests-under-eua.

[12] 360dx, "APHL Asks FDA to Make Own Tests as CDC Struggles to Provide SARS-CoV-2 Test Kits," February 25, 2020, https://www.360dx.com/clinical-lab-management/aphl-asks-fda-make-own-tests-cdc-struggles-provide-sars-cov-2-test-kits?trendmd-shared=0&utm_medium=TrendMD&utm_campaign=0&utm_source= TrendMD#.XmKIwqhKiUm.

allowing certain laboratories that have developed and validated COVID-19 LDTs to begin to use the test clinically *prior* to it receiving an EUA from the agency but *after* validation of the test and notification of the agency (see "What Steps Did FDA Take to Expand Testing Capacity in Response to the Problems with CDC's Test?").[13]

THE CDC 2019-NOVEL CORONAVIRUS (2019-NCOV) REAL-TIME REVERSE TRANSCRIPTASE (RT)-PCR DIAGNOSTIC PANEL

How Does the CDC's COVID-19 Diagnostic Test Work?

The diagnostic test developed by the CDC, called the 2019-Novel Coronavirus (2019-nCoV) Real-Time Reverse Transcriptase (RT)-PCR Diagnostic Panel, is a complex molecular diagnostic test that relies on generally standard molecular biology laboratory techniques. Specifically, the test uses a technique called Polymerase Chain Reaction (PCR), a standard in vitro technique for amplification of DNA. Because the SARS-CoV-2 virus—the virus that causes COVID-19—is an RNA[14] virus, the RNA must be first reverse transcribed to generate copy DNA, or cDNA, which is then amplified (multiple copies are generated) using PCR. PCR relies on primers—very short single stranded pieces of DNA that are complementary to and bind with specific regions of the viral genome and thus define the specific genomic region to be amplified. The test then relies on a probe, or a single-stranded piece of DNA that is chemically or radioactively labelled, that can bind to and thus detect the amplified target portion of the viral genetic material.

---

[13] See generally FDA, "Policy for Diagnostics Testing in Laboratories Certified to Perform High Complexity Testing under CLIA prior to Emergency Use Authorization for Coronavirus Disease-2019 during the Public Health Emergency," February 29, 2020, https://www.fda.gov/media/135659/download.

[14] RNA stands for ribonucleic acid. RNA is genetic material with a slightly different chemical composition from DNA, or deoxyribonucleic acid.

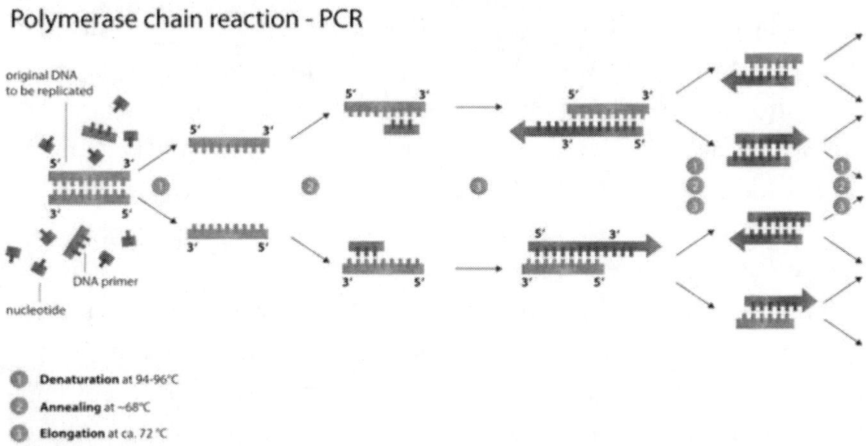

Source: https://upload.wikimedia.org/wikipedia/commons/thumb/9/96/Polymerase_chain_reaction.svg/835px- Polymerase_chain_reaction.svg.png, accessed March 3, 2020.

Figure 1. Polymerase Chain Reaction Overview.

CDC's original test used three sets of primers and probes: two to target specific regions of a designated gene within the SARS-CoV-2 viral genome, and a third that was specific to all SARS- like coronaviruses (see "What Quality Problems Did the CDC's Test Experience on Rollout to the State and Local Public Health Laboratories?"). The test also includes a number of authorized control samples, including a positive control for SARS-CoV-2 and a "no template control" to test for system contamination. Together, these controls help ensure that the test is functioning properly.

What Type of IVD Is the CDC's Test and Who May Carry It Out?

The CDC's test is being developed by the agency as a test kit and is generally authorized to be distributed to state and local public health laboratories to augment public health testing capacity. The test received an EUA from the FDA on February 4, 2020, under which "authorized laboratories" may receive and carry out the test despite the fact that it is not

FDA-approved or FDA-cleared, and that it does not meet all related regulatory requirements for marketing.[15] The EUA notes that "[t]esting is limited to qualified laboratories designated by CDC and, in the United States, certified under the Clinical Laboratory Improvement Amendments of 1988 (CLIA), (42 U.S.C. §263a), to perform high complexity tests."[16] CDC-qualified laboratories with a CLIA certification for high-complexity testing able to receive the test kits include U.S. state and local public health laboratories, Department of Defense (DOD) laboratories, and select international laboratories. The public health laboratories must verify the test themselves prior to using it, and are currently required to send presumptive positive cases back to the CDC in Atlanta for confirmatory testing by the agency.

What Is the Role of the Commercial Manufacturer IDT in the Development and Distribution of the CDC's Test Kit?

The Trump Administration had estimated that approximately 1 million tests would be broadly available imminently, facilitated by leveraging manufacturing of the CDC test kit by a private company, Integrated DNA Technologies (IDT), a manufacturer that has been working with CDC.[17] According to HHS Secretary Azar on March 5, 2020, IDT will send the CDC test kit to "hospitals, other labs around the country, commercial, public health ... labs" by the end of the week of March 2.[18] The test kit being manufactured by IDT, identical to the CDC test kit and referred to as "IDT 2019-novel coronavirus kit," is being qualified by CDC in lots, and FDA reports that these CDC-qualified, IDT-manufactured test kits are covered by the CDC's EUA authorization of February 4, 2020.[19]

---

[15] EUA Letter from FDA to CDC, dated February 4, 2020, https://www.fda.gov/media/134919/download.

[16] Ibid.

[17] RAPS, "FDA's Hahn Addresses Coronavirus Test Capacity, Drug Shortages at Senate Hearing," March 3, 2020, https://www.raps.org/news-and-articles/news-articles/2020/3/fdas-hahn-addresses-coronavirus-test-capacity-dr.

[18] Secretary of HHS Alex Azar, Coronavirus Press Briefing, March 5, 2020, https://www.c-span.org/video/?470068-2/ secretary-azar-federal-health-officials-coronavirus-briefing.

[19] Stenzel, Timothy, FDA Office of In Vitro Diagnostics Webinar, "Policy for Diagnostics Testing in Laboratories Certified to Perform High Complexity Testing under CLIA prior to Emergency Use Authorization for Coronavirus Disease-2019 during the Public Health

FDA notes that if a lab purchases a test kit from IDT, the laboratory does not need its own EUA to carry it out, but that "[t]esting using CDC's EUA-authorized protocol and CDC qualified lots of reagents is considered to be testing done under the CDC's EUA. Labs performing such testing should follow any applicable conditions set forth in the EUA."[20] LabCorp, a large commercial laboratory, is already reporting that it can perform the CDC test "if needed to meet testing demand" and that the test is only for use with "authorized specimens collected from individuals who meet CDC criteria for COVID-19 testing."[21] IDT is manufacturing test kits in two sizes, with the largest having a capacity of 500 reactions (approximately 250 individual patients).[22]

What Quality Problems Did the CDC's Test Experience on Rollout to the State and Local Public Health Laboratories?

As noted above, the CDC's test kit used three sets of probes and primers—or reagents—to detect and identify viral DNA beyond that specific to COVID-19. One of these reagents, the one meant to detect any SARS-like coronavirus including SARS-CoV-2, was returning inconclusive results. In response, the CDC validated a new protocol for their test that allows it to be run excluding the faulty reagent, running the test with only the other two diagnostic components. CDC has the authority to modify the test through enforcement discretion granted by FDA.[23] The agency determined that the exclusion of this reagent does not affect the accuracy or the sensitivity and specificity of the test.

Emergency" Immediately in Effect Guidance," March 2, 2020; see slide 13, https://www.fda.gov/media/135707/download.

[20] FDA, "FAQs on Diagnostic Testing for SARS-CoV-2," https://www.fda.gov/medical-devices/emergency-situations- medical-devices/faqs-diagnostic-testing-sars-cov-2.

[21] LabCorp, "Information from LabCorp about Coronavirus Disease 2019 (COVID-19)," March 5, 2020, https://www.labcorp.com/information-labcorp-about-coronavirus-disease-2019-covid-19.

[22] IDT, https://www.idtdna.com/pages/landing/coronavirus-research-reagents.

[23] CDC, "Revision to Test Instructions: CDC 2019 Novel Coronavirus (nCoV) Real-Time RT-PCR Diagnostic Panel (EUA200001)," February 26, 2020, https://www.aphl.org/Materials/Signed_CDC_Letter_to_PHLs- N3_Removal_Instructions_26Feb2020.pdf.

Certain laboratories have continued to experience problems running the test, even when using the modified protocol, with at least one laboratory reporting that the first reagent was also returning inconclusive results. This problem severely limited the state and local public health laboratories' ability to carry out the CDC's test.

In response to these issues, the New York State Department of Health requested and was granted the FDA's second EUA for its own laboratory-developed test, the New York SARS-CoV-2 Real- time RT-PCR Diagnostic Panel.[24] Testing is limited under the EUA to two laboratories in New York—the Wadsworth Center, New York State Department of Public Health, and the New York City Department of Health and Mental Hygiene, Public Health Laboratories. New York was one of the states that had continued difficulty implementing CDC's original test kit, even with the modified protocol.

In response, CDC is also manufacturing new test kits after reportedly resolving the manufacturing issue that affected the original test kit. This time, however, CDC is manufacturing test kits with only the two reagents that were unaffected by the quality issue—that are specific to SARS-CoV-2—and those kits are being made available to qualified CDC labs through the International Reagent Resource.[25,26] These test kits are expected to result in the public health laboratories having capacity to test up to 75,000 patients.[27]

Some believe that the CDC's choice to develop and mitigate quality problems with its own COVID-19 diagnostic when an accepted diagnostic was available through the World Health Organization (WHO), which was efficiently distributing a German-developed test globally early in the

---

[24] FDA Letter to NYSDOH, February 29, 2020, https://www.fda.gov/media/135661/download.

[25] GenomeWeb, Johnson, Madeline, "CDC Revises SARS-CoV-2 Assay Protocol; Surveillance Testing on Track to Start Next Week," February 28, 2020, https://www.genomeweb.com/pcr/cdc-revises-sars-cov-2-assay-protocol-surveillance-testing-track-start-next-week#.Xl63kqhKiUk.

[26] "The International Reagent Resource (IRR) was established by the Centers for Disease Control and Prevention (CDC) to provide registered users with reagents, tools and information for studying and detection of Influenza Virus," see https://www.internationalreagentresource.org/About/IRR.aspx.

[27] CDC, "Coronavirus Disease 2019 (COVID-19) Situation Summary," Updated March 3, 2020, https://www.cdc.gov/ coronavirus/2019-ncov/summary.html.

outbreak, was a decision that cost the United States time in its response to the virus's introduction and spread in the country.[28] Some speculated about the use of the third reagent—that was to detect SARS-like coronaviruses—and whether it had been strictly necessary if the test was still accurate at diagnosing COVID-19 without that reagent included in the test at all, or if it had instead overcomplicated the test.[29] In general, there have been questions raised about the CDC's handling of the development and distribution of its test, and its response to the quality problems that occurred, and the impact this may have had on the country's ability to detect community spread of the disease before it occurred more widely.[30]

What Steps Did FDA Take to Expand Testing Capacity in Response to the Problems with CDC's Test?

On February 29, 2020, as problems with the rollout of the CDC-developed diagnostic test continued, FDA announced a new policy to immediately leverage LDTs developed in high- complexity commercial, reference, and clinical laboratories nationwide to expand testing capacity. Specifically, the new agency guidance allows CLIA-certified high-complexity laboratories that have developed and validated their own COVID-19 diagnostics to use the tests while the laboratory is preparing, and FDA is reviewing, their EUA submission.[31],[32]

---

[28] Sheridan, Cormac, "Coronavirus and the Race to Distribute Reliable Diagnostics," *Nature*, February 19, 2020, https://www.nature.com/articles/d41587-020-00002-2.

[29] ProPublica, "Key Missteps at the CDC Have Set Back its Ability to Detect the Potential Spread of Coronavirus," February 28, 2020, https://www.propublica.org/article/cdc-coronavirus-covid-19-test.

[30] Politico, "How testing failures allowed the coronavirus to sweep the United States," March 6, 2020, https://www.politico.com/news/2020/03/06/coronavirus-testing-failure-123166.

[31] GenomeWeb, "FDA Provides SARS-CoV-2 Test Validation Guidance for High-Complexity Labs Seeking EUA," March 3, 2020, https://www.genomeweb.com/pcr/fda-provides-sars-cov-2-test-validation-guidance-high-complexity- labs-seeking-eua#.Xl7JFqhKiUk.

[32] FDA, "Policy for Diagnostics Testing in Laboratories Certified to Perform High Complexity Testing under CLIA prior to Emergency Use Authorization for Coronavirus Disease-2019 during the Public Health Emergency," February 29, 2020, https://www.fda.gov/media/135659/download.

The FDA guidance states that laboratories have 15 days after validating their test to submit an EUA application to FDA, and the guidance recommends confirming the test's first five negative and positive results against an EUA-authorized diagnostic. According to FDA, it "does not intend to object to the use of these tests for clinical testing while the laboratories are pursuing an EUA with the FDA. Importantly, this policy only applies to laboratories that are certified to perform high-complexity testing consistent with requirements under Clinical Laboratory Improvement Amendments."[33] The guidance includes detailed information about FDA's expected methods for test validation.

Pursuant to this FDA guidance, on March 5, 2020, LabCorp announced that it had begun offering its LDT, the LabCorp 2019 Novel Coronavirus (COVID-19), NAA test "for ordering by physicians or other authorized healthcare providers anywhere in the U.S.," and that it is currently pursuing an EUA with the agency for the test.[34] This test is to take between three to four days to return results, and a health care provider must order and authorize it, and obtain the required specimen from the patient. Under the FDA's new guidance, Quest has also announced that it will begin testing for coronavirus with its own LDT, beginning March 9, 2020, and that it plans to pursue an EUA with the agency within 15 days, as required by the guidance.[35]

---

[33] FDA, "Coronavirus (COVID-19) Update: FDA Issues New Policy to Help Expedite Availability of Diagnostics," press release with link to guidance, February 29, 2020, https://www.fda.gov/news-events/press-announcements/ coronavirus-covid-19-update-fda-issues-new-policy-help-expedite-availability-diagnostics. See also CRS In Focus IF11389, *FDA Regulation of Laboratory-Developed Tests (LDTs)*.

[34] LabCorp, "Information from LabCorp about Coronavirus Disease 2019 (COVID-19)," March 5, 2020, https://www.labcorp.com/information-labcorp-about-coronavirus-disease-2019-covid-19.

[35] QuestDiagnostics, "Quest Diagnostics to Launch Coronavirus Disease 2019 (COVID019) Test," March 5, 2020, https://newsroom.questdiagnostics.com/2020-03-05-Quest-Diagnostics-to-Launch-Coronavirus-Disease-2019-COVID- 19-Test.

In: Testing and Contract Tracing …
Editor: Ernesto M. Batista
ISBN: 978-1-53618-857-8
© 2020 Nova Science Publishers, Inc.

Chapter 4

COVID-19 TESTING*

United States Government Accountability Office

WHY THIS MATTERS

As the nation works to save lives and flatten the curve of COVID-19 cases, widespread testing could help reduce the death rate, help identify those who should self-isolate, and help businesses recover. There are challenges, however, associated with the use and availability of tests, as well as with determining their accuracy.

THE TECHNOLOGY

What is it? There are currently three types of tests for COVID-19: molecular, antigen, and serology. Molecular tests and a new antigen test help

* This is an edited, reformatted and augmented accessible version of the United States Government Accountability Office Report of Science, Technology Assessment, and Analytics, Publication No. GAO-20-584SP COVID-19 Testing, dated May 2020.

diagnose active COVID-19 infections, and serology tests help determine whether someone was previously exposed to the novel coronavirus, which causes COVID-19.

How does it work? While each kind of test takes a different approach, they all collect vital information about exposure to the virus.

Molecular tests amplify and detect genetic material from novel coronavirus in a sample taken from a patient's saliva, nose, or throat to determine whether there is an active infection (Figure 1). For example, molecular tests based on the polymerase chain reaction (PCR) use a genetic photocopier, copying a unique portion of the coronavirus genetic material, if present, until there are enough copies to detect.

Antigen tests can detect the virus by binding parts of the virus, called antigens, to a membrane. Antibodies that can fluoresce are also added to the membrane. If enough antigen is present to bind to the antibodies, the total fluorescence from the antibodies becomes high enough to indicate a positive result.

Serology tests, which typically require a sample of blood from a patient, can detect the presence of antibodies produced by a patient's immune system in response to the coronavirus (Figure 1). Such antibodies can persist in the blood after a patient recovers from an infection. Thus, a positive serology test result indicates prior exposure to the novel coronavirus but does not necessarily mean that the patient is still infected.

How mature is it? All three kinds of COVID-19 tests are commercially available under the Food and Drug Administration's (FDA's) emergency use authorization (EUA), which allows for the use of certain unapproved medical products or unapproved uses of approved medical products under certain circumstances during a public health emergency. As of May 13, 2020, FDA has authorized at least 56 molecular tests for COVID-19 via EUA; these tests generally rely on PCR technology. Devices used for administering molecular tests range in size from larger equipment to smaller, portable devices that can be used on-site near the patient.

On May 8, 2020, FDA authorized the first antigen test for COVID-19 via EUA. According to FDA, antigen tests, which can be run in minutes, have a higher chance of false negatives compared to molecular tests. FDA states that negative antigen test results may need to be confirmed with a molecular test before making treatment decisions.

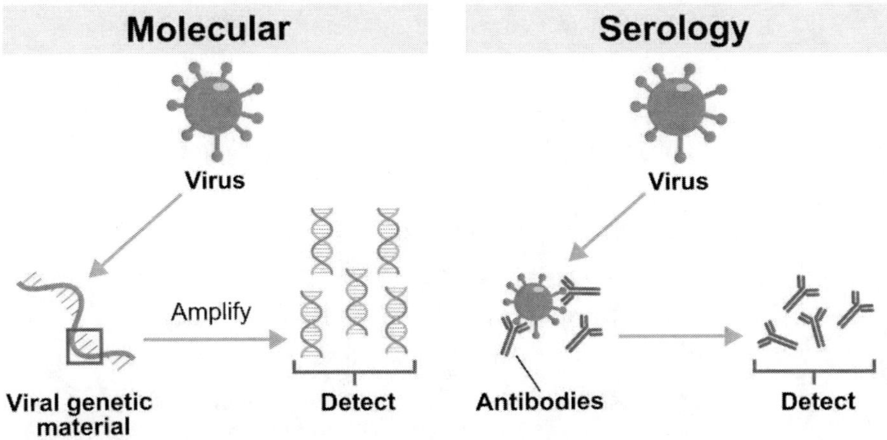

Source: GAO.| GAO-20-584SP.

Figure 1. Most Common COVID-19 Test Types. Molecular tests detect viral genetic material. Serology tests detect antibodies against the virus.

As of May 13, 2020, FDA has authorized at least 12 serology tests for COVID-19 via EUA. For COVID-19, serology tests were first authorized by FDA about a month after molecular tests were authorized. Devices used to administer serology tests also range in size, with some about the size of an over-the-counter pregnancy test.

OPPORTUNITIES

Testing provides critical information for a variety of purposes, including medical care, policymaking, and business. For example:

- *Determining risk.* Serology tests can help establish the percentage of the population previously exposed to the virus. Such information can help improve the accuracy of statistics on infection rates, among other things.

- *Understanding disease impact.* Testing can help establish the impact of the disease, including identifying those who may have been exposed to the virus but did not show symptoms and those who recovered. This is important for characterizing the risk of the disease to the elderly and other subpopulations.
- *Guiding treatment and resource allocation.* Molecular and antigen tests can provide information on the rate and geographic location of active infections. This can help guide patient treatment and inform decisions about the distribution of medical supplies and equipment.
- *Informing responses.* Testing is also important for informing decisions on quarantine and isolation, including decisions related to health care workers. Additionally, testing can help inform public responses such as school closures and reopenings.

CHALLENGES

Although widespread testing offers a number of opportunities, there are also challenges in implementation. For example:

- *Limited information on test accuracy.* The performance characteristics of some COVID-19 tests have raised concerns about test accuracy. In particular, available data suggest variability hin the rates of false positive and false negative results. This uncertainty can complicate patient treatment and public health decisions.
- *Number and timing of test results.* Centralized laboratories generally have higher reported testing throughput, but may take days to report test results. Point-of-care testing conducted on-site can return results more quickly, sometimes within an hour. However, the throughput of these tests can be lower than that of central laboratories. It may be challenging to balance the need for fast results and the need for large numbers of tests (Figure 2).

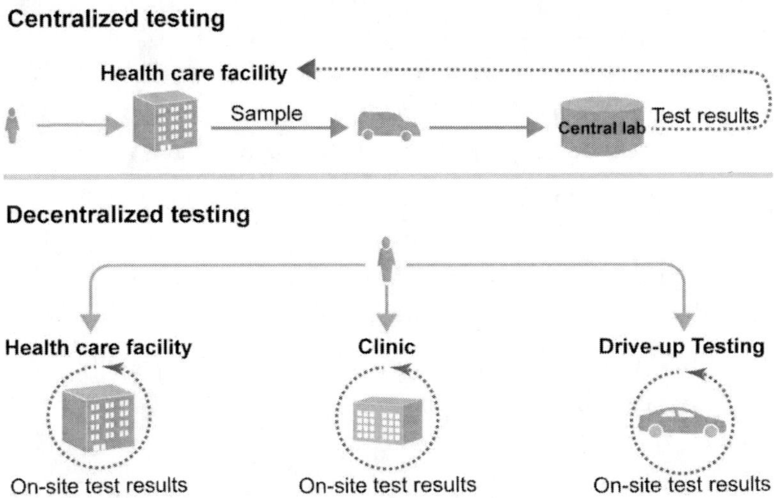

Source: GAO.| GAO-20-584SP.

Figure 2. Types of test processing based on site location. Decentralized testing, including testing at the point-of-care, reduces the time to obtain test results but can have limited throughput and other challenges. Centralized testing can have higher throughput, but may take longer to provide test results.

- *Scalability.* Expanding testing to reach more people would require greater availability of resources such as personal protective equipment needed by health care workers. Another option for expanding testing may be for FDA to authorize the use of additional at-home sample collection kits. Allowing consumers to take their own samples, however, could result in reduced test accuracy, due to sample contamination or other issues.

POLICY CONTEXT AND QUESTIONS

There are a number of important policy issues related to COVID-19 testing. For example:

- What are the barriers, if any, to FDA's and CDC's ability to help facilitate the development and use of tests during an early stage of an outbreak, and how could any barriers be addressed?
- What actions could help the general public and health care workers understand and assess the accuracy and reliability of different tests?
- What information could help decision-makers determine the number and distribution of tests to most effectively respond to outbreaks such as the COVID-19 pandemic?
- How can federal, state, and local health departments coordinate to facilitate accurate and timely testing and reporting of test results?

SELECTED REFERENCES

Library of Congress. Congressional Research Service. *COVID-19 Testing: Key Issues.*

IF11516. Washington, D.C.: Apr. 23, 2020.

Sharfstein, Joshua M., Scott J. Becker, and Michelle M. Mello. "Diagnostic Testing for the Novel Coronavirus," *Journal of the American Medical Association*, vol. 323, no. 15 (2020): pp. 1437-1438.

In: Testing and Contract Tracing …
Editor: Ernesto M. Batista
ISBN: 978-1-53618-857-8
© 2020 Nova Science Publishers, Inc.

Chapter 5

INTERIM GUIDANCE ON DEVELOPING A COVID-19 CASE INVESTIGATION AND CONTACT TRACING PLAN*

U.S. Department of Health and Human Services
Centers for Disease Control and Prevention

INTRODUCTION

Case investigation[1] and contact tracing are fundamental activities that involve working with a client (symptomatic and asymptomatic) who has been diagnosed with an infectious disease to identify and provide support to people (contacts) who may have been infected through exposure to the patient. This process prevents further transmission of disease by separating people who have (or may have) an infectious disease from people who do

---

* This is an edited, reformatted and augmented version of U.S. Department of Health and Human Services; Centers for Desease Control and Prevention, Publication No. CS317074-A, dated May 16, 2020.

[1] *Investigation* in this context refers to a public health/infectious disease investigation and should in no way be interpreted as a criminal investigation.

not. It is a core disease control measure that has been employed by public health agency personnel for decades. Case investigation and contact tracing are most effective when part of a multifaceted response to an outbreak.

Key Considerations for COVID-19

- Since COVID-19 can be spread before symptoms occur or when no symptoms are present, case investigation and contact tracing activities must be swift and thorough.
- The complete clinical picture of COVID-19 is not fully known. As scientists learn more, updates may be made to recommendations for testing priorities and the contact initiation window (when the patient was infectious and not under isolation) in which contacts should be elicited.
- Remote communications for the purposes of case investigation and contact tracing should be prioritized; in-person communication may be considered only after remote options have been exhausted.
- Given the potentially large number of cases and contacts, jurisdictions may need to prioritize case investigation and contact tracing activities. Prioritization should be based on vulnerability, congregate settings/workplaces and healthcare facilities, including long-term care facilities and confined spaces (prisons).
- Depending on jurisdictional testing capacity, case investigations may be considered for clients with a probable diagnosis of COVID-19, not just confirmed COVID-19 cases.
- Broad community engagement is needed to foster an understanding and acceptance of local case investigation and contact tracing efforts within each community.
- Significant social support may be necessary to allow clients with probable and confirmed COVID-19 diagnoses to safely self-isolate and close contacts to safely self-quarantine.
- Due to the magnitude of the pandemic, jurisdictions will likely need to build up their workforce, recruit from new applicant pools, and train individuals from varied backgrounds.
- The use of digital contact tracing tools may help with certain case investigation and contact tracing activities but will not replace the need for a large public health workforce.

Case investigation is the identification and investigation of clients with confirmed and probable diagnoses of COVID-19, and contact tracing is the subsequent identification, monitoring, and support of their contacts who have been exposed to, and possibly infected with, the virus. Prompt identification, voluntary quarantine (hereby referred to as *self-quarantine* in this document unless otherwise noted), and monitoring of these COVID-19 contacts can effectively break the chain of disease transmission and prevent further spread of the virus in a community. While case investigation and contact tracing for COVID-19 may be new, health departments and frontline public health professionals who perform these activities have experience conducting these activities for tuberculosis, sexually transmitted infections, HIV, and other infectious diseases. Case investigation and contact tracing are well-honed skills that adapt easily to new public health demands and are effective tools to slow the spread of COVID-19 in a community.

This guidance aims to provide a foundation for state, territorial, local, and tribal development of case investigation and contact tracing plans. It is important to note that COVID-19 case investigation and contact tracing activities will vary based on the level of community transmission, characteristics of the community and their populations, and the local capacity to implement case investigation, contact tracing, and COVID-19 testing.

Scaling up Staffing Roles Involved in Case Investigation and Contact Tracing

Successful case investigation and contact tracing for COVID-19 is dependent on a robust and well-trained public health workforce. Many are familiar with case investigation and contact tracing as a core strategy used in outbreak investigations (CDC Field Epidemiology Manual). It has also been implemented for decades by Communicable Disease Investigators (CDI) or Disease Intervention Specialists (DIS) in health departments throughout the United States to prevent and control tuberculosis, sexually transmitted infections, HIV, and other infectious diseases, as well as to respond to outbreaks.

To be effective, case investigation and contact tracing requires staff with adequate training, language skills, cultural sensitivity, supervision, and access to social and medical support for clients and their contacts.

One way to quickly scale up surge capacity for case investigation and contact tracing is to specify two explicit job tasks for designated staff:

Job Task 1. *Case Investigation*—Interviewing clients with COVID-19, eliciting their close contacts, monitoring the clients for COVID-19 symptoms, connecting clients to resources to support self-isolation

Job Task 2. *Contact Tracing*—Notifying close contacts of their potential exposure, referring them to testing, monitoring them for COVID-19 symptoms, connecting contacts to resources to support self-quarantine

Case investigation and contact tracing can be handled by one properly trained person when the number of clients diagnosed with COVID-19 and their close contacts can be interviewed by the staff member within 24 hours of being reported to the health department. When the number of reported daily cases does not allow for case interviews within 24 hours, a divided approach employing several staff can provide a focused scope of activity and streamlines the training competencies for the surge workforce. One staff member (case investigator) interviews and elicits contacts from a patient with COVID-19, and additional staff members (contact tracers) notify and follow-up with the patient's contacts. This approach requires excellent communication between staff to ensure clarity and prompt transfer of information, limited redundancy, and cohesive messaging to clients with COVID-19 and their contacts. Given each patient with COVID-19 will likely have multiple close contacts, staffing plans should include a greater number of contact tracers to meet this demand.

Public health personnel with infection control, worker safety, and health expertise will be required to support case investigation and contact tracing within healthcare facilities (e.g., hospitals, acute care centers), critical infrastructure settings (e.g., meat and poultry processing facilities, grocery stores), and other congregate living or workplace settings (e.g., long-term care facilities, correctional facilities). These complex investigations require the application of infection control principles to make appropriate recommendations and protect additional residents and workers from infection. Occupational health specialists should also be engaged to assess COVID-19-related protocols in place to promote workers' health and safety.

Scaling up case investigation and contact tracing efforts ideally involves a large multidisciplinary workforce under the daily oversight and management of a leadership team with subject matter expertise. The table below outlines the various roles of key public health staff needed. There may be variability in the title and classification of staff conducting these activities; however, the roles appear to be fairly consistent across jurisdictions. Depending on the jurisdiction, each role may be assigned to an individual staff member or one staff member may cover several roles.

Roles and Responsibilities of Key Public Health Staff to Support COVID-19 Case Investigation and Contact Tracing

Role	Description	Existing Public Health Classifications Performing these Activities	Surge Capacity Workforce* with Required Training
Surveillance Triage and Support	Processes incoming laboratory and provider reports in surveillance system. Follows-up to obtain relevant medical and demographic information. Acts as a resource for interjurisdictional communication & transfer of patient and contact information. Responsible for gathering relevant locating information (e.g., "people-searches") for clients and contacts.	Surveillance Data Clerks, Disease Intervention Specialists (DIS)***	Administrative Support Staff, Data Entry Technicians
Case Investigator	Conducts interviews of clients with confirmed or probable COVID-19, with a focus on motivational interviewing and cultural competency.	Disease Intervention Specialists (DIS),*** Public Health Associate Program (PHAP) Assignees, Public Health Nurses, Epidemiologists	Public Health Graduates or Current Students (MPH and Bachelors), Retired Registered Nurses, Health Educators, Social Workers,

(Continued)

Role	Description	Existing Public Health Classifications Performing these Activities	Surge Capacity Workforce* with Required Training
	Interviews should be guided by standard protocols and include: providing disease-specific information; assessing signs and symptoms, and underlying health conditions; discussing symptom onset to determine window period for contact elicitation and exposure risk for close contacts; discussing work, social, recreational, and community activities to identify who may have been exposed; eliciting information on close contacts, including names, exposure dates and locating information; and assessing support needs to maintain health and compliance during self-isolation. Facilitates testing and referral to healthcare services and resource care coordination, as indicated. May conduct home-based specimen collection. Provides recommendations for self-isolation and review of daily monitoring procedures. Conducts daily monitoring during self-isolation—temperature, signs/symptoms, use of fever-reducing medications—via electronic tool (e.g.,		Medical or Nursing Students, Patient Navigators, Community Health Outreach Workers/Promotores, Community Members with emotional intelligence, good communication and problem-solving skills. Ideally, they have language skills or similar cultural/social background as clients.

Role	Description	Existing Public Health Classifications Performing these Activities	Surge Capacity Workforce* with Required Training
	smartphone app, case management software) or other designated mechanism until patient is no longer infectious.**		
Contact Tracer	Communicates with contacts to notify them of exposure, provides disease and transmission information, gathers data on demographics, living arrangements, and daily activities. Asks about signs/symptoms and underlying medical conditions. Provides referrals for testing (if appropriate). May conduct home-based specimen collection. Provides recommendations for self-quarantine and reviews daily monitoring procedures. Assesses supports necessary to maintain compliance during self-quarantine. Conversations with contacts should be guided by standard protocols. Conducts daily monitoring during self-quarantine—temperature, signs/symptoms, use of fever-reducing medications— via electronic tool (e.g., smartphone, case management software) or other designated mechanism, until 14 days after last potential exposure, and referral to healthcare if contact becomes symptomatic.**	Disease Intervention Specialists (DIS),*** Public Health Investigators, Public Health Associate Program (PHAP) Assignees, Public Health Nurses, Epidemiologists	Community Health Outreach Workers/ Promotores, Medical Assistants, Teachers, Librarians, College Students, Customer Service-Oriented Professionals such as Flight Attendants, Call Center Employees, Restaurant and Other Service Industry Employees

(Continued)

Role	Description	Existing Public Health Classifications Performing these Activities	Surge Capacity Workforce* with Required Training
Case Investigation & Contact Tracing Lead	Directly oversees the work of the Case Investigator and/or Contact Tracer and others who may work as part of a team. Assigns work and oversees the quality of work. Ensures completion of case interviews and contact follow-up according to established standards. Reviews work for missing information, inconsistencies, or areas that need further exploration and directs staff follow-up to seek clarification and obtain additional information. Addresses complex issues with cases or contacts that have been escalated by staff. Uses qualitative (interview audits) and quantitative (review of statistical outputs) methods to review performance and determine areas for formal or informal professional development, training, coaching, and mentoring. When necessary, uses progressive discipline to address performance or conduct issues. Recognizes staff for exceptional and outstanding performance. Maintains employee personnel files.	Supervisory Public Health Nurses, Senior Epidemiologist	Supervisory Public Health Nurses, STD Program Front Line Supervisors, Public Health Investigator Supervisors, Communicable Disease Investigator Supervisors, TB Case Investigators/Outreach Worker Supervisors

Role	**Description**	**Existing Public Health Classifications Performing these Activities**	**Surge Capacity Workforce* with Required Training**
Care Resource Manager	Assesses social support that clients and contacts need to maintain healthy living in self-isolation or self-quarantine. Identifies housing needs and facilitates transition to appropriate housing supports. Provides tools (e.g., thermometer) to assist with daily monitoring and prevent further spread in home. Coordinates other support services such as delivery of food or medications, and referral to programs that provide financial assistance.	Patient Navigators, Linkage to Care Specialists, Disease Intervention Specialists	Social Workers, Medical Assistants, Community Health Outreach Workers/ Promotores, Medical Case Managers, Medical Care Coordinators
Self-Isolation & Self-Quarantine Monitor	Daily monitoring (ideally) of clients with COVID-19 during self-isolation and contacts during self-quarantine—temperature, signs/ symptoms—via electronic tool (e.g., smartphone app, case management software) or other designated mechanism. Assesses changes (initiation or increase in severity) in COVID-19 signs and symptoms. Facilitates prompt medical attention, as necessary. Tracks when clients or contacts are eligible to discontinue self-isolation/ self-quarantine and refers them to testing when available to assess their readiness for discontinuation.**	Community Health Outreach Workers	Certified Medical Assistants, Health Educators, Patient Navigators, Community Members with emotional intelligence, good communication and problem-solving skills, language skills

(Continued)

Role	Description	Existing Public Health Classifications Performing these Activities	Surge Capacity Workforce* with Required Training
High-Risk Medical Monitor	Interactive daily monitoring of clients with COVID-19 during self-isolation and contacts during self-quarantine who are at higher risk for severe disease. Assesses changes (initiation or increase in severity) in signs and symptoms. Facilitates prompt medical attention, as necessary. Tracks when clients or contacts are eligible to discontinue self-isolation or self-quarantine.	Public Health Nurses	Nurse Practitioners, Physician Assistants, Registered Nurses, Licensed Vocational Nurses
Infection Control Personnel	Conducts investigation of congregate living facilities (e.g., skilled nursing facilities, hospitals, acute care settings, long-term care facilities, group homes, homeless shelters, prisons, jails) and workplaces that have a patient (either resident/ patient or staff member) with COVID-19 to assess potential exposure of other staff and residents/ clients at the site and recommend infection control procedures.	Infection Control Practitioners (Nurses or Physicians), Hospital Acquired Infection Practitioners (Nurses or Physicians), Hospital Epidemiologists, Occupational Health Liaisons, Field Epidemiologists	Public Health Nurses, Registered Nurses, Physicians
Data Manager	Manages digital infrastructure for surveillance and contact investigation. Abstracts data from surveillance system for import into appropriate contact investigation platform and visa-versa, when automated data synchronization is not	Epidemiologists, Data Managers, Public Health Informatics Specialists	Software Developers, Systems Engineers, Data Engineers, Data Integration Specialists

Role	Description	Existing Public Health Classifications Performing these Activities	Surge Capacity Workforce* with Required Training
	available. Assesses and improves data quality and interoperability of data systems. Supports the development and modification of data systems to appropriately capture, integrate and report multiple data streams necessary to monitor response progress and outcomes.		
Epidemiologist	Analyzes data on cases and contact outcomes in order to identify outbreaks and priority populations. Monitors and evaluates the response in order to shift program efforts appropriately.	Epidemiologists, Epidemic Intelligence Service Officers (EISOs), Career Epidemiology Field Officers (CEFOs), Statisticians, Research Scientists, Data Scientists	Epidemiologists, Statisticians, Research Scientists, Data Scientists, Epidemic Intelligence Service Officers (EISOs), Epidemiology and Statistics Graduate Students, and other fellows
Clinical Consultant	Provides clinical support to the case investigation team, provides consultation for complex cases, and collaborates with healthcare providers, hospitals, and other facilities regarding clinical recommendations.	Practicing Registered Nurses, Public Health Nurses, Nurse Practitioners, Physician Assistants, Physicians	Practicing and Retired Registered Nurses, Public Health Nurses, Nurse Practitioners, Physician Assistants, Physicians, Medical Epidemiologists

(Continued)

Role	Description	Existing Public Health Classifications Performing these Activities	Surge Capacity Workforce* with Required Training
Servers of Public Health Orders****	Serves public health orders for isolation (clients with COVID-19) or quarantine (contacts) as necessary for people who are noncompliant with public health recommendations to self-isolate or self-quarantine—either in-person or electronically.**	Public Health Investigators or other public health personnel with delegated authority	Public Health Personnel and other staff with delegated authority

*Suggested surge capacity workforce does not include all potential job classifications.

**Per jurisdictional protocols

***Also known as Communicable Disease Investigator, Communicable Disease Representative, Disease Intervention Technician.

****Jurisdiction-specific laws that provide authority for the local health department to issue legal orders for isolation of people diagnosed with infectious disease and quarantine of people who have been exposed to infectious disease. Local policies and procedures dictate the delegation of authority (e.g., officially deputized, acting on behalf of local health officer) and type of personnel who can serve legal orders.

Knowledge and Skills Needed for Case Investigation and Contact Tracing Staff

Case investigation and contact tracing are specialized skills. Knowledge and skills that staff may need include:

- A keen understanding of the need for patient confidentiality and the ability to conduct case interviews without violating confidentiality and to conduct contact tracing without disclosing the identity of the patient (case).
- Understanding of, and ability to explain, the medical terms associated with COVID-19 and principles of exposure, infection, infectious period, potentially infectious interactions, symptoms of disease, pre-symptomatic and asymptomatic infection, types of tests

used to diagnose infection, and available prevention and control interventions (e.g., isolation/quarantine, social distancing, environmental surface cleaning).

- Excellent and tactful interpersonal skills, cultural sensitivity, and language and interviewing skills that allow them to build and maintain trust with clients and contacts.
- Basic skills of crisis counseling and the ability to confidently refer clients and contacts for further care, if needed.
- Resourcefulness in locating and communicating with clients and contacts who may be difficult to reach or reluctant to engage in conversation.
- Awareness of the sensitivities surrounding immigration status and how this can be a barrier to case investigation and contact tracing activities. Understanding that assurances should be made to clients and contacts that all information collected will be used exclusively for public health purposes and not shared with immigration authorities.
- Understanding of when to refer individuals or situations to medical, social, or supervisory resources.
- Ability to conduct environmental assessments of a patient's or contact's home, including the need for any social support during self-isolation/self-quarantine.
- Ability to collect basic standardized surveillance data per protocols.
- Understanding of when the use of public health legal authorities may be necessary and how to notify the appropriate public health officer for authorization.

The following cross-cutting knowledge, skills and abilities support the successful practice of case investigation and contact tracing. Recruitment for case investigators and contact tracers should focus on identifying people with these attributes:

- Ethical and professional conduct
- Active listening
- Open communication
- Critical thinking
- Negotiating skills
- Problem solving
- Cultural humility and competency
- Fluency in non-English languages for communities where English is not the primary language
- Emotional intelligence
- Flexibility and adaptability

Strong interpersonal skills are important, but the role of the case investigator also requires a higher level of acuity and training. The case investigator must be able to conduct a conversation-based investigation (as opposed to reading a script or data collection form) to obtain information on close contacts and to assess healthcare and support needs for people diagnosed with COVID-19.

Case Investigation & Contact Tracing Training

CDC has trained case investigators and contact tracers for over 40 years. Typically, training includes a blend of knowledge-based and skills-based coursework. Initial knowledge-based training covers disease-specific information, client-centered counseling and motivational interviewing techniques, assessment of risk and other social support needs, and approaches to facilitate confidential client communication. Initial skills-based training uses interview technique modeling, scripted language, case scenarios, and role-playing. These trainings are followed by on-the-job learning supported by experienced staff.

Similar techniques can be applied to the training of the COVID-19 surge workforce. All new staff mobilized to support case investigation and contact

ien to Suspend Case Investigation & ntact Tracing Activities

When a jurisdiction does not have the capacity to investigate a majority its new COVID-19 cases, case investigation and contact tracing may not the most effective approach. At that point, jurisdictions should consider spending or scaling down contact tracing activities and reimplementing ict mitigation measures (such as stay-at-home orders, business closures, d school closures) until transmission begins to decline.

INVESTIGATING A COVID-19 CASE

Comprehensive information on a patient diagnosed with COVID-19 is he foundation of case investigation and contact tracing. This information ncludes the socio-demographic information, date of symptom onset or date f specimen collection for SARS-CoV-2 (the virus that causes COVID-19) esting, source of illness, list of close contacts and their locating information, duration of exposure, activity history during the contact elicitation window (when the patient was infectious and not under isolation), and exposure locations (including events/gatherings with unknown contacts).

Health departments are responsible for conducting COVID-19 case investigations and contact tracing and often have legal mandates to investigate cases of communicable disease and a duty to notify contacts of exposure. Health departments should initiate investigations as quickly as possible. Having written policies and procedures for investigations, including interview guides and call scripts, improves the efficiency and uniformity of investigations. In certain circumstances, it may take more than one interview with a patient to obtain all necessary and accurate informatio to complete the investigation.

Establishing trust and rapport between a case investigator and a p diagnosed with COVID-19 is necessary to obtain information an cooperation throughout the investigation. Good interview ski taught and will improve with practice. Public health personne

tracing will need a comprehensive overview of COVID-19 and the investigative process. Training for each of the case investigation and contact tracing roles should cover disease-specific information, interview guides, and protocols that include referral of high-risk individuals and complex cases to clinical staff, guidance on maintaining privacy/confidentiality, and referrals to support services, and should also include interactive skills-based training. CDC's website provides COVID-19 Contact Tracing Training Guidance and Resources. Given the more nuanced work of the case investigator, staff conducting follow-up with clients with COVID-19 should be provided with a more intensive skills-based training. This should include special emphasis on enhancing their ability to navigate difficult conversations.

The urgency in standing-up the case investigation and contact tracing workforce requires that the training for COVID-19 be abbreviated. Therefore, supervisory structures should be put in place in state, territorial, local, and tribal health jurisdictions to provide guidance and mentorship for new trainees to ensure quality of practice.

Identifying Case Investigation & Contact Tracing Resources

Efforts are under way across the nation to recruit and train a case investigation and contact tracing workforce. This will take the coordination of federal, state, and local organizations as well as public-private partnerships where possible. Resources from each level will need to be woven together to create a blanket of support for case investigation and contact tracing within each community. Guidance and resources for state, tribal, local, and territorial health departments on staffing the public health workforce are available from CDC.

The estimated number of case investigators and contact tracers needed in each community may be large and will vary depending on a number of factors, including the number of COVID-19 cases reported each day, number of close contacts elicited per patient, languages spoken in the community, and the amount of time and resources needed to notify and monitor clients and contacts. Local jurisdictions can review the guidance in Appendix D to estimate the number of case investigators/contact tracers needed in their community.

The surge workforce will likely come from a variety of sources:

- There may be local, state, and federal employees whose job can no longer be done due to COVID-19 who are available for redirection.
- Additionally, some local communities have identified volunteers who are willing and eager to support the COVID-19 response. Matching their knowledge, skills, and abilities with key roles in the COVID-19 response effort and providing relevant training can expand the workforce.
- Partnerships between public health and philanthropic entities can also expand the case investigation and contact tracing workforce by hiring and training individuals from local communities.
- Partnerships between public health and the technology sector can aid in the development of data management systems and innovations in communication.
- Finally, partnerships across all sectors can help support clients and contacts in need of housing and other support services during self-isolation and self-quarantine.

Alignment of Case Investigation & Contact Tracing Staff with Workflow

Combining large numbers of staff from different sources (e.g., local, state, federal) and varying categories (e.g., employees, contractors, temporary hires, volunteers) will be a challenge unique to the COVID-19 surge workforce. Consideration should be given to the alignment of staff assignments and supervision with workflow. For instance, those activities requiring knowledge of and access to public health surveillance systems (e.g., surveillance triage, case investigation) may be better integrated into the health department's workflow. Some jurisdictions have found it useful

to mobilize a cadre of state case investigators to bolster lo event of clusters or outbreaks.

When to Initiate Case Investigat & Contact Tracing Activities

Case investigation and contact tracing activities should be at two distinct points in an epidemic:

- First, early on in an epidemic, during the containmen investigation and contact tracing are needed to stop trans prevent a large outbreak from occurring. If efforts to epidemic are unsuccessful and widespread transmissio the community, then stricter community mitigation mea as stay-at-home orders, business closures, etc.) implemented. If the strict mitigation measures are transmission will begin to decline, and the community w suppression phase.
- Second, once the community enters the suppression pha epidemic, the jurisdiction should begin to implement or case investigation and contact tracing activities bef mitigation measures are fully lifted, in order to continue to community transmission.

The decision to initiate or scale up COVID-19 case investigati contact tracing activities will be unique to each area and will depend level of community transmission, characteristics of the community and populations, and the local capacity to implement case investigation contact tracing. It is critical that case investigation and contact tr activities be adequately resourced and widely accepted in any commu where they are implemented.

investigate clients with COVID-19 should be trained in interview methods and mentored by experienced employees. Case investigation and contact tracing training guidance and resources are available, including suggestions for role-playing exercises for trainees.

A patient will ideally be interviewed by a case investigator who is fluent in their primary language. If this is not possible, health departments should provide interpretation services, ideally by an individual with an understanding of the patient's cultural background.

When possible and appropriate, case interviews and contact elicitation should be conducted via phone call or another distance-based application to ensure the safety of the case investigator and efficient use of program resources.

Step 1: Case Identification & Prioritization

COVID-19 case investigations are typically initiated when a health department receives a report from a laboratory of a positive SARS-CoV-2 test result or a report from a healthcare provider of a patient with a confirmed or probable diagnosis of COVID-19.

Ideally, jurisdictions will have ample testing available to facilitate laboratory confirmation of all COVID-19 cases within the community and the public health capacity to investigate all symptomatic and asymptomatic clients with a confirmed diagnosis of COVID-19.

Considerations when Laboratory Testing Capacity is Limited

For areas that have limited laboratory testing capacity, prioritization of testing resources should take into consideration the following factors: 1) ensuring optimal care for hospitalized clients and reducing the risk of healthcare-associated infections, 2) ensuring those at higher risk for severe disease are rapidly identified and triaged, 3) identifying individuals in communities experiencing high numbers of COVID-19 hospitalizations to decrease community spread and ensure the health of critical infrastructure workers.

CDC provides recommended priorities for COVID-19 testing that can be adapted by health departments to respond to rapidly changing local circumstances. CDC's testing recommendations reinforce the role of case investigation and contact tracing as an effective strategy to decrease community transmission.

Once a COVID-19 laboratory or provider report is received, this information will be entered into the health department surveillance system. With expanded laboratory testing in both public and private sectors, it is important to establish electronic laboratory reporting systems to enhance the timeliness of data to inform public health action.

The health department should use a triage system to use any information known about a patient diagnosed with COVID-19, prior to case interview, to delegate the investigation to either a case investigator or special infection control team (specific settings where a special team is needed are included in Section VI).

Health departments can communicate with healthcare providers by phone when a positive laboratory test is reported to obtain information necessary for triaging. Conversely, health departments could request that providers phone-in case information on the same day that a provider receives a positive SARS-CoV-2 test result in a Priority 1 or Priority 2 patient (see Box 1).

In addition to identifying potential outbreaks, information to assist in case prioritization includes a patient's COVID-19 symptoms, underlying health conditions, patient locating information (residence type/location/ contact information), workplace role and location, confirmation that patient was notified of test result, and initiation of self-isolation.

Triage staff should have rapid turn-around times with provider queries (within 24 hours). Triage staff should then prioritize cases for investigation to either a case investigator or special infection control team based on known information. These strategies are only feasible with adequate staff to provide triage support and sufficient patient information available to allow for prioritizing.

For areas that have limited public health resources to investigate all cases, the following case investigation hierarchy (Box 1) can be used to help guide prioritization when information is known about the case.

Box 1. COVID -19 case investigation hierarchy

All confirmed and probable COVID-19 cases should be investigated. When resources are limited, priorities for who should be investigated are listed below. Priority 1 clients are likely to have exposed a larger number of people and/or are likely to have close contacts who could potentially expose: many people, those at higher risk for severe disease, or critical infrastructure workers. Priority 2 clients may be at higher risk for severe disease and will need prompt risk assessment and linkage to any needed medical and support services.

Investigate Clients with a Confirmed or Probable Diagnosis Who Are:

Priority 1

- Hospitalized clients
- Healthcare personnel (HCP)
- First responders (e.g., Emergency Medical Services (EMS) personnel, law enforcement, firefighters)
- Individuals living, working or visiting acute care, skilled nursing, mental health, and long-term care facilities
- Individuals living, working or visiting community congregate settings (e.g., correctional facilities, homeless shelters, educational institutions, mass gatherings, and crowded workplaces including production plants)
- Members of a large household living in close quarters especially with a resident with co-morbidities
- Individuals known to live in households with a higher risk individual or to provide care in a household with a higher risk individual

Priority 2

- Critical infrastructure workers[2]
- Individuals 65 years of age and older
- Individuals at higher risk for severe disease
- Pregnant women

Priority 3

- Individuals with symptoms who do not meet any of the above categories
- Deceased cases

Priority 4

- Individuals without symptoms who do not meet any of the above categories

[2] Consider moving to Priority 1 any critical infrastructure worker who works closely with other critical infrastructure workers and/or is in close contact with large numbers of people (e.g., transportation, food service).

Operational Questions to Consider

- How are reports received and how are they entered into the database? How complete are the reports?
- Can electronic laboratory reporting for COVID-19 cases be easily implemented?
- How will the time between a patient's symptom onset and self-isolation be assessed? How can delays in laboratory or case reporting, assignment to case investigator, time to patient interview and subsequent isolation be monitored?
- How will non-laboratory-confirmed cases be reported by providers and managed by the health department? Will this require a modification of provider reporting requirements and confidential morbidity report forms?
- How will public health staff coordinate with healthcare providers to facilitate testing of probable cases?
- Can laboratory and provider reporting requirements be altered to alert local and state health departments of critical data elements to aid in prioritization?
- Can you develop public health alerts to request that providers report probable cases and cases in Priority 1 clients (Box 1) within 24 hours?
- What type of collaborative agreements can be set in place for data sharing between public health and healthcare providers (e.g., access to electronic health records)?
- For areas with blended state, regional and/or local health department authorities, which entity will be responsible for case prioritization?
- How will investigations be handled for a patient who regularly travels between jurisdictions?

The hierarchy is based on the assumption that clients with a confirmed or probable diagnosis of COVID-19 in Priority 1 are likely to have exposed a larger number of people and/or are likely to have close contacts who could potentially expose many people, those at higher risk for severe disease, or critical infrastructure workers. Priority 2 includes clients who may be at higher risk for severe disease and will need prompt risk assessment and linkage to any needed medical and support services. Clients should be prioritized based on the highest priority category they fall into. When prioritizing clients with a positive SARS-CoV-2 test result or a probable diagnosis of COVID-19 to investigate, jurisdictions should be guided by the local characteristics of disease transmission, demographics, and public health and healthcare system capacity. Decisions should be supported by local guidance and circumstances.

Step 2: Rapid Notification of Results or Diagnosis

- Some clients will have been notified of their positive SARS-CoV-2 test result or probable case diagnosis by their healthcare provider and already received instructions for self-isolation.
- When communication with the patient about their positive SARS-CoV-2 test result or probable diagnosis is unclear or has not be taken place, the health department should notify the patient as soon as possible (within 24 hours of reporting to the health department).
- Ideally, a patient with a probable COVID-19 diagnosis will be linked to testing (if available and appropriate).
- If there is a need for testing and the case investigator plans to collect the specimen in person, case investigators need to have had appropriate training on infection prevention and control practices. They must also obtain any necessary personal protective equipment (PPE) prior to conducting in-person activities.
- The first connection can be made through different channels such as phone, text, email or in-person (if appropriate) in the primary language of the individual. This process can be manual, automated, or semi-automated based on jurisdictional capacity. Protocol should clearly outline the primary and secondary means of reaching a patient and address confidentiality at the start of communication.
- Special considerations should be given to ensure culturally and linguistically appropriate communication.
- Protocols should be in place to provide services to people who are deaf or who have hearing loss.
- Depending on the source of the case report, information for locating a patient may be insufficient. Tips on additional resources that may be used to obtain missing locating information can be found in Appendix B. Every effort should be made to reach the patient remotely before attempting in-person communication.

Operational Questions to Consider

- How can your jurisdiction incorporate existing or new technology into a case investigator's workflow to expedite patient notification?
- What technological precautions can be taken to ensure the confidentiality of clients and case investigators?
- What process will be followed when the patient is a minor? *Review jurisdiction-specific laws and consult with legal counsel if uncertain.*
- When is in-person notification needed? *Case investigators expected to perform in person notification need appropriate training on infection prevention and control practices and must obtain any necessary personal protective equipment (PPE) prior to conducting in-person activities.*
- How will positive test notifications be handled in congregate facilities (e.g., correctional facilities, skilled nursing facilities, assisted care facilities, mental health facilities, various workplaces) where a positive test has implications for the patient, other residents, staff and visitors?
- How will investigations be handled for clients who are hospitalized and unable to be interviewed or deceased?
- What are local policies regarding interviewing of surrogates/proxies?

Step 3: Case Interview

- Every effort should be made to interview the patient by telephone or video conference instead of in-person. For in-person interviews, guidance on recommended infection prevention and control practices at a home or non-home residential setting can be found on CDC's Evaluating PUIs Residential page.
- Clients in special populations and/or congregate settings may require additional considerations and should be triaged and assigned to a special infection control team. See Section VI for additional information.
- Appendix C includes critical data elements that can be incorporated into a jurisdiction's paper form or electronic system used to elicit detailed information about a patient's close contacts and activity history, including any household contacts during self-isolation.

Operational Questions to Consider

- If the patient needs to be interviewed via an interpreter, how will those services be accessed?
- What steps will be taken if the patient is unwilling to communicate remotely (e.g., phone, video conference)?
- What procedures will be established to interview clients in correctional facilities? Hospitalized clients? Minors?
- What procedures will be established to locate and interview people experiencing homelessness?

Step 3a: Monitoring and Isolation Instructions

- Clients with probable or confirmed COVID-19 should be advised to self-isolate immediately, if they are not doing so already. Self-isolation is recommended for people with probable or confirmed COVID-19 who have mild illness and are able to recover at home.
- It should be made clear to the patient whether the isolation instructions are voluntary or mandatory.
- If a patient refuses to comply with voluntary isolation instructions, state and local jurisdictions have the authority to mandate isolation.
- The patient should be informed of COVID-19 symptoms to monitor for and be instructed to get medical attention immediately if he/she has any emergency warning signs (including trouble breathing). Clients with no primary healthcare provider will need linkage to telemedicine or phone consultation.
- The patient should also be informed of ways to prevent infection among those living in their household.
- Additional self-isolation guidance should be reviewed with the patient and instructional materials provided. Sample materials can be found on the CDC website:
    - 10 things you can do to manage your COVID-19 symptoms at home
    - What to Do If You Are Sick
- All instructions should be provided in a patient's primary language.

Operational Questions to Consider

- Under what circumstances will isolation be mandatory (under public health orders) as opposed to voluntary? How will this distinction be made clear to a patient?
- How will clients be monitored for isolation compliance?
- In the event that self-isolation is not feasible, what alternative supports exist, and/or what risk-reduction measures can be taken?

Step 3b: Assessing Self-Isolation Support Needs

Emphasis should be placed on conducting an environmental assessment of the patient's self-isolation location, as this will identify any need for social support during self-isolation.

Self-Isolation of clients with a diagnosis of COVID-19 prevents transmission to others and is critical to the success of any case investigation and contact tracing efforts. For most clients diagnosed with COVID-19 (i.e., those in an outpatient setting who are medically stable or discharged home following diagnosis at hospital), self-isolation can take place at home. If possible, clients should be asked to voluntarily stay home, monitor themselves, and maintain social distance from others. The timeframe for self-isolation varies by case but, in general, people should isolate until the risk of secondary transmission is considered low. Adherence to self-isolation instructions mainly depends on the clients' needs and their living situation, as well as on the support provided by the case investigation and contact tracing team.

Self-isolation requires that clients remain separate from others in the home, staying in a specific room away from other people and pets, and ideally with access to a separate bathroom. First and foremost, a case investigator should assess a patient's ability to self-isolate in a safe environment that provides access to a private room and bathroom, as well as access to adequate food and water, among other considerations. For a portion of the US population, self-isolation at home will be a challenge. It may be particularly difficult for some of the most vulnerable populations. Considerations must also be made for clients who express fear of abuse or violence if they must self-isolate at home. Additionally, some clients (e.g., single parents, nursing mothers, parents with children and toddlers, and other primary caregivers) may face other challenges, such as childcare or dependent adult care, that may affect their ability to self-isolate. Social services, housing and other supportive services will be needed for those clients who are unable to separate themselves from others in their current living situation. See Section XI of this guidance for further considerations.

Clients will also need to be supported with health coaching to ensure daily monitoring of temperature and COVID-19 symptoms, and have access to clinical services for medical concerns. Coordination of access to tele-health services may be needed for clients without virtual access to a primary care provider. Reminding clients about the emergency warning signs and contact information for healthcare providers is imperative to ensure early medical management in the event that they develop new symptoms or their symptoms worsen.

All clients with a confirmed or probable diagnosis of COVID-19 who are entering self-isolation in a non-healthcare setting ideally would be provided a COVID-19 kit with the following resources:[3]

- Washable cloth face covering
- Gloves
- Digital thermometer
- Alcohol-based hand sanitizer, soap, EPA-registered household disinfectant
- COVID-19 health education materials (translated into the appropriate language)
- Instructions for cleaning and disinfecting your home for those sharing space with others
- A hotline/warmline to address any support needs during the self-isolation period, including medical support

[3] The composition of the COVID-19 kit will depend on the jurisdiction's resources.

Operational Questions to Consider
• Are there other resources that your jurisdiction can share to provide health advice and answer questions? (e.g., mobile app, CDC Coronavirus Symptom Self-Checker, CDC-INFO) • Who can you partner with to provide other services to support clients during self-isolation?

Step 3c: Eliciting Contacts

- Contact elicitation is a voluntary and critical part of the case interview.
- The case investigator can use information from any reports received by the health department, along with the patient's symptom history gathered earlier in the case interview, to determine the contact elicitation window (the timeframe when the patient was infectious and not under isolation). See Box 2 below for additional guidance on determining the contact elicitation window.
- A close contact is defined as someone who was within 6 feet of an infected person for at least 15 minutes starting from 48 hours before illness onset (or, for asymptomatic clients, 10 days prior to positive specimen collection) until the time the patient is isolated.
- It will be important that the case investigator clearly explain why close contacts are being elicited and assure the patient that their identity will not be disclosed to any close contacts that they identify.
- The trust and rapport built earlier in the case interview, combined with open-ended and probing questions, will help facilitate the contact elicitation portion of the interview.
- Information to be gathered for each close contact can be found in the Contact Elicitation Investigation data elements table in Appendix C and includes the contact's name and locating information, the setting of the exposure, contact's work setting and occupation, and any underlying health conditions or other risk factors the contact may have (if known by the patient).

- In communities near international land borders, specific interview questions should be asked to identify relevant contacts across the border.
- The case investigator should also confirm the best way to reach the patient for any follow-up discussion.
- Proxy interviews are essential when the patient cannot be interviewed (e.g., patient is deceased, intubated, unconscious, a minor, cognitively impaired). Key proxy informants are those likely to know the patient's practices, habits, and behaviors. However, because proxy interviews jeopardize patient confidentiality, jurisdictions should establish clear guidelines for these interviews that recognize the challenge of maintaining confidentiality.

Box 2. Determining the contact elicitation window

In order to elicit contacts from a confirmed or probable COVID-19 patient, a case investigator will first need to determine the appropriate contact elicitation window. An assessment of the patient's COVID-19 symptoms will help identify their infectious period. Building on that information, the contact elicitation window is the timeframe when the patient was infectious and not under isolation. If there are additional contacts during isolation (such as household contacts), those contacts should also be elicited.

Patient with Confirmed or Probable COVID-19—Symptomatic

When interviewing a symptomatic patient, a case investigator should elicit all close contacts from 48 hours prior to onset of any symptoms through the beginning of isolation.

Start date: 48 hours before symptom* onset

End date: Beginning of isolation period OR until discontinuation of home isolation (to elicit household contacts of clients recovering at home)

*All possible symptoms should be considered, with particular attention to those that may be mild and/or nonspecific (e.g., fatigue, muscle pain) and those less common.

Patient with Confirmed or Probable COVID-19—Asymptomatic

Determining the contact elicitation window for an asymptomatic patient is challenging and should be considered an estimate instead of a precise timeframe. Rather than focusing on the suggested start date, a case investigator may want to prioritize eliciting any recent close contacts in higher priority groups (as listed in Box 4).

Start date: 10 days before the date of specimen collection for confirmed laboratory test

End date: Beginning of isolation period OR discontinuation of home isolation (to elicit household contacts of clients recovering at home)

Operational Questions to Consider

- How can your jurisdiction use technology to facilitate contact elicitation (e.g., download contact list from a patient's phone)?
- What types of data tools would help increase efficiency?
- How will case investigators document and transfer the list of contacts to the contract tracer?
- Will clients be asked to notify household contacts or close contacts themselves? How will patient-notified contacts be managed and dispositioned?
- If an employer knows the identity of an employee diagnosed with COVID-19, how can a list of close contacts from the worksite best be gathered?

Step 4: Case Follow-Up & Medical Monitoring

- The initial patient interview covers a great deal of material, which can be overwhelming for a patient.
- In some instances, the case investigator may need to follow-up with the patient to clarify details from the conversation including:
    - Onset of symptoms, particularly the nonspecific symptoms (e.g., fatigue, muscle pain);
    - Further exploration of occupation and interactions in the workplace or last day at work;
    - Transportation to and from work, social and recreational activities;
    - Additional locating information for close contacts or additional contacts from their self-isolation period;
    - Home, family, and other factors that could impact compliance with self-isolation.
- Ideally, all clients diagnosed with COVID-19 will be monitored using real-time communication methods (e.g., telephone call, video conferencing) to share daily reports on their temperature and COVID-19 symptoms throughout the length of their self-isolation.

- Prioritizing which clients to monitor closely and which may be able to adequately self-monitor should be determined in the context of existing resources. In some instances, clients with underlying health conditions and other special circumstances (such as pregnancy) may present complex medical challenges. While these may not require hospitalization, these clients may need in-home medical monitoring by a healthcare provider until their COVID-19 symptoms resolve.
- If a jurisdiction's resources do not allow for active daily monitoring, clients will be asked to self-monitor and communicate remotely (e.g., email, recorded video, telephone message, text, monitoring apps) to notify public health authorities of their health status and promptly communicate any new symptoms or symptoms of increasing severity.
- For those individuals self-monitoring and sharing reports remotely, reports must be received by the agreed upon time each day, and protocol must address follow-up actions for clients who do not report out.

Operational Questions to Consider

- What types of tools and schedules will be used for medical monitoring?
- Which staff in the jurisdiction will conduct medical monitoring? Will certain cases be delegated to a staff member with clinical expertise (e.g., complex or high-risk cases)?
- What social support is necessary for a patient to maintain self-isolation? What support may a patient's family need?
- What criteria will your jurisdiction use to refer clients to healthcare or emergency services?
- What steps will be taken for self-monitoring clients who do not comply with reporting requirements?
  How intensive will the outreach be (e.g., same-day home visit)?

Step 5: Additional Case Follow-Up

- Additional follow-up may be needed for clients with COVID-19 who are transitioning from one facility to another—for example, from a hospital to a long-term care facility or to home isolation. Care coordination plans should be put in place to maintain proper infection control and isolation procedures.

- Additional coordination will also be necessary to support clients with COVID-19 who are discharged from a correctional facility (e.g., prisons, jails, youth detention centers). These individuals will be transitioning to self-isolation in their home communities and will need assessment for social supports to ensure adequate housing, food, and medical care throughout the remainder of their self-isolation.
- Transitional case management plans are incredibly important to ensure continuity of care for clients with COVID-19 and protect the community from further transmission.

Step 6: Discontinuation of Self-Isolation

- The decision to discontinue self-isolation is made on a case-by-case basis, taking into consideration a patient's COVID-19 test results, symptom history and other factors, including occupation.
- CDC guidance included in Box 3 provides a framework for decision-making. However, decisions are determined at the local level and should be communicated clearly to a patient.
- Decisions about return to work for healthcare providers with confirmed or suspected COVID-19 should be made in the context of local circumstances. CDC guidance is available to help occupational health programs and public health officials make these decisions.

Box 3. Criteria for ending isolation if not in a healthcare setting

People with COVID-19 or its symptoms who are recovering at home (or other non-hospital setting), and

will not be tested	will be tested
to determine if they are no longer contagious, can leave their "sick room" and home when:	
• They have had no fever for at least 72 hours (that is 3 full days of no fever) without the use of medicine that reduces fevers AND • Other symptoms have improved (for example, when their cough or shortness of breath have improved) AND • At least 10 days have passed since their symptoms first appeared	• They no longer have a fever (without the use of medicine that reduces fevers) AND • Other symptoms have improved (for example, when their cough or shortness of breath have improved) AND • They received two negative tests in a row, 24 hours apart

People who DID NOT have COVID-19 symptoms, but tested positive who:

will not be tested again	will be tested again
to determine if they are no longer contagious, can leave their "sick room" and home when:	
• At least 10 days have passed since the date of the first positive test AND • They continue to have no symptoms (no cough or shortness of breath) since the test	• They received two negative tests in a row, at least 24 hours apart

Operational Questions to Consider

- Will a "return to work" letter be available to clients who request one after completing their self-isolation period?
- Will a warmline be offered to address any follow-up issues?

Contact Tracing for COVID-19

Summary of COVID-19 Specific Practices

- Contact tracing will be conducted for close contacts (any individual within 6 feet of an infected person for at least 15 minutes) of confirmed or probable COVID-19 clients.
- Remote communications for the purposes of case investigation and contact tracing should be prioritized; in-person communication may be considered only after remote options have been exhausted.
- Testing is recommended for all close contacts of confirmed or probable COVID-19 clients.
- Those contacts who test positive (symptomatic or asymptomatic) should be managed as a confirmed COVID-19 case.
- Asymptomatic contacts testing negative should self-quarantine for 14 days from their last exposure (i.e., close encounter with confirmed or probable COVID-19 case)
- If testing is not available, symptomatic close contacts should self-isolate and be managed as a probable COVID-19 case.
- If testing is not available, asymptomatic close contacts should self-quarantine and be monitored for 14 days after their last exposure, with linkage to clinical care for those who develop symptoms.

For COVID-19, a close contact is defined as any individual who was within 6 feet of an infected person for at least 15 minutes starting from 48 hours before illness onset until the time the patient is isolated.

The public health evaluation of close contacts to clients with confirmed or probable COVID-19 may vary depending on the exposure setting. Contacts in special populations and/or congregate settings require additional considerations and may need handoff to a senior health department investigator or special team. Additional guidance on managing these contacts can be found in Section VI of this guidance.

Close Contact Evaluation and Monitoring Priorities

In jurisdictions with testing capacity, symptomatic and asymptomatic close contacts to clients with confirmed and probable COVID-19 should be evaluated and monitored. For areas with insufficient testing support and/or limited public health resources, the following evaluation and monitoring hierarchy (Box 4) can be used to help guide prioritization. The hierarchy is based on the assumption that if close contacts listed in Priority 1 become infected, they could potentially expose many people, those at higher risk for severe disease, or critical infrastructure workers. If close contacts in Priority 2 become infected, they may be at higher risk for severe disease, so prompt notification, monitoring, and linkage to needed medical and support services is important.

Box 4. Close contact evaluation and monitoring hierarchy

Evaluate/Monitor Close Contacts Who Are:

Priority 1

- Hospitalized clients
- Healthcare personnel (HCP)
- First responders (e.g., EMS, law enforcement, firefighters)
- Individuals living, working or visiting acute care, skilled nursing, mental health, and long-term care facilities
- Individuals living, working or visiting community congregate settings (e.g., correctional facilities, homeless shelters, educational institutions, mass gatherings, and workplaces including production plants)
- Member of a large household living in close quarters
- Individuals who live in households with a higher risk individual or who provide care in a household with a higher risk individual (Note: Household members who likely had extensive contact with a patient with COVID-19 should constitute the highest risk close contacts.)

Priority 2

- Critical infrastructure workers[4]
- Individuals 65 years of age and older
- Individuals at higher risk for severe disease
- Pregnant women

Priority 3

- Individuals with symptoms who do not meet any of the above categories

Priority 4

- Individuals without symptoms who do not meet any of the above categories

---

[4] *Consider moving to Priority 1 any critical infrastructure worker who works closely with other critical infrastructure workers and/or is in close contact with large numbers of people (e.g., transportation, food service).*

When prioritizing close contacts to evaluate and monitor, jurisdictions should be guided by the local characteristics of disease transmission, demographics, and public health and healthcare system capacity. Some states require mandatory testing for specific circumstances. Local decisions depend on local guidance and circumstances.

Contact tracers use clear protocols to notify, interview, and advise close contacts to clients with confirmed or probable COVID-19. Jurisdictions can use the following steps and considerations as a framework when developing a protocol for the tracing of close contacts.

Step 1: Rapid Notification of Exposure

For contacts in your health department's jurisdiction:

- A close contact to a patient with confirmed or probable COVID-19 should be notified of their exposure as soon as possible (within 24 hours of contact elicitation). The patient may elect to notify some or all of their close contacts before the contact tracer.
- *The identity of the patient will not be revealed or confirmed by the contact tracer, even if asked by a contact.*
- Contacts can be notified through different channels such as phone, text, email, or in-person (if appropriate) in the primary language of the individual. Special consideration should be given to ensure culturally and linguistically appropriate communications. The protocol should clearly outline the primary and secondary means of notifying a contact.
- Protocols should be in place to provide services to people who are deaf or who have hearing loss.
- Depending on the information elicited during the case investigation, locating information for the contact may be insufficient. Tips on additional resources that may be used to obtain missing locating information can be found in Appendix B. Every effort should be

made to reach the contact remotely before attempting in-person communication.

Operational Questions to Consider

- Who will conduct contact notification in your jurisdiction? (e.g., case investigators, other public health staff, volunteers, contracted staff)
- How will you collaborate to transfer contact information from one jurisdiction to another to ensure notification of exposure for contacts outside of your jurisdiction?
- How can your jurisdiction incorporate existing or new technology (e.g., mobile app) into a contact tracer's workflow to speed up contact notification?
- When is in-person notification needed? *Contact tracers expected to perform in-person notification need appropriate training on infection prevention and control practices and must obtain any necessary PPE prior to conducting in-person activities.*
- Will contact tracers be asked to notify a patient's household contacts/known contacts, or will the patient be asked to make these notifications?
- How will notification of exposure be handled for minors?
- If an entire household is exposed, will there be one point of contact for the household or separate contacts for every household member?
- How will a contact tracer follow up with a contact if the patient makes the notification?
- How will you work with employers when many contacts are within a work setting?

Step 2: Contact Interview

- Every effort should be made to interview the close contact by telephone, text, or video conference instead of in-person. The interview should be conducted in the individual's primary language (through interpretation services, if necessary). For in-person interviews, guidance on recommended infection prevention and control practices at a home or non-home residential setting can be found on CDC's Evaluating PUIs Residential page.
- Appendix C includes critical data elements that can be incorporated into a jurisdiction's form used to interview contacts to assess symptoms, better characterize their underlying risk for infection, and assess home and social factors that could impact compliance with self-quarantine.

Operational Questions to Consider

- If a contact needs to be interviewed via an interpreter, how will those services be accessed?
- How will your jurisdiction navigate confidentiality challenges when the calendar date of an exposure easily reveals who may have exposed a contact to COVID-19?
- What steps will be taken if a contact is unwilling or unable to be interviewed or cannot be located?

Step 2a: Testing and Quarantine/Isolation Instructions

- Close contacts with symptoms should immediately self-isolate and be referred for testing and medical care. Contacts with no primary healthcare provider will need linkage to telemedicine or phone consultation.
- Close contacts with no symptoms will be asked to self-quarantine for 14 days from their last potential exposure. The last potential exposure would initially be determined by the case investigator.
- If resources permit, jurisdictions should arrange for the testing of all close contacts, as appropriate.
    - If positive, the contact will be referred to a case investigator.
    - If negative, asymptomatic close contacts should continue to self-quarantine for a full 14 days after last exposure and follow all recommendations of public health authorities.
    - If negative, symptomatic close contacts should continue to self-quarantine and follow all recommendations of public health authorities. A second test and additional medical consultation may be needed if symptoms do not improve.
    - If testing is not available, symptomatic close contacts should be advised to self-isolate and be managed as a probable case. *Self-isolation is recommended for people with probable or confirmed COVID-19 who have mild illness and are able to recover at home.*

- Contacts should be educated about COVID-19 symptoms to monitor for and be instructed to promptly report any new symptoms to public health authorities and seek medical care when necessary.
- CDC guidance is available on critical infrastructure workers who may have had exposure to a person with suspected or confirmed COVID-19. To ensure continuity of operations of essential functions, CDC advises that critical infrastructure workers may be permitted to continue working following potential exposure to COVID-19, provided they remain asymptomatic and additional precautions are implemented to protect them and the community. Any decisions should be made in the context of local circumstances.
- CDC guidance is also available on asymptomatic healthcare providers with a recognized COVID-19 exposure. They might be permitted to work in a crisis capacity strategy to address staffing shortages if they wear a facemask for source control for 14 days after the exposure. Any decisions should be made in the context of local circumstances.

Sample Instructions for Close Contacts

- Self-quarantine, preferably at home, until 14 days after last potential exposure and maintain social distance (at least 6 feet) from others at all times.
- Follow CDC guidance on self-quarantine.
- Self-monitor daily for symptoms *[NOTE: Include instructions on how close contacts can report symptoms to the health department and agreed upon reporting times.]*
    - If you have a thermometer, check and record your temperature twice a day.
    - Contact a healthcare provider immediately if you:
        - Feel feverish or have a temperature of 100.4ºF or higher
        - Develop a cough or shortness of breath
        - Develop mild symptoms like sore throat, muscle aches, tiredness, or diarrhea
- Avoid contact with people at higher risk for severe illness (unless they live in the same home and had same exposure as you).
- Follow CDC guidance if you develop symptoms.

Operational Questions to Consider

- Under what circumstances will quarantine be mandatory (under public health orders) as opposed to voluntary?
- Who will be referred for testing (e.g., symptomatic, asymptomatic) and how (e.g., testing site, home test kit)?
- How will contacts be checked against databases of already confirmed cases to ensure they are not already in self-isolation?
- Will contact tracers be collecting diagnostic respiratory specimens?
- How will contacts be monitored for self-quarantine compliance?
- What services are available in the community to support workers who need to stay home and self-quarantine?
- How can your jurisdiction incorporate technology, such as a mobile app or online tool, to assist with active monitoring of close contacts (e.g., symptom reporting, temperature checks)?
- Can your jurisdiction supply a letter/email to close contacts documenting their need to self-quarantine for a specified date range? Contacts could provide this to their employers to verify the reason for a work absence.

Step 2b: Assessing Self-Quarantine Support Needs

Emphasis should be placed on conducting an environmental assessment of the contact's self-quarantine location, as this will identify any need for social support during self-quarantine.

Self-quarantine of close contacts exposed to COVID-19 prevents transmission to others and is critical to the success of case investigation and contact tracing efforts. For most, self-quarantine can take place at home. If possible, contacts should be asked to voluntarily stay home, monitor themselves, and maintain social distance from others. The timeframe for self-quarantine is 14 days following the last day of exposure to a patient with COVID-19, to ensure that the contact does not get sick themselves and spread the virus to others. Adherence to self-quarantine instructions may depend on the support provided to contacts.

Self-quarantine requires that a contact remain in a specific room separate from other non-exposed people and pets in the home, and ideally with access to a separate bathroom. First and foremost, the contact tracer should assess an individual's ability to self-quarantine in a safe environment that provides access to a private room and bathroom, as well as access to adequate food and water among other considerations. For a portion of the US population, self-quarantine at home will be a challenge. It will be particularly difficult for some of the most vulnerable populations.

Considerations must also be made for close contacts who express fear of abuse or violence if they must self-quarantine at home. Additionally, some contacts (e.g., single parents, nursing mothers, parents with children and toddlers, and other primary caregivers) may face other challenges, such as childcare or dependent adult care, that may affect their ability to self-quarantine. Social services, housing and other supportive services will be needed for those contacts who are unable to separate themselves from others in their current living situation. See Section XI of this guidance for further considerations.

Close contacts will also need to be supported with health coaching to ensure daily monitoring of temperature and the onset of any COVID-19 symptoms and have access to clinical services should symptoms appear. Coordination of access to telehealth services may be needed for contacts without virtual access to a primary care provider. All close contacts entering a 14-day self-quarantine period should be provided a COVID-19 kit with the following resources:[5]

- Washable cloth face covering
- Gloves
- Digital thermometer
- Alcohol-based hand sanitizer, soap, EPA-registered household disinfectant
- COVID-19 health education materials (translated into the appropriate language)
- Instructions for cleaning and disinfecting your home for those sharing space with others
- A hotline/warmline to address any support needs during the self-quarantine period, including medical support

[5] The composition of the COVID-19 kit will depend on the jurisdiction's resources.

Operational Questions to Consider

- Are there other resources that your jurisdiction can share to provide health advice and answer questions? (e.g., mobile app, hotline/call center, CDC Coronavirus Symptom Self-Checker, CDC-INFO)

Step 3: Medical Monitoring

- Contacts who agree to self-quarantine will ideally receive active daily monitoring through real-time communication methods (e.g., telephone calls, video conferencing) to check-in on their temperature and COVID-19 symptoms throughout the length of their self-quarantine.
- If a jurisdiction's resources do not allow for active daily monitoring, contacts will be asked to self-monitor and communicate remotely (e.g., email, recorded video, telephone message, text, monitoring apps) to notify public health authorities of their health status and promptly communicate any new symptoms or symptoms of increasing severity.
- For those individuals self-monitoring and sharing reports remotely, reports must be received by the agreed upon time each day, and protocol must address follow-up actions for contacts who do not report out.
- Contacts who develop and report symptoms will be linked to clinical care and testing. For contacts who report testing, follow up to confirm results.
    - If positive, the contact will be referred to a case investigator.
    - If negative, symptomatic contacts should continue to self-quarantine and follow all recommendations of public health authorities. A second test and additional medical consultation may be needed if symptoms do not improve.
    - If testing is not available, symptomatic close contacts should be advised to self-isolate and be managed as a probable case. *Self-isolation is recommended for people with probable or*

confirmed COVID-19 who have mild illness and are able to recover at home.

Operational Questions to Consider
• What steps will be taken for contacts under self-monitoring who do not report as required? How intensive will the outreach be (e.g., same-day home visit)?

Step 4: Contact Close Out

- Contacts who remain asymptomatic for 14 days after last exposure can be notified of their release from monitoring and provided general health education in their primary language.
- Contacts who develop symptoms but test negative during their monitoring period should continue to self-quarantine and follow all recommendations of public health authorities. A second test and additional medical consultation may be needed if symptoms do not improve. The decision to release a contact from self-quarantine should be determined at the local level and should be communicated clearly to the contact.

Operational Questions to Consider
• Will the health department send an alert notification to the individual one day prior to the end of self-quarantine to double-check signs/symptoms and authorize return to work?
• Will a "return to work" letter be available to contacts who request one after completing the monitoring period?
• Will a warmline be offered to address any post-monitoring issues?

OUTBREAKS

Most jurisdictions will create a special investigation team to take over outbreaks as they require expertise and resources beyond typical case investigation and contact tracing efforts. CDC has developed specific guidance for investigating clients with COVID-19 in a number of settings. When relevant, the CDC guidance is highlighted below.

A COVID-19 outbreak indicates potentially extensive transmission within a setting or organization. An outbreak investigation involves several overlapping epidemiologic, case, and contact investigations, with a surge in the need for public health resources. More emphasis on active case finding is recommended, which can result in more contacts than usual needing testing and monitoring.

Definitions for COVID-19 outbreaks are relative to the local context. A working definition of "outbreak" is recommended for planning investigations. A recommended definition is a situation that is consistent with either of two sets of criteria:

- During (and because of) a case investigation and contact tracing, two or more contacts are identified as having active COVID-19, regardless of their assigned priority.
  OR
- Two or more clients with COVID-19 are discovered to be linked, and the linkage is established outside of a case investigation and contact tracing (e.g., two clients who received a diagnosis of COVID-19 are found to work in the same office, and only one or neither of the them was listed as a contact to the other).

Typically, jurisdictions will require potential outbreaks to be investigated by a special team of experts. An outbreak increases the urgency of investigations and places greater demands on the health department. In an outbreak, contacts can be exposed to more than one patient diagnosed with COVID-19, and clients and contacts can be interrelated through multiple social connections, which complicate efforts to set priorities.

Congregate Settings

For congregate settings, the types of information for designating priorities are site-specific, and therefore a customized algorithm is required for each situation. The general concepts of patient characteristics, duration and proximity of exposure, environmental factors that affect transmission, and susceptibility of contacts to COVID-19 should be considered. These investigations are extremely complex and will require collaboration with multiple partners in order to assess risk for both facility residents, staff, and external contractors who provide services in those facilities. Symptom screening, testing, and isolation and quarantine recommended may vary based on the facility (e.g., healthcare facility versus others), the environmental constructs, and the number of clients with COVID-19 and contacts under consideration.

In some instances, case investigation and contact tracing conducted within facilities will need to be undertaken by specially trained staff (e.g., infection control practitioners, industrial hygienists) in collaboration with facility leadership, occupational health liaisons and other relevant SMEs. Interruption of transmission within the facilities will also require complementary community case investigation and contact tracing efforts, so planning for these activities should be a joint endeavor involving community leadership and other key stakeholders.

The information below provides a snapshot of areas for consideration and links to available CDC guidance.

Correctional Facilities

CDC has issued guidance on preventing and controlling COVID-19 in correctional facilities. Jails, prisons, and immigrant detention centers have reported COVID-19 outbreaks. Multiple factors can hinder contact tracing in correctional facilities. The best preparation for conducting case investigation and contact tracing in jails, prisons, and immigration centers is a preexisting formal collaboration between correctional and public health officials. Health department TB, HIV, and STD programs have long-standing relationships with correctional facilities and can be seen as a resource. If a collaboration has not been established prior to an outbreak, quickly developing relationships with correctional partners will be critical. Building trust with people held in the facilities will also be necessary to successfully investigate the outbreak.

Investigations in jails can be particularly challenging because of rapid turnover of inmates and crowding. The number of contacts in close proximity to a patient/inmate can be large. Contacts who are transferred, released, or paroled from a correctional facility before being evaluated for COVID-19 should be traced.

Workplaces

CDC has resources for businesses and workplaces, including guidance on how to prevent COVID-19 in the work-place. Duration and proximity of exposure can be greater than for other settings. Details regarding employment, hours, working conditions, and workplace contacts should be obtained during the initial interview with the patient, and the workplace should be toured after accounting for confidentiality and permission from workplace administrators or managers. If the employer has occupational health professionals/program, they should be included in the walkthrough and engaged throughout the investigative process.

Employee lists are helpful for identifying contacts, but certain employees might have left the workplace and thus been omitted from current employee lists. Also consider contractual personnel who may not be on workplace rosters but could also be exposed (e.g., housekeeping, cafeteria, business associates for meetings/conference, etc.). Investigators need to be aware of the sensitivities surrounding the immigration status of workers and how this can be a barrier to case investigation and contact tracing activities. Assurances should be made that all information collected will be used exclusively for public health purposes and not shared with immigration authorities.

Workplace administrators or managers are likely to express concern regarding liability, lost productivity, sick leave policies, responsibility for testing and screening, and media coverage. In addition, they might have limited obligations to protect patient confidentiality. All of these issues can be addressed during planning. For example, the assistance of the health department's media relations specialist can be offered to the workplace. For questions of liability and requirements under law, discussions between the health department's and the workplace's legal counsels are recommended.

Unions may also be engaged and have concerns about worker safety and other issues.

Multiple outbreaks of COVID-19 among meat and poultry processing facility workers have occurred in the United States recently. CDC provides guidance for meat and poultry processing workers and employers—including those involved in beef, pork, and poultry operations.

Hospitals and Other Healthcare Settings

Nearly every type of healthcare setting has been impacted by transmission of SARS-CoV-2, and guidance on preventing transmission has been provided by CDC. State governments have different degrees of regulatory authority over healthcare settings. Personnel collaborating with hospitals and other healthcare entities should have knowledge of applicable legal requirements.

Nursing homes and other long-term care facilities (LTCF) have been especially vulnerable to COVID-19 outbreaks. Recent experience with outbreaks in nursing homes has also reinforced that residents with COVID-19 may not be willing or able to report typical symptoms such as fever or respiratory symptoms; some may not report any symptoms. CDC has guidance on how LTCF and nursing homes can be prepared to prevent COVID-19. The Centers for Medicare and Medicaid Services (CMS) also provides guidance for nursing homes.

Infection control practitioners may or may not be familiar with COVID-19 case investigations and contact tracing. An investigation should be planned jointly as a collaboration between the facility and the health department, including the facility's occupational health services and infection protection and control staff. Initial discussions should cover data sharing and division of responsibilities.

Liability, regulations, confidentiality, media coverage, and occupational safety are complex for healthcare settings. Occupational Safety and Health Administration (OSHA) rules, which are interpreted differently by different jurisdictions, might require hospital administrators to report when employees have been diagnosed with COVID-19 from occupational exposure. Public health officials should consider inviting legal counsel to the initial planning sessions with healthcare administrators.

Schools and Child Care Settings

This category includes childcare centers, preschools, primary through secondary schools, vocational schools that replace or immediately follow secondary school, and colleges and universities. CDC issued guidance for administrators of public and private child care programs and K-12 schools, as well as guidance for administrators of public and private institutions of higher education (IHE) and guidance for child care programs that remain open.

During an outbreak in these settings, a coordinated investigation that includes communication and collaborative decision making with education agencies and parents can increase the efficiency and success of the process. Consent, assent, and disclosure of information are more complex for non-emancipated minors than for adults. Each interaction with a minor is also a potential interaction with the family. The health department typically has limited alternatives for evaluating a minor if permission is not granted. Anticipatory legal consultation is recommended.

The presence of COVID-19 in schools often generates publicity. Ideally, the health department should communicate with the school and parents/guardians before any media coverage occurs. Public health officials should anticipate media coverage and plan a collaborative strategy.

Public health officials should consider extramural activities add other exposure sites and contacts. Clubs, sports, and certain classes require the case investigator to obtain additional information when interviewing the patient, the patient's parents/guardians, and school personnel. For clients with COVID-19 who ride school buses, a bus company might keep a roster of riders with addresses.

The strategy for case investigation and contact tracing in child care centers, preschools, and primary schools depends on whether the person diagnosed with COVID-19 is a child or an adult (e.g., a teacher or caregiver). In a case investigation of a child aged <5 years who has COVID-19 and who attends preschool or child care, all adults in these settings should be included if the source of the child's infection has not been located in the family or household. Certain home-based child care centers include adults who do not provide child care but still share space or interact with the children.

School breaks, vacations, graduations, and transfers can disrupt the case investigation and contact tracing. In collaboration with school officials, the health department can notify students and other contacts who will be unavailable at the school. These contacts should be referred for testing.

Shelters and Other Settings Providing Services for People Experiencing Homelessness

CDC has guidance on how to investigate potential cases of COVID-19 among people living in a homeless shelter or living in an unsheltered situation. In addition, CDC has provided guidance for homeless service providers to plan and respond to COVID-19. Please access these guidance documents for detailed information.

SPECIAL CONSIDERATIONS

This section provides general guidance and highlights key issues that may need thoughtful attention.

Special Sites Not under Jurisdiction

Examples of sites that are not under the jurisdiction of the state, territorial, or local health department are those under the jurisdiction of the US government (e.g., military bases and federal correctional facilities), diplomatic missions, or reservations for American Indian/Alaska Native tribes. If these sites have their own healthcare systems, the health department can offer technical consultation and can share and request data from case investigations and contact tracing. At sites that do not have healthcare systems, agreements can be made between local infection control officials and the onsite authorities to delegate the public health response to the health department.

Clients Unable to Participate

There may be instances when COVID-19 clients have difficulty recalling close contacts (e.g., substance use or cognitive impairment) or they are unavailable for inquiry (e.g., died before an interview could be conducted, are intubated, unconscious, a minor, mentally incapacitated, or intellectually disabled). Social-network information, setting-based investigations, and proxy interview methods are recommended to supplement the contact list. In lieu of the ability to speak to the patient, details to inform case investigation and contact tracing may be gleaned from healthcare providers or legal proxies.

Culturally and Linguistically Diverse Minority Populations

Culturally and linguistically diverse minority populations are growing in the United States. These populations include racial and ethnic minorities, members of tribal nations, immigrants (i.e., those born outside the United States) and refugees. They may be at higher risk for COVID-19 or worse health outcomes due to a number of reasons including living conditions, work circumstances, underlying health conditions, and limited access to care.

It is important that case investigations and contact tracing are conducted in a culturally appropriate manner, which includes meaningfully engaging community representatives from affected communities, collaborating with community-serving organizations, respecting the cultural practices in the community, and taking into consideration the social, economic and immigration contexts in which these communities live and work.

To help build trust, jurisdictions should try to employ public health staff who are of the same racial and ethnic background as the affected community and are fluent in their preferred language. When that is not possible, it is important to provide interpreters for individuals who have limited English proficiency and consider translating the data collection instruments. Core demographic variables should be included in case investigation and contact tracing forms, including detailed race and ethnicity, as well as preferred language. Finally, given that minority populations experience discrimination and may be stigmatized or otherwise harmed for their participation, it is important to ensure the privacy and confidentiality of data collected and to ensure that the participant is aware of these safeguards.

Interjurisdictional Case Investigation and Contact Tracing

Clients diagnosed with COVID-19 may live in one jurisdiction and work in another, so collaboration between jurisdictions to synchronize community messaging can be helpful. Timely and confidential transfer of patient and close contact information to facilitate testing (if available), self-isolation/self-quarantine, and clearance to return to work are essential to keeping communities healthy.

Ideally, each jurisdiction will assign a person or team to send and receive reports from other jurisdictions of any clients diagnosed with COVID-19 and close contacts who reside in their jurisdiction. The jurisdiction where the patient resides is responsible for leading the investigation and notifying other health departments of any close contacts and/or congregate settings needing investigation in their area. Bi-directional confidential communication between health departments should include COVID-19 test results related to the investigation and confirmation of clients and contacts being released from self-isolation/self-quarantine.

There are nuances to each situation, and joint planning and problem-solving is recommended. A team of representatives from multiple health departments can increase the efficiency of larger investigations by planning the overall strategy together and monitoring the progress. Health department TB, HIV, and STD programs have established protocols to transfer confidential data between jurisdictions and can be a resource. Developing systems to share information about new or ongoing case investigations and contact tracing across jurisdictional boundaries is critical to ensure that appropriate COVID-19 clients and close contacts are being interviewed and monitored.

Clients with COVID-19 Traveling within the United States or Internationally

Our nation's population is mobile, with people traveling between states and internationally for work and leisure on a daily basis. Interjurisdictional communication is essential to the success of case investigations and contact tracing spanning multiple jurisdictions. Officials from the health department that initially encounter the patient with a positive SARS-CoV-2 laboratory result or probable diagnosis should interview the patient to gather as much identifying and locating information as possible for the patient, any close contacts visited, and events attended during the patient's travels, as well as information about the mode of travel. These data should be shared with the jurisdictions in which the close contacts are located. If the patient is initially interviewed in a jurisdiction other than his or her residence, information should be transferred between jurisdictions for continuity of case management. If a person becomes symptomatic after they have returned home from their trip, it will be important to assess whether the flight (or other mode of transportation) was within the contact elicitation window. If so, flight information should be obtained and appropriate authorities informed, and close contacts participating in the journey notified. The jurisdiction where the patient resides is assigned responsibility for managing the overall investigation.

Case investigations and contact tracing for flights arriving in the United States or between US states, or cruise ships arriving at a US port, are coordinated by CDC. To initiate case investigation and contact tracing of an aircraft or ship, the health department managing the overall investigation should notify the CDC quarantine station with jurisdiction for their area. CDC will obtain identifying and locating information for potentially exposed passengers and provide that information to health departments with jurisdiction for where the contacts reside. These health departments then follow-up with contacts within their jurisdiction and report outcomes to the relevant CDC quarantine station. For international flights departing the United States, CDC will notify public health authorities at destinations who will be responsible for conducting the aircraft case investigation and contact tracing.

BUILDING COMMUNITY SUPPORT

The success of a case investigation and contact tracing program hinges on a community's level of participation. For many community members, this may be the first time they've engaged with public health personnel. Jurisdictions will need to communicate clearly with the public to generate an understanding and acceptance of case investigation and contact tracing as an important way to protect friends, family, and community members from future potential infections.

A jurisdiction's case investigation and contact tracing plan should include a communication strategy that engages community leaders and key public officials. Local community leaders, public officials, and influencers can amplify clear, empowering messages that support case investigation and contact tracing activities and encourage community members to take responsibility for their health and the health of their community by following guidance from public health agencies. Jurisdictions should consider using all available communication channels to regularly reinforce these messages including television, radio, and social media, along with official websites.

In addition to case investigation and contact tracing awareness messages, jurisdictions should develop and share messages that dispel misinformation in their community and direct the public to reliable sources. There may be concerns about COVID-19 scams, so it will be particularly important that community members know where to go for verified information. Consideration should be made to cultural sensitivity and language diversity when developing messages and outreach materials.

Messages should also be tailored to reach specific audiences, including vulnerable populations within the community.

DATA MANAGEMENT

The development and implementation of a robust data management infrastructure will be critical for assigning and managing investigations, linking clients with confirmed and probable COVID-19 to their contacts, and evaluating success and opportunities for improvement in a case investigation and contact tracing program. COVID-19 case investigations will likely be triggered by one of three events:

1) A positive SARS-CoV-2 laboratory test or
2) A provider report of a confirmed or probable COVID-19 diagnosis or
3) Identification of a contact as having COVID-19 through contact tracing

Data management systems should be able to capture these three types of events electronically. Ideally laboratory, provider, and contact case reports should be transmitted to the local health authority electronically and then seamlessly imported into the system in an automated fashion.

Upon receipt of a triggering event, the case investigation and contact tracing system should assign an auto-generated, unique patient identifier to the patient report. The unique IDs should not include a component of personal identifying information (e.g., date of birth, patient initials). The system should allow for the assignment of new investigations to contact tracing staff with clear modules for the investigation. Module components that should be considered include:

- Patient locating and sociodemographic information (e.g., date of birth, race/ethnicity, residential address) and COVID-19-specific information (e.g., symptoms, date of symptom onset, date of SARS-CoV-2 testing, test results, hospitalizations, co-morbid conditions).

- Patient risk assessment (e.g., specific people the patient had close contact with during the contact elicitation window, community locations where the patient visited and may have exposed others (e.g., supermarket, workplace, public transportation). Greater specificity in the information collected can greatly improve the effectiveness of contact tracing, so the system should be flexible enough to allow for text field entry but structured enough that frequency distributions of locations and people can be quickly obtained.
- Named contacts should be captured on a separate module which includes all information provided by the patient, as well as additional risk assessment information for the contact (e.g., location and close contacts they may have had during their contact elicitation window). This module should allow for the entry of specific people (Jane Doe), people with partial contact information (Doug from the neighborhood BBQ) and locations (bus or train routes, neighborhood grocery store). This module should also create a unique identifier that can be assigned to each contact using the same conventions as above, and that will allow for a contact to be linked to the case and to also turn into a patient if they are in fact infected with SARS-CoV-2. Additional information to collect from the contacts include any symptoms of COVID-19, symptom onset dates, and dates and results of SARS-CoV-2 tests, as well as whether they were previously aware or informed of their exposure.

In addition, every case and contact form should have a public health ID variable for program evaluation purposes. Management of COVID-19 investigations will quickly become complicated as the number of case reports increases. The data system must be relational in nature and be able to link multiple individuals to many other individuals in the system. Assigning each individual in the system a unique ID will help support this.

However, separate tables will be needed to account for the complex interconnectedness of many of the investigations.

Ideally, the data system should facilitate many-to-many relationship mapping between identified cases and contacts in order to support data analysis and source-spread mapping of COVID-19 transmission. The data system should be user-friendly, flexible and accessible by mobile device, as well as a laptop or desktop computer. A cloud-based system will allow the greatest flexibility and ensure routine data storage, protection and updating, but unique jurisdictional laws and regulations may necessitate on-premises data storage.

Additionally, the system should be able to be manipulated by public health informatics, data management and epidemiologic staff, without the need for support from the vendor or contractors. This will allow for rapid updates of modules as new data collection needs are identified, the ability to produce both canned and ad-hoc reports for management of investigations, and the ability to seamlessly integrate with other modules to perform quality assurance and more complicated network and epidemiologic analyses. The data system should also be interoperable with existing surveillance systems.

Ensuring local health authority IT and informatics support is critical. Involving relevant IT, informatics, fiscal, and leadership entities early can help overcome delays and cost over-runs in implementation and maintenance of the system. Additionally, consideration should be made to who has ultimate responsibility for the maintenance and upkeep of the system early to ensure the correct partners are engaged in system developments. Data security and confidentiality standards should be considered and incorporated into all plans related to case investigation and contact tracing activities.

EVALUATING SUCCESS

Routine review of both process and outcome metrics will also be crucial for case investigation and contact tracing success. By examining these data regularly, issues can be identified and rapidly addressed, changes to internal case investigation and contact tracing processes can be made, and the local health authority can more easily pivot when new high-risk populations are identified. The uses of data related to case investigation and contact tracing fit broadly into four main domains:

1. Individual case investigation and contact tracing supervision and management
2. Programmatic process measures
3. Programmatic outcome measures
4. Ad-hoc epidemiologic and other public health analyses

Here we will focus on the first three mentioned above.

During case investigations and contact tracing, it takes time to identify and interview clients and then counsel and test all contacts. Examining "live" data for evaluation can lead to spurious or false inferences as there has not been enough time to finish and close out open or pending investigations.

Consider adding a lag period to all reports or data runs to ensure that partial or ongoing investigations are not being included in reports and metrics.

Also consider setting targets for select process and outcome metrics (especially for timeliness of patient and contact notification and self-isolation/self-quarantine) to guide adjustments to policies and protocols.

Individual Case Investigation and Contact Tracing Supervision and Management

To support supervision of case investigation and contact tracing staff, canned reports at the level of the individual case investigator and contact tracer will help ensure that staff are meeting expectations and identify areas for additional training. Reports can be produced for a 2-week review period and could include:

- Number of case investigations assigned during review period
- Number of clients interviewed during review period

- Number and percentage of clients interviewed ≤24 hours from report to health authority during review period
- Number of case investigations closed during review period
- Number and percent of case investigations in which at least one close contact was elicited during review period
- Median number of days from assignment of investigations to interview during review period
- Total number of contacts elicited from case investigations during review period
- Median number of contacts elicited from clients per case interview during review period, among cases where at least one contact was elicited
- Number of contacts notified during review period and percent out of total number of contacts named
- Total number of contacts interviewed/total number of contacts named by cases during review period
- Median number of days from initiation/assignment of contact to notification during review period
- Number of cases who completed isolation/total number of cases advised to isolate during review period
- Number of contacts who completed quarantine/total number of contacts advised to quarantine during review period
- Number of referrals to social support
- Number of referrals for clinical consultation

Programmatic Process Measures

Data examined among all case investigation and contact tracing staff will help provide leadership with insights into program successes and possible opportunities for additional training, resources or focus areas. These can be canned reports that are produced regularly (bi-weekly or monthly). These measures could include:

- Number of case investigations assigned during review period
- Number of clients interviewed during review period
- Number and percentage of clients interviewed ≤24 hours from report to health authority during review period
- Number of case investigations closed during review period
- Number and percentage of clients who named at least one close contact during review period
- Median days from receipt of report to interview during review period
- Total number of contacts elicited among case investigations during review period
- Total number of contacts interviewed/total number of contacts named by cases during review period
- Median number of contacts named per patient interview during review period
- Number of clients who completed isolation/total number of clients advised to isolate during review period
- Number of contacts who completed quarantine/total number of contacts advised to quarantine during review period
- Number of referrals to social support
- Number of referrals for clinical consultation

Programmatic Outcome Measures

- Number of clients interviewed/Number of case investigations
- Number of contacts tested for SARS-CoV-2/Number of contacts interviewed
- Number and percentage of new confirmed COVID-19 cases arising from quarantined contacts
- Number of contacts self-quarantined as a result of contact tracing
- Number and percentage of clients who completed full self-isolation period

- Number of contacts who completed 14-day self-quarantine/notified contacts

Confidentiality and Consent

All aspects of case investigation and contact tracing must be voluntary, confidential, and culturally appropriate. Minimum professional standards for any agency handling confidential information should include providing employees with appropriate information and/or training regarding confidential guidelines and legal regulations. All public health staff involved in case investigation and contact tracing activities with access to such information should sign a confidentiality statement acknowledging the legal requirements not to disclose COVID-19 information. Efforts to locate and communicate with clients and close contacts must be carried out in a manner that preserves the confidentiality and privacy of all involved. This includes never revealing the name of the patient to a close contact unless permission has been given (preferably in writing), and not giving confidential information to third parties (e.g., roommates, neighbors, family members).

Maintaining confidentiality during COVID-19 case investigations and contact tracing can be particularly difficult in congregate settings. Prior discussions with the patient can generate solutions for safeguarding confidentiality. Onsite administrators/employers who already know confidential information regarding a patient or contacts can be asked to respect confidentiality, even if they are not legally bound to do so.

Legal and ethical concerns for privacy and confidentiality extend beyond COVID-19. All personal information regarding any COVID-19 clients and contacts should be afforded the same protections. This includes any and all patient records. Data and security protocols should include recommendations for password-protected computer access, as well as locked, confidential storage cabinets and proper shredding and disposal of notes and other paper records. Protocols should include instructions for the protection of confidential data and confidential conversations in a working-from-home setting (e.g., make telephone or video-conferencing calls from private room to avoid the conversation being overheard). Approaches to ensuring confidentiality and data security should also be included in training of staff.

SUPPORT SERVICES TO CONSIDER

Significant social support may be necessary to allow clients to safely self-isolate and contacts to safely self-quarantine. For some of the most vulnerable populations in the United States, self-isolation or self-quarantine will be a hardship that may be impossible without additional assistance. Adherence to isolation and quarantine instructions will greatly depend on each individual's safety, comfort, and health during this period. Social support services must be an integral component of a jurisdiction's case investigation and contact tracing activities. In developing jurisdictional protocols, programs must define their social support services package and eligibility criteria.

Many clients with COVID-19 and close contacts will be able to self-isolate and self-quarantine at home with a basic kit of resources, such as cloth face coverings, gloves, thermometers, hand sanitizer, disinfectants, and health education materials. Others may need additional wrap-around services, such as food and pharmacy delivery, laundry services, and garbage removal. Also, financial considerations must be made for those whose employment will be affected by their need to self-isolate or self-quarantine. There may be additional needs that persons with disabilities may require to successfully self-isolate or self-quarantine.

Care resource coordinators will be essential in this process, acting as a bridge between the patient and key service providers. The case resource coordinator will assist the patient in identifying services available to meet their needs. It will be essential that these staff be able to communicate in a culturally and linguistically appropriate manner. In some instances, care resource managers may be reflective of the affected communities and viewed as a trusted resource. Jurisdictions are encouraged to engage community leadership and community-based organizations that have strong ties to specific groups in the community with unique needs such as members of tribal nations, refugees, migrants and recent immigrants. This is particularly important during case investigation and contact tracing associated with clusters or outbreaks. If jurisdictions are unable to employ a care coordinator, they should ensure that case investigation and contact tracing staff are appropriately trained to evaluate patient and contact needs, assess their eligibility, and link them to the appropriate resources.

Social support services include:

- Basic social support such as food, household supplies, laundry, pharmacy, and garbage removal services. Internet access should also be considered.
- Provision of a telemedicine safety net pool of providers for on-call clinical consultations with clients and contacts who do not have a primary healthcare provider. Transportation to medical care should also be considered.
- Health insurance navigation, Medicare/Medicaid assistance, mental health treatment services, substance abuse and misuse services.
- Childcare and/or dependent adult care services support should also be considered for those who are the primary caregivers for family and other household members.
- Economic support to recover income lost during the self-isolation/self-quarantine period, including working with employers to provide paid time off, unemployment assistance, and negotiations with landlords.

Success in this area will require assessment of individual needs and cultural factors within communities, in addition to multi-sector partnerships to bring resources together for comprehensive support for individuals, their families and their communities. Jurisdictions should take inventory of the existing resources available to assist clients and contacts who are self-isolating/self-quarantining, as well as their families, and find ways to fill any critical service gaps.

Once social support services are in place, jurisdictions will need to determine how to rapidly triage requests and assess eligibility. It will be essential to have mechanisms in place to ensure that people under self-isolation/self-quarantine orders receive expedited waivers for eligibility criteria or an alternative source of support for basic psychosocial needs. Absence of timely support may cause hardship and a break in self-isolation/self-quarantine.

Out-of-Home Isolation and Quarantine

Throughout the nation, there are many close-knit families with multiple generations living in the same household. Clients and contacts in these living situations may need to be supported with alternative living arrangements in order to protect their families and other household members. Others who may need alternate housing support include people being released from correctional institutions and those experiencing homelessness.

To address these situations, jurisdictions should identify facilities that can be used for alternative housing, as well as criteria to determine eligibility and access to out-of-home isolation and quarantine accommodations. Public health departments will need to engage other local government agencies and community organizations to partner for locally relevant housing solutions. Alternative housing may be necessary for people self-isolating/self-quarantining who are healthcare workers, living in group housing, living with individuals at high risk for severe disease, discharged from hospitals or correctional facilities, and experiencing homelessness and others in need. Behavioral health teams should be involved in the planning for these sites to facilitate continued access to support for people with substance use or mental health disorders.

Some states have established emergency orders to use hotels in order to support the isolation and quarantine of COVID-19 clients. Other states have engaged in cooperative agreements with facilities on an as-needed basis. Jurisdictions are using local hotels, dormitories, and disaster relief housing units for individuals who need to be relocated from their homes. Some jurisdictions are establishing large shelters in public buildings to house and monitor people experiencing homelessness. Others are setting up outreach systems for check-ins to monitor clients and contacts at tent encampments. It is important that facilities that are used for out-of-home isolation and quarantine be able to provide basic services and resources to those temporarily housed there.

Digital Contact Tracing Tools

There will be emerging information on smartphone-based exposure notifications from proximity tracking tools that could significantly increase the number of contacts that health departments are alerted to. As these tools are implemented, they should be used to initiate contact notification.

Case Management Tools

Case management tools for case investigation and contact tracing capture data on cases and contacts and can help improve the efficiency of manual contact tracing and medical monitoring methodologies. A case management tool should generally have the following capabilities:

1. Ability to ensure data security and confidentiality of patient information, which is critical to consider in the development of any case management tool.
2. Interoperability capabilities to receive input from the public health authorities (PHA) (including local, state, tribal, and territorial public health departments), information systems and/or laboratory systems, either via import or real-time synchronization.
3. Ability to facilitate identification/elicitation and documentation of known contacts of clients with COVID-19, both through manual entry by the PHA and via self-report from cases.

4. Ability to send notifications to users (clients and contacts) via manual and/or automated means. These messages will include:
   a. Notification to contacts of their exposure and time window when exposure may have occurred.
   b. Initial survey about their symptoms and clear instructions on how to regularly monitor their symptoms and health status and report that information every day. (This will ensure their data reaches the contact management team at the PHA and that aggregate data reach relevant state and federal partners.)
   c. Public safety messages to identified contacts to educate them about COVID-19, its common signs and symptoms, and reinforcing prevention messages defined by the government, such as self-quarantine and social distancing. (This messaging should be repeated daily throughout the contact's self-quarantine period with new information supportive of the evolving stage of isolation.)
5. Ability to send notifications in multiple formats, such as voice messages, emails, and SMS.
6. Capability for contact-generated and system-generated alerts or workflows (e.g., contact failed to follow-up, presence of symptoms, contact request for information).
7. Ability to produce individual-level and aggregate data supporting worker and PHA-level process metrics as described above.

Preliminary evaluations were conducted on ready-to-implement tools (e.g., proximity contact tracing, medical monitoring aids, data management systems) based on a standard set of criteria (Preliminary Criteria for the Evaluation of Digital Contact Tracing Tools for COVID-19). CDC continues to evaluate tools and assess their suitability for use to facilitate specific activities in the case investigation, contact tracing, and monitoring workflows.

Medical Monitoring Tools

A variety of medical monitoring tools are currently in use by health departments to communicate with clients and contacts for TB, and other infectious diseases. These tools can help improve the efficiency in medical monitoring in both active engagement (e.g., Skype, Facetime, Zoom) of high-risk individuals, and self-report of daily temperature check, signs and symptoms (e.g., recorded video) for others diagnosed or exposed to COVID-19. In addition, some case management systems have built in technology to push system-generated alerts (e.g., request to check-in the day prior to end of patient self-isolation or contact self-quarantine). Ensuring data security and confidentiality of patient information is critical to consider in the development of any case management tool.

Proximity Tracking Tools

There are numerous initiatives that propose to use smartphones as "sensors" to detect proximity and exposure to individuals who may have COVID-19. Proximity-tracking tools propose to relieve several challenges associated with traditional case investigation and contact tracing and have been implemented in several countries. Several ongoing efforts in the United States and internationally seek to develop privacy-preserving, accurate, and energy-efficient applications for use on mobile devices. There are currently very limited data on the performance of these applications in US communities; particularly the sensitivity and specificity of these methods as it pertains to identifying true close contacts. Many tools are not yet widely available, and there remain critical gaps that could pose challenges to their implementation.

There are two major technologies that are under discussion in the United States—Bluetooth and GPS. At present, many consider Bluetooth to be more promising than GPS. There are currently little published empirical data showing the capabilities of either technology. Some preliminary advantages, disadvantages, and implementation challenges are listed below. It is assumed that people would voluntarily agree to participate and would have an opt-in option.

Potential Advantages of Bluetooth and GPS-Enabled Tools for Case Investigation and Contact Tracing

1. Preserves the patient's or contact's ownership of their health information and preserves their agency to optin to sharing relevant information with public health authorities.
2. Augments capacity of case investigator and contact tracer workforce (e.g., may decrease burden of manual contact elicitation, help to identify contacts in a timelier manner, facilitate communication with contacts, and help ensure rapid isolation of contacts to interrupt the chain of transmission).
3. Augments contact identification by identifying potentially unknown contacts.
4. Provides more comprehensive mobility history, which serves as a mnemonic to elicit potential aggregate setting and community exposures (GPS).
5. Provides granularity of proximity and associated temporal data that may be useful in stratifying contacts into different exposure risk categories that PHAs can match with differing levels of tracing, notification and monitoring.

Potential Disadvantages

1. Has inherent socioeconomic and technology literacy biases—requires that clients and contacts have access to a smartphone, knowledge of how to install apps, and literacy to navigate app menus.
2. May not be effective until a "critical mass" of users in a community are using the apps.

3. Requires individuals to keep their smartphones on them at all times with the appropriate functions enabled and depends on users to elect to share their information with PHAs.
4. Disparate data formats from multiple apps may not be interoperable and could add burden on PHAs for integrating data seamlessly into their case management and contact tracing systems and workflows.
5. May require more consultation on the ethical and legal issues related to electronic tracking.
6. Hacking and other unauthorized access or use of data may compromise data security and confidentiality.

Implementation Challenges

1. Social mobilization and mass marketing media campaigns are required to gain a critical mass behind one or more application for broad public usage.
2. Building and sustaining public trust in PHA's ability and intention to preserve the privacy of individuals is crucial to widespread adoption of new technologies.
3. Systems are needed to integrate disparate data streams into PHA information systems without compromising the integrity of existing workflows and to safeguard against false-positive alerts.

For more information on digital contact tracing, visit the following resources:

- Digital Contact Tracing Tools for COVID-19
- Preliminary Criteria for the Evaluation of Digital Contact Tracing Tools for COVID-19

RESOURCES

These additional resources may be of use as jurisdictions plan and operationalize their contact tracing efforts. Resources from CDC and Other Federal Agencies

- CDC Support for States, Tribes, Localities and Territories
- Principles of Contact Tracing to Stop COVID-19
- Sample Contact Tracing Training Plan
- Implementation of Mitigation Strategies for Communities with Local COVID-19 Transmission
- Guidelines for Opening Up America Again
- Opening Up America Again Testing Overview and Blueprint

Resources from other agencies and organizations. These resources are cited for informational purposes only, and their inclusion in this document does not indicate *an actual or implied endorsement by CDC.*

- A National Plan to Enable Comprehensive COVID-19 Case Finding and Contact Tracing—Johns Hopkins Center for Health Security and ASTHO
- ASTHO COVID-19 Resources—Association of State and Territorial Health Officers
- Box It In Strategy—Resolve to Save Lives
- Considerations for Loosening and Tightening Mitigation Measures—Resolve to Save Lives
- Contact Tracing Overview—Resolve to Save Lives
- Contact Tracing Staffing Calculator—Resolve to Save Lives
- COVID-19 Command Center—National Coalition of STD Directors
- NACCHO COVID Response Effort—National Association of County and City Health Officers
- National Coronavirus Response: A Road Map to Reopening—American Enterprise Institute

APPENDIX A — GLOSSARY OF KEY TERMS

Term	Definition
Case Investigation & Contact Tracing	Fundamental activities that involve working with a patient who has been diagnosed with an infectious disease to identify and provide support to people (contacts) who may have been infected through exposure to the patient. This process prevents further transmission of disease by separating people who have (or may have) an infectious disease from people who do not.
Close Contact	*Someone who was within 6 feet of an infected person for at least 15 minutes starting from 48 hours before illness onset until the time the patient is isolated.* Data are limited to precisely define the "prolonged exposure" to determine "close contact," however 15 minutes of close exposure can be used as an operational definition for contact investigation. Factors to consider when defining close contact include proximity, the duration of exposure (e.g., longer exposure time likely increases exposure risk), whether the individual has symptoms (e.g., coughing likely increases exposure risk) and whether either the case patient or contact were wearing an N95 respirator (which can efficiently block respiratory secretions from contaminating others and the environment).
	At this time, differential determination of close contact for those using fabric face coverings is not recommended at this time. In healthcare settings, it is reasonable to define a prolonged exposure as any exposure greater than 10 minutes because the contact is someone who is ill. Brief interactions are less likely to result in transmission; however, symptoms and the type of interaction (e.g., did the person cough directly into the face of the individual) remain important. https:// www.cdc.gov/coronavirus/2019-ncov/php/public-health-recommendations.html
Confirmed COVID-19 Case	Report of person with COVID-19 and meeting confirmatory laboratory evidence https://wwwn.cdc.gov/nndss/conditions/coronavirus-disease-2019-covid-19/case-definition/2020/
Contact Elicitation Window	The timeframe when the case was likely infectious and not under isolation. This is the time period for which possible contacts should be elicited.
Critical Infrastructure Worker	Workers in 16 different sectors including Chemical, Commercial Facilities, Communications, Critical Manufacturing, Dams, Defense Industrial Base, Emergency Services, Energy, Financial Services, Food and Agriculture, Government Facilities, Healthcare and Public Health, Information Technology, Nuclear Reactors, Materials, and Waste, Transportation Systems, and Water and Wastewater Systems. These workers include: (a) federal, state and local law enforcement; (b) 911 call center employees; (c) fusion center employees; (d)

Term	Definition
	public and private hazardous material responders; (e) janitorial and custodial staff; (f) workers and contractors in the food and agriculture, critical manufacturing, informational technology, transportation, energy, and government facilities industries. https://www.cdc. gov/coronavirus/2019-ncov/downloads/critical-workers-implementing-safety-practices.pdf
Exposure	Having come into contact with a cause of, or possessing a characteristic that is a determinant of, a particular health problem https://www.cdc.gov/csels/dsepd/ss1978/ glossary.html
First-responder	Law enforcement, fire services, emergency medical services, and emergency management officials. https://www.cdc.gov/coronavirus/2019-ncov/hcp/guidance-for-ems.html
Healthcare personnel	All paid and unpaid people serving in healthcare settings who have the potential for direct or indirect exposure to clients or infectious materials, including body substances; contaminated medical supplies, devices, and equipment; contaminated environmental surfaces; or contaminated air. https://www.cdc.gov/coronavirus/2019-ncov/hcp/guidance-risk-assesment-hcp.html
Incubation period	Period of time between exposure to an infection and onset of symptoms
Isolation	The separation of a person or group of people known or reasonably believed to be infected with a communicable disease and potentially infectious from those who are not infected to prevent spread of the communicable disease. Isolation for public health purposes may be voluntary or compelled by federal, state, or local public health order. https://www.cdc. gov/quarantine/quarantineisolation.html
Multi-generational Household	Households that consist of more than two generations living under the same roof. Many researchers also include households with a grandparent and at least one other generation. https://www.census.gov/library/publications/2012/acs/acsbr11-03.html
Probable COVID-19 Case	Report of person meeting clinical AND epidemiologic evidence of COVID-19 but without confirmatory laboratory evidence https://cdn.ymaws.com/www.cste.org/resource/ resmgr/2020ps/interim-20-id-01_covid-19.pdf
Quarantine	The separation of a person or group of people reasonably believed to have been exposed to a communicable disease but not yet symptomatic from others who have not been so exposed to prevent the possible spread of the communicable disease. Quarantine may be voluntary or compelled by federal, state, or local public health order. https://www.cdc.gov/ quarantine/quarantineisolation.html

Appendix B—Tips for Locating COVID-19 Cases and Contacts

When the locating information provided for a patient or close contact is insufficient, case investigation and contact tracing may come to an abrupt halt. The following list includes additional resources that may be used to obtain missing locating information and keep the investigation moving forward.

- State DMV records
- Online people search engines (may incur additional costs)
- Health department records
- Social media/mobile apps
- Following up with the index case to ask for additional locating information on a contact
- Jail and other correctional facility records
- Property tax records
- Frequent shopper cards
- Women Infants and Children Program, Food Stamps and other social services records
- Online white pages
- Google maps
- Employment records

APPENDIX C—DATA ELEMENTS FOR CASE INVESTIGATION AND CONTACT TRACING FORMS

Case Investigation

Data Element	Type	Codes	Notes
Contact Information			
Investigator	Open Text		Name of investigator
Investigator ID	Numeric		
Date Assigned for Investigation	Date		
Index patient ID	Numeric		Autogenerated
Lot Number (to link related cases and contacts)	Numeric		To track clusters
Patient Last Name	Open Text		
Patient First Name	Open Text		
Patient Preferred Name	Open Text		
DOB	Date		
Gender	Categorical	M/F/Other/Unk	
Primary Language	Open Text/Categorical		
Interpreter used	Categorical	Y/N/U/R	
Residential Street Address	Open Text		
City of Residence	Open Text		
County of Residence	Open Text		
State of Residence	Open Text		
Zip code	Numeric		
Tribal Affiliation	Open Text		
Born in the United States	Categorical	Y/N/U/R	
Phone Number 1	Numeric		
Phone Number 2	Numeric		
Email 1	Open Text		
Email 2	Open Text		
Ok to Text	Categorical	Yes, No, Partial, Refused	
Ok to Email	Categorical	Yes, No, Partial, Refused	
Race	Categorical	Check all apply	Use Census or HHS categories
Ethnicity	Categorical	Check box	Use Census or HHS categories
Date of interview Attempt 1	Date		
Interview 1 occurred	Categorical	Yes, No, Partial, Refused	

(Continued)

Data Element	Type	Codes	Notes
Date of interview Attempt 2	Date		
Interview 2 occurred	Categorical	Yes, No, Partial, Refused	
Date of interview Attempt 3	Date		
Interview 3 occurred	Categorical	Yes, No, Partial, Refused	
Symptoms and Clinical Course			
Fever	Categorical	Check Box (Y/N/U/R)	
Cough	Categorical	Check Box (Y/N/U/R)	
Shortness of Breath	Categorical	Check Box (Y/N/U/R)	
Diarrhea/GI	Categorical	Check Box (Y/N/U/R)	
Headache	Categorical	Check Box (Y/N/U/R)	
Muscle ache	Categorical	Check Box (Y/N/U/R)	
Chills	Categorical	Check Box (Y/N/U/R)	
Sore throat	Categorical	Check Box (Y/N/U/R)	
Vomiting	Categorical	Check Box (Y/N/U/R)	
Abdominal Pain	Categorical	Check Box (Y/N/U/R)	
Nasal congestion	Categorical	Check Box (Y/N/U/R)	
Loss of sense of smell	Categorical	Check Box (Y/N/U/R)	
Loss of sense of taste	Categorical	Check Box (Y/N/U/R)	
Malaise	Categorical	Check Box (Y/N/U/R)	
Fatigue	Categorical	Check Box (Y/N/U/R)	
Other symptom	Categorical		
Other symptom description	Open Text		
Date of symptom onset	Date		
SARS-CoV-2 testing	Categorical	Check Box (Y/N/U/R)	
Date of first SARS-CoV-2 test	Date		
Results of first SARS-CoV-2 test	Categorical	Pos/Neg/Equi/Unk	
Date of last SARS-CoV-2 test	Date		
Results of last SARS-CoV-2 test	Categorical	Pos/Neg/Equi/Unk	
Hospitalized	Categorical	Yes, No, Partial, Refused	
Pneumonia	Categorical	Yes, No, Partial, Refused	
ECMO			
ICU	Categorical	Yes, No, Partial, Refused	
Death	Categorical	Yes, No, Partial, Refused	
Stroke	Categorical	Yes, No, Partial, Refused	
MI	Categorical	Yes, No, Partial, Refused	
Pre-existing conditions			
Chronic lung disease	Categorical	Yes, No, Partial, Refused	
Diabetes	Categorical	Yes, No, Partial, Refused	
Severe Obesity (BMI>=40)	Categorical	Yes, No, Partial, Refused	
CVD	Categorical	Yes, No, Partial, Refused	
Chronic renal disease	Categorical	Yes, No, Partial, Refused	

Data Element	Type	Codes	Notes
Chronic liver disease	Categorical	Yes, No, Partial, Refused	
Immunocompromised	Categorical	Yes, No, Partial, Refused	
Pregnant (if Female)	Categorical	Yes, No, Partial, Refused	
Risk Factors			
Contact with confirmed COVID case	Categorical	Y/N/U/R	
Employed	Categorical	Yes/No-unemployed/ No-retired/No-unable to work/No-student	
If employed, what occupation	Open text		
If employed, what kind of workplace	Open text		
HCP	Categorical	Y/N/U/R	Work or volunteer in a healthcare setting
If HCP, what kind of setting			
Hospital	Categorical	Check box	
Ambulatory care	Categorical	Check box	
EMS/Fire/Law Enforcement/1st responder	Categorical	Check box	
Urgent care	Categorical	Check box	
Long term care	Categorical	Check box	
Hospice	Categorical	Check box	
Name of HCP setting	Open Text		
Address of HCP setting	Open Text		
Congregate setting	Categorical	Y/N/U/R	Do you live or work in congregate setting
If Congregate, what kind			
Corrections	Categorical	Check box	
Dorm	Categorical	Check box	
Group home	Categorical	Check box	
Multi-family household	Categorical	Check box	
Multi-generational household	Categorical	Check box	
Name of congregate setting	Open Text		
Address of congregate setting	Open Text		
Contact Tracing (during contact elicitation window)			
Any household contact	Categorical	Y/N/U/R	
Total Number of household contacts	Numeric		

(Continued)

Data Element	Type	Codes	Notes
Can you self-isolate	Categorical	Y/N/U/R	Add in script what this means (use of bedroom and bathroom away from others)
Do you need assistance to self-isolate	Categorical	Y/N/U/R	
Any intimate partners	Categorical	Y/N/U/R	Partners you do not reside with
Total Number of Intimate Partners	Numeric		
Any other people in close-contact with, including coworkers	Categorical	Y/N/U/R	

Contact Elicitation Investigation

Data Element	Type	Codes	Notes
Contact Information			Collected on the index
Investigator	Open Text		Name of investigator
Investigator ID	Numeric		
Date Assigned for Investigation	Date		
Index patient ID	Numeric		Autogenerated
Lot Number	Numeric		To track clusters
Date of contact elicitation	Date		
Start date of Contact Elicitation Window	Date		
End date of Contact Elicitation Window	Date		
Information about contacts			Ask for each identified contact
Contact Last Name	Open Text		
Contact First Name	Open Text		
Contact AKA	Open Text		

Data Element	Type	Codes	Notes
Contact Phone 1	Open Text		
Contact Phone 2	Open Text		
Contact email 1	Open Text		
Contact email 2	Open Text		
Contact social media handle 1	Open Text		Twitter, Grindr, etc.
Contact social media handle 2	Open Text		
Contact Address	Open Text		
Contact setting	Check all that apply		
Home	Check box		
School	Check box		
Day Care	Check box		
Workplace	Check box		includes customers/clients/clients and coworkers
Place of Worship	Check box		
Shelter	Check box		
Hospital/Medical Care	Check box		
Travel or Transit	Check box		
Retail setting	Check box		includes, supermarkets, gas stations, farmers markets, etc.
Duration of Exposure (minutes)	Numeric		
Pre-existing conditions			If known
Chronic lung disease	Categorical	Y/N/U/R	
Diabetes	Categorical	Y/N/U/R	
Severe Obesity (BMI>=40)	Categorical	Y/N/U/R	
CVD	Categorical	Y/N/U/R	
Chronic renal disease	Categorical	Y/N/U/R	
Chronic liver disease	Categorical	Y/N/U/R	
Immunocompromised	Categorical	Y/N/U/R	
Pregnant (if Female)	Categorical	Y/N/U/R	
Risk Factors			If known
HCP	Categorical	Y/N/U/R	Work or volunteer in a healthcare setting
If HCP, what kind of setting			
Hospital	Categorical	Check box	
Ambulatory care	Categorical	Check box	
EMT/Fire/1st responder	Categorical	Check box	
Urgent care	Categorical	Check box	
Long term care	Categorical	Check box	

(Continued)

Data Element	Type	Codes	Notes
Hospice	Categorical	Check box	
Congregate setting	Categorical	Y/N/U/R	Do you live or work in congregate setting
If Congregate, what kind			
Corrections	Categorical	Check box	
Dorm	Categorical	Check box	
Group home	Categorical	Check box	
Multi-family household	Categorical	Check box	
Multi-generational household	Categorical	Check box	
Community Settings			
Travel risk	Categorical	Y/N/U/R	Train, plane, public transit
Specify travel	Open Text		List specific flights, routes, etc.
Workplace	Categorical	Y/N/U/R	
Specify workplace	Open Text		Specific work locations
Retail	Categorical	Y/N/U/R	
Specify retail	Open Text		
Large community social event	Categorical	Y/N/U/R	
Specify	Open Text		
Recreational activity	Categorical	Y/N/U/R	
Specify	Open Text		
Places of Worship	Categorical	Y/N/U/R	
Specify	Open Text		

Contact Investigation

Data Element	Type	Codes	Notes
Contact Information			
Investigator	Open Text		Name of investigator
Investigator ID	Numeric		
Date Assigned for Investigation	Date		
Index patient ID	Numeric		Autogenerated
Lot Number	Numeric		To track clusters
Contact patient ID	Numeric		
Contact Last Name	Open Text		
Contact First Name	Open Text		

Data Element	Type	Codes	Notes
Contact Preferred Name	Open Text		
DOB	Date		
Gender	Categorical	M/F/Other/Unk	
Primary Language	Open Text/ Categorical		
Interpreter used	Categorical	Y/N/U/R	
Residential Street Address	Open		
City of Residence	Open Text		
County of Residence	Open Text		
State of Residence	Open Text		
Zip code	Numeric		
Tribal Affiliation	Open Text		
Born in the United States	Categorical	Y/N/U/R	
Phone Number 1	Numeric		
Phone Number 2	Numeric		
Email 1	Open Text		
Email 2	Open Text		
Ok to Text	Categorical	Yes, No, Partial, Refused	
Ok to Email	Categorical	Yes, No, Partial, Refused	
Race	Categorical	Check all apply	Use Census or HHS categories
Ethnicity	Categorical	Check box	Use Census or HHS categories
Date of interview Attempt 1	Date		
Interview 1 occurred	Categorical	Yes, No, Partial, Refused	
Date of interview Attempt 2	Date		
Interview 2 occurred	Categorical	Yes, No, Partial, Refused	
Date of interview Attempt 3	Date		
Interview 3 occurred	Categorical	Yes, No, Partial, Refused	
Any household contact	Categorical	Y/N/U/R	
Total Number of household contacts	Numeric		

(Continued)

Data Element	Type	Codes	Notes
Can you self-isolate	Categorical	Y/N/U/R	Add in script what this means (use of bedroom and bathroom away from others)
Do you need assistance to self-isolate	Categorical	Y/N/U/R	
Symptoms and Clinical Course			
Fever	Categorical	Check Box (Y/N/U/R)	
Cough	Categorical	Check Box (Y/N/U/R)	
Shortness of Breath	Categorical	Check Box (Y/N/U/R)	
Diarrhea/GI	Categorical	Check Box (Y/N/U/R)	
Headache	Categorical	Check Box (Y/N/U/R)	
Muscle ache	Categorical	Check Box (Y/N/U/R)	
Chills	Categorical	Check Box (Y/N/U/R)	
Sore throat	Categorical	Check Box (Y/N/U/R)	
Vomiting	Categorical	Check Box (Y/N/U/R)	
Abdominal Pain	Categorical	Check Box (Y/N/U/R)	
Nasal congestion	Categorical	Check Box (Y/N/U/R)	
Loss of sense of smell	Categorical	Check Box (Y/N/U/R)	
Loss of sense of taste	Categorical	Check Box (Y/N/U/R)	
Other symptom	Categorical		
Other symptom description			
Date of symptom onset	Date		
SARS-CoV-2 testing	Categorical	Check Box (Y/N/U/R)	
Date of first SARS-CoV-2 test	Date		
Results of first SARS-CoV-2 test	Categorical	Pos/Neg/Equi/Unk	

Data Element	Type	Codes	Notes
Date of last SARS-CoV-2 test	Date		
Results of last SARS-CoV-2 test	Categorical	Pos/Neg/Equi/Unk	
Pre-existing conditions			
Chronic lung disease	Categorical	Yes, No, Partial, Refused	
Diabetes	Categorical	Yes, No, Partial, Refused	
Severe Obesity (BMI>=40)	Categorical	Yes, No, Partial, Refused	
CVD	Categorical	Yes, No, Partial, Refused	
Chronic renal disease	Categorical	Yes, No, Partial, Refused	
Chronic liver disease	Categorical	Yes, No, Partial, Refused	
Immunocompromised	Categorical	Yes, No, Partial, Refused	
Pregnant (if Female)	Categorical	Yes, No, Partial, Refused	
Risk Factors			
Contact with confirmed COVID case	Categorical	Y/N/U/R	
Employed	Categorical	Yes/No-unemployed/No-retired/No-unable to work/No-student	
If employed, what occupation	Open text		
If employed, what kind of workplace	Open text		
HCP	Categorical	Y/N/U/R	Work or volunteer in a healthcare setting
If HCP, what kind of setting			
Hospital	Categorical	Check box	
Ambulatory care	Categorical	Check box	
EMS/Fire/Law Enforcement/1st responder	Categorical	Check box	
Urgent care	Categorical	Check box	
Long term care	Categorical	Check box	

(Continued)

Data Element	Type	Codes	Notes
Hospice	Categorical	Check box	
Name of HCP setting	Open Text		
Address of HCP setting	Open Text		
Congregate setting	Categorical	Y/N/U/R	Do you live or work in congregate setting
If Congregate, what kind			
Corrections	Categorical	Check box	
Dorm	Categorical	Check box	
Group home	Categorical	Check box	
Multi-family household	Categorical	Check box	
Multi-generational household	Categorical	Check box	
Name of congregate setting	Open Text		
Address of congregate setting	Open Text		

Appendix D—Tool for Estimating the Number of Contact Tracers Needed

Once states have lower COVID-19 case rates for at least 14 days, widely available testing, and adequate medical/ hospital resources, contact tracing becomes an important strategy to eliminate transmission of SARS-CoV-2, the virus that causes COVID-19. Contact tracing involves multiple steps, including case investigation of COVID-19 clients, notification of close contacts, and daily monitoring of close contacts. This process can be labor-intensive, and communities have different circumstances that affect contact tracing activities. These factors include the number of persons diagnosed with COVID-19 each day, number of contacts per patient, and the amount of time and resources needed to reach and follow the clients and contacts.

The number of contact tracers needed is large and will vary by community. Each community will need to examine local case load and other factors to estimate how many contact tracers will be needed.

Mathematical modeling tools can be used to help estimate the number of contact tracers needed. These models require data to quantify each part of the process. The data used may differ among communities and over the course of the pandemic, which may lead to large differences in estimates from different models—or from the same model if using different values. Each community will need to determine some key parameters to be in the model. Local tuberculosis/sexually transmitted disease contact tracers are likely familiar with community-specific "inputs" regarding the average number of contacts per case and how difficult contacts are to find.

CDC does not endorse the use of a specific model; however, these tools may be used to guide planning and calculate resources needed under different scenarios. Each community should carefully incorporate as much knowledge about its situation as possible to estimate the number of contact tracers needed.

Content describing non-CDC tools in this document is provided for informational purposes only and is not intended to indicate endorsement, actual or implied, of the tools. Additionally, information on this site is provided "as is," for users to evaluate and make their own determination as to their effectiveness.

Example Using an Available Tool: Contact Tracing Staffing Tool—Resolve to Save Lives

This model is built into an Excel workbook and requires input on the following values:

- # new COVID-19 clients/day
- # close contacts/COVID-19 patient

- Proportion of clients who are easy/hard/hardest to reach (and never reached). The amount of time needed to arrange and conduct the initial interview with the index patient can vary.
    - Average time needed for patient investigation for each patient category
- Proportion of contacts who are household/easy/hard/hardest to reach (and never reached). Some contacts might live with the patient; other contacts might lack contact information and require fieldwork to identify.
    - Average time spent on contact notification for each contact category
- Proportion of contacts who can be followed in a mostly automated way versus those who need more staff time. For instance, contacts self-reporting their symptoms via email or text messages require much less time than contacts requiring daily telephone calls.
    - Average amount of time spent on contacts for each day in each category
- Days spent following contacts (e.g., 14 days after exposure)
- Staffing considerations:
    - Hours of daily productive work per contact tracer
    - Number of workdays per week per contact tracer
    - Number of contact tracers per manager

Changing the parameters in the model will change the estimated total staffing needed, even when keeping the number of daily new COVID-19 clients constant. (Note that this model does not specify overall population size. The total amount of work is proportional to the number of COVID-19 clients and contacts identified in each community rather than the total number of people living in the community.)

Estimates of Contact Tracers Needed Based on Different Assumptions in the Model

Model developed by Resolve to Save Lives	Assumed daily COVID-19 Incidence/100,000 persons	Contact tracing staff needed/100,000 persons	Notes or assumptions
Contact Tracing Staffing Calculator—Lower estimate (See below)	9*	33	5 contacts per patient; contact tracers work 8 hours/day; contacts easy-to-reach; many contacts use app/email to report daily.
Contact Tracing Staffing Calculator—Higher estimate (See below)	136**	3,739	20 contacts per patient; contact tracers work 7-hour days; contacts harder to reach, take longer to interview, most require calls each day.

*Between April 15-23, 2020, the daily incidence of COVID-19 in the United States ranged between approximately 8 and 9 per 100,000 (between 25,858 and 29,916 new COVID-19 clients per day; assume US population of 328M).

**Approximate peak daily incidence of COVID-19 in New York City (approx. 11,400 incident new clients on 4/15/2020, assume NYC population of 8.4M).

Additional Considerations for Estimating Contact Tracing Resources

There are numerous factors that could affect contact tracer staffing needs that should be accounted for when estimating contact tracer needs:

- These estimates do not necessarily include all managers or additional professions needed.
- Increased case finding and testing efforts, as well as relaxing mobility restrictions could lead to more daily COVID-19 clients and/or contacts, which would require tracing resources.
- Effective contact tracing could reduce the number of new COVID-19 clients and contacts over time.
- Time from diagnosis to isolation for the index patient with COVID-19 will affect the number of contacts exposed and needing follow-up.

- Use of digital contact tracing tools could improve workflow efficiency or allow automated messages/contact self-report of symptoms to save contact tracer effort.
- These models do not necessarily apply to special populations such as people in prisons or long-term care facilities.

This information will be updated as more tools become available.

Parameter Values Used for High and Low Estimates (These Are for Illustrative Purposes Only)

Low Estimate Values—daily incident cases based on approximate average national daily incidence

	Number
	5
acts per case	5

nvestigation (locating and interviewing index case, determining infectious period, eliciting contacts, providing instructions for isolation, referring to social/medical services)

	Proportion of all index cases	Number	Hours on case investigation	Total hours
hone number etc available)	0.7	6.3	4	25.2
o info initially available)	0.1	0.9	6	5.4
requiring field outreach	0.1	0.9	6	5.4
t to follow up	0.1	0.9	4	3.6
check: add to 1?	1.00		Sum	39.6

tification (notifying contacts about exposure, providing instructions re: quarantine, referral for testing, referral for social/medical services)

40.5	Proportion of all contacts	Number	Hours on contact notification	Total hours
	0.7	28.35	0.5	14.175
to reach (phone num available)	0.1	4.05	0.5	2.025
to reach (no info initially available)	0.05	2.025	1	2.025
:h - requiring field outreach	0.05	2.025	4	8.1
lost to follow up	0.1	4.05	4	16.2
check: add to 1?	1.00		Sum	42.525

f cases and contacts (daily check-in, responding to questions, referral to services)

ontacts in follow-up	44.55				
	Proportion of all follow-ups	Number	Daily hours on follow up	Total Daily Hours	Days of follow up
automated follow up and minimal Q&A throughout	0.70	31	0.1	3	14
tomated follow up or lots of Q&A throughout	0.30	13	0.25	3	

umptions

ours per workday (eg 8, or fewer to account for average non-tracing activities, time off, etc)
r week (eg 5)
taff per Supervisor/Manager

ults

	Staff needed	Hours (from above)	Proportion of all hours
	7	40	0.23
	7	43	0.25
up	16	90	0.52
Sum staff	30		
sors/Managers	3		
Total staff	33		

High Estimate Values—daily incident cases based on peak daily incidence from NYC (approx. 11,400 cases among 8.4M persons)

	Number
	136
: per case	20

stigation (locating and interviewing index case, determining infectious period, eliciting contacts, providing instructions for isolation, referring to social/medical services)

	Proportion of all index cases	Number	Hours on case investigation	Total hours
e number etc available)	0.5	68	4	272
fo initially available)	0.2	27.2	6	163.2
uiring field outreach	0.2	27.2	8	217.6
follow up	0.1	13.6	8	108.8
check: add to 1?	1.00		Sum	761.6

ation (notifying contacts about exposure, providing instructions re: quarantine, referral for testing, referral for social/medical services)

	Proportion of all contacts	Number	Hours on contact notification	Total hours
2448				
	0.4	979.2	1	979.2
each (phone num available)	0.1	244.8	1	244.8
each (no info initially available)	0.2	489.6	2	979.2
equiring field outreach	0.2	489.6	8	3916.8
to follow up	0.1	244.8	4	979.2
check: add to 1?	1.00		Sum	7099.2

ses and contacts (daily check-in, responding to questions, referral to services)

acts in follow-up 2325.6

	Proportion of all follow-ups	Number	Daily hours on follow up	Total Daily Hours	Days of follov
mated follow up and minimal Q&A throughout	0.30	698	0.1	70	14
ated follow up or lots of Q&A throughout	0.70	1628	0.33	537	

tions

s per workday (eg 8, or fewer to account for average non-tracing activities, time off, etc)
eek (eg 5)
per Supervisor/Manager

	Staff needed	Hours (from above)	Proportion of all hours
	152	762	0.05
	1420	7099	0.43
	1700	8498	0.52
Sum staff	3272		
/Managers	467		
tal staff	3739		

In: Testing and Contract Tracing …
Editor: Ernesto M. Batista
ISBN: 978-1-53618-857-8
© 2020 Nova Science Publishers, Inc.

Chapter 6

CASE INVESTIGATION AND CONTACT TRACING: PART OF A MULTIPRONGED APPROACH TO FIGHT THE COVID-19 PANDEMIC*

U.S. Department of Health and Human Services
Centers for Disease Control and Prevention

COVID-19 CASE INVESTIGATION AND CONTACT TRACING FOR HEALTH DEPARTMENTS

This web page highlights basic principles of case investigation and contact tracing to stop COVID-19 transmission; detailed guidance for health departments is available.

Case investigation and contact tracing, a core disease control measure employed by local and state health department personnel for decades, is a

* This is an edited, reformatted and augmented version of the US Department of Health and Human Services publication No. 316704A, dated May 27.2020.

key strategy for preventing further spread of COVID-19. Immediate action is needed. Communities must scale up and train a large workforce and work collaboratively across public and private agencies to stop the transmission of COVID-19.

Certain Core Principles of Case Investigation and Contact Tracing Must Always Be Adhered to

- Case investigation is part of the process of supporting patients with suspected or confirmed infection.
- In case investigation, public health staff work with a patient to help them recall everyone with whom they have had close contact during the timeframe while they may have been infectious.
- Public health staff then begin contract tracing by warning these exposed individuals (contacts) of their potential exposure as rapidly and sensitively as possible.
- To protect patient privacy, contacts are only informed that they may have been exposed to a patient with the infection. They are not told the identity of the patient who may have exposed them.
- Contacts are provided with education, information, and support to understand their risk, what they should do to separate themselves from others who are not exposed, monitor themselves for illness, and the possibility that they could spread the infection to others even if they themselves do not feel ill.
- Contacts are encouraged to stay home and maintain social distance from others (at least 6 feet) until 14 days after their last exposure, in case they also become ill. They should monitor themselves by checking their temperature twice daily and watching for cough or shortness of breath. To the extent possible, public health staff should check in with contacts to make sure they are self-monitoring and have not developed symptoms. Contacts who develop symptoms should promptly isolate themselves and notify public health staff.

They should be promptly evaluated for infection and for the need for medical care.

Case Investigation and Contact Tracing Is a Specialized Skill

To be done effectively, it requires people with the training, supervision, and access to social and medical support for patients and contacts. Requisite knowledge and skills for case investigators and contact tracers include:

- An understanding of patient confidentiality, including the ability to conduct interviews without violating confidentiality (e.g., to those who might overhear their conversations)
- Understanding of the medical terms and principles of exposure, infection, infectious period, potentially infectious interactions, symptoms of disease, pre-symptomatic and asymptomatic infection
- Excellent and sensitive interpersonal, cultural sensitivity, and interviewing skills such that they can build and maintain trust with patients and contacts
- Basic skills of crisis counseling, and the ability to confidently refer patients and contacts for further care if needed
- Resourcefulness in locating patients and contacts who may be difficult to reach or reluctant to engage in conversation
- Understanding of when to refer individuals or situations to medical, social, or supervisory resources

- Cultural competency appropriate to the local community

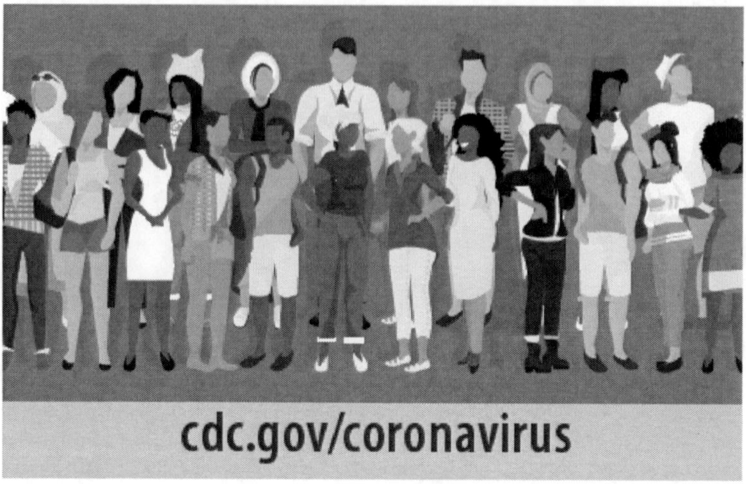

Case Investigators and Contact Tracing Is Part of the Process of Supporting Patients and Warning Contacts of Exposure in Order to Stop Chains of Transmission

Given the magnitude of COVID-19 cases and plans to eventually relax mitigation efforts such as stay at home orders and social distancing, communities need a large number of trained case investigators and contact tracers. Case investigators need to quickly locate and talk with the patients, assist in arranging for patients to isolate themselves, and work with patients to identify people with whom the patients have been in close contact so the contact tracer can locate them. The actual number of staff needed is large and varies depending on a number of factors including but not limited to:

- The daily number of cases
- The number of contacts identified
- How quickly patients are isolated, and contacts are notified and advised to stay home, self-monitor, and maintain social distance from others

The Time to Start Building the Trained Workforce Is Now

Time Is of the Essence

Identifying contacts and ensuring they do not interact with others is critical to protect communities from further spread. If communities are unable to effectively isolate patients and ensure contacts can separate themselves from others, rapid community spread of COVID-19 is likely to increase to the point that strict mitigation strategies will again be needed to contain the virus.

Case investigators and contact tracers need to:

- Immediately identify and interview people with SARS CoV-2 infections and COVID-19 (i.e., disease)
- Support isolation of those who are infected
- Warn contacts of their exposure, assess their symptoms and risk, and provide instructions for next steps
- Link those with symptoms to testing and care

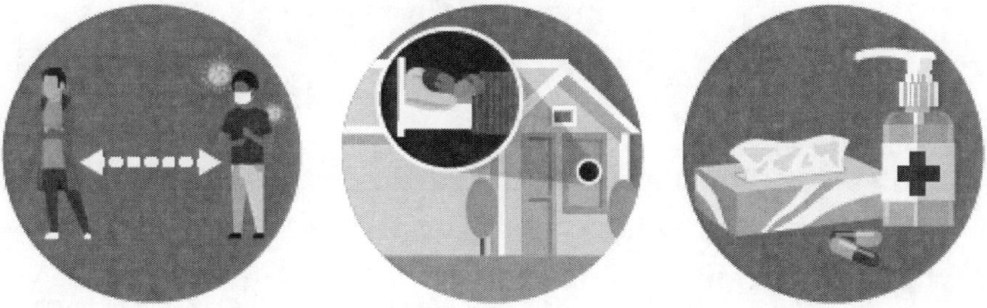

Based on our current knowledge, a close contact is someone who was within 6 feet of an infected person for at least 15 minutes starting from 48 hours before illness onset until the time the patient is isolated. They should stay home, maintain social distancing, and self-monitor until 14 days from the last date of exposure.

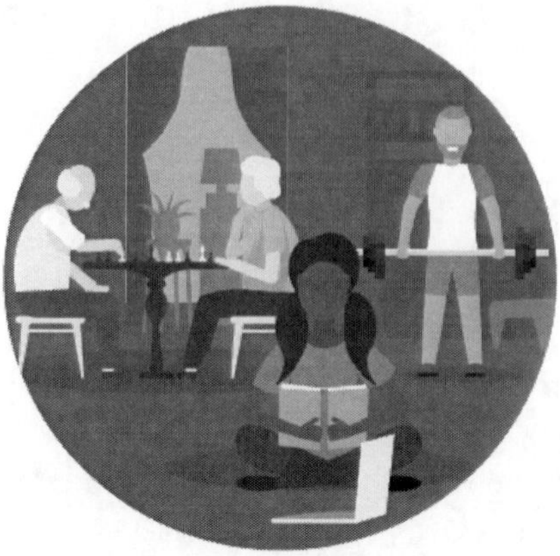

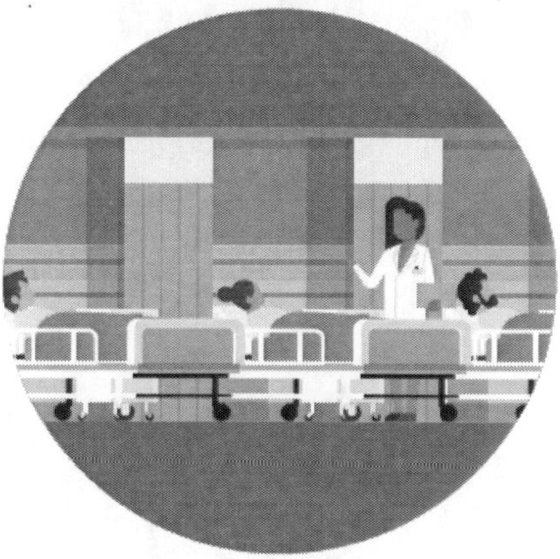

Case Investigation and Contact Tracing in Care Facilities, Other Congregate Living Settings and Households with Many People Living in One House Is a Priority

Case investigation and contact tracing of patients with COVID-19 potentially exposed at work and patients in healthcare facilities, congregate living settings or housing with many people is complex. Appropriate engagement with infection control and occupational health programs is recommended. Priority settings include:

- Healthcare facilities including long-term care facilities
- Group home/board
- Homeless shelters
- Federal, state and local correctional facilities
- Crowded, multigenerational housing

In addition to healthcare workers, it is important to assess interactions between residents and all staff, including but not limited to activity coordinators, food service staff, and sanitation management. Transitional case management plans should be put in place for patients in isolation and contacts who are separated for monitoring. Management plans should also be created for transitioning from one setting to another, such as transitions from hospitals to acute or long-term care facilities or home isolation, or from prison and jail to parole and probation.

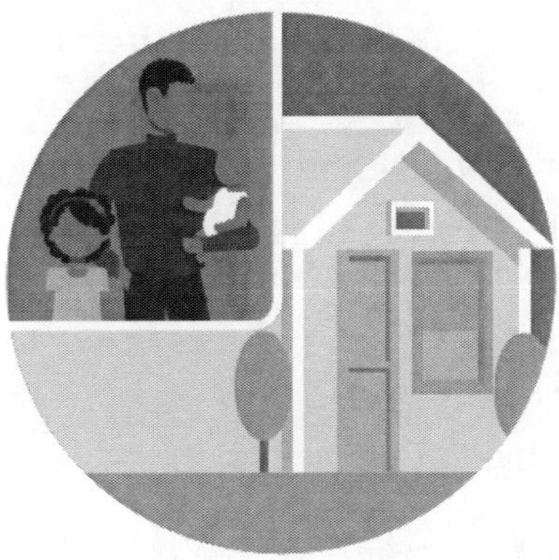

Social Services and Housing Will Be Needed for Contacts Unable to Separate Themselves from Others in Their Current Living Situation

Separating contacts from people who are not exposed is critical to the success of any contact tracing effort and requires social supports for individual compliance and medical monitoring. First and foremost is the assessment of an individual's ability to stay home and maintain social distance from others, a safe environment that provides the necessary supports (private room and bathroom, adequate food and water, and access to medication) and the ability to practice adequate infection control. For a portion of the U.S. population this will be a challenge, particularly for some of the most vulnerable populations. Support services for consideration include housing, food, medicine, and economic supports. For contacts without a primary care provider, linkage to clinical care may be needed. Support for medical monitoring includes patient care packages (e.g., thermometers, sanitizers, mask, gloves) and technological supports for medical monitoring (e.g., mobile phone apps). If possible, contacts should be asked to voluntarily stay home, monitor themselves, and maintain social distancing from others. However, health departments have the authority to issue legal orders of quarantine, should the situation warrant that measure.

Communication with the Public Is Crucial

Engagement of the public with case investigators and contact tracers must be widely accepted in order to protect friends, family, and community members from future potential infections. Key public officials and community leaders will need to be engaged and supportive of case investigation and contact tracing efforts. Consider reaching out to community leaders as part of the neighborhood-level case investigation and contact tracing team.

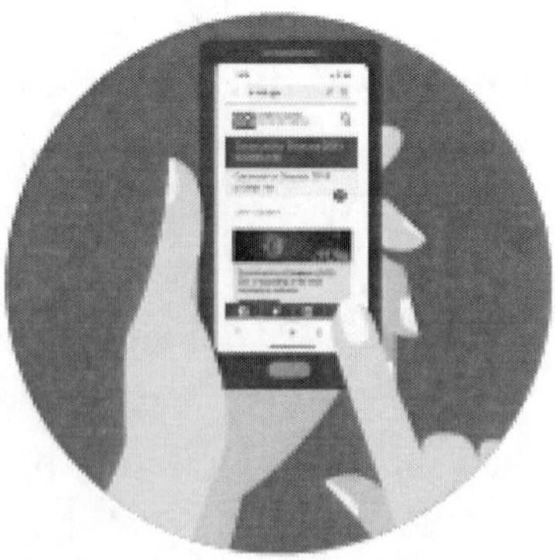

To be successful, a community will need public awareness, and understanding and acceptance of case investigation and contact tracing and the need for contacts to separate themselves from others who are not exposed. Community members need to take responsibility to follow the guidance from public health agencies.

Data Management and Technology Will Be Needed

Case investigation, contact tracing, and contact follow-up and monitoring will need to be linked with timely testing, clinical services, and agile data management systems to facilitate real-time electronic transmission of laboratory and case data for public health action. Technology partners are key in the modification of existing systems and the development of new user-friendly data interfaces to manage multiple data streams with seamless interoperability. Case management tools can help automate key pieces of the case investigation and contact tracing process, making the overall process more efficient. Ideally, data systems would also include automated reports to aid in monitoring progress and outcomes of case investigation and contact tracing. Data sharing agreements between local, tribal and state, and federal jurisdictions need to be established or augmented to ensure timely and accurate data collection and sharing. The adoption of emerging technologies that can assist private and public health practitioners with client communication, medical monitoring, and strategies to amplify case investigation and contact tracing may greatly help with scaling up these activities as needed. Digital Contact Tracing Tools for COVID-19.

Ongoing Monitoring and Assessment of Case Investigation and Contact Tracing Efforts Will Be Needed

Public health agencies and their partners will need to monitor some key components of their programs to improve performance as needed. Potential metrics routinely reviewed could include the following process and outcome measures:

- Case interviewing: Time to interview from symptom onset and from diagnosis; proportion interviewed; median number of contacts elicited; proportion with no contacts elicited.
- Contact notification: Proportion of contacts notified; time from first potential exposure to notification.
- Contact follow-up: Daily proportion of contacts whose status is evaluated; proportion of contacts with symptoms evaluated within 24 hours of onset of symptoms; proportion of contacts who complete their full self-monitoring period.
- Contact tracing efficacy: Percent of new COVID-19 cases arising among contacts during self-monitoring period.

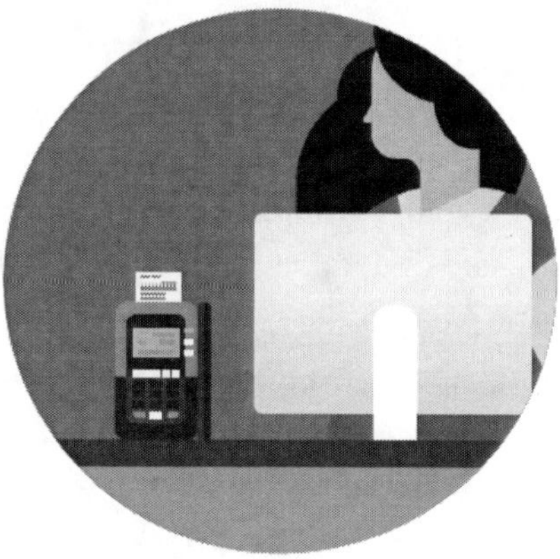

In: Testing and Contract Tracing … ISBN: 978-1-53618-857-8
Editor: Ernesto M. Batista © 2020 Nova Science Publishers, Inc.

Chapter 7

CONTACT TRACING FOR COVID-19: DOMESTIC POLICY ISSUES*

Kavya Sekar and Laurie A. Harris

Contact tracing is a classic tool of public health investigation used to identify the close contacts of persons infected with a communicable disease, notify themof potential exposure, and enable control measures such as quarantining exposed persons. Contact tracing programs are generally subject to state, territorial, tribal, and local laws and policies. The U.S. Centers for Disease Control and Prevention (CDC) assists jurisdictions' programs by providing guidance, technical assistance, and funding.

Several public health experts affiliated with universities (e.g., Johns Hopkins University), policy research organizations (e.g., American Enterprise Institute), and state associations (e.g., National Governors Association) have posited that contact tracing (combined with adequate diagnostic testing) could help prevent surges in infections, particularly when case counts are low. Contact tracing to control Coronavirus Disease 2019 (COVID-19) has been

* This is an edited, reformatted and augmented version of Congressional Research Service Publication No. IF11609, dated August 3, 2020.

used with arguable success in countries such as South Korea, Taiwan, Iceland, and New Zealand—many attribute their relatively low reported case counts, in part, to successful contact tracing. However, several experts assert that a successful contact tracing effort in the United States would require additional workforce and possibly the use of new technologies by jurisdictions. Federalism has led to heterogeneous contact tracing efforts across states. As the pandemic progresses, Congress may consider whether and how to guide U.S. contact tracing efforts.

WHAT IS CONTACT TRACING?

Contact tracing, a component of *public health investigation,* is a core tool of communicable disease control. U.S. jurisdictions' public health departments have used contact tracing to help control the spread of diseases like HIV and tuberculosis. Typically, when a confirmed case of a disease is identified and determined to require a case investigation, public health departments contact the patient and conduct extensive interviews to acquire information about persons with whom the patient may have been in contact and therefore possibly exposed to the disease. Those individuals are then notified by either the patient or the health department and then referred for testing, prophylaxis, and/or treatment (if available) or asked/required to self-quarantine (depending on the applicable jurisdiction's laws and policies). Contacts are usually informed by health departments of a potential disease exposure, but are not given the identity of the individual who exposed them.

COVID-19 SPECIFIC CONSIDERATIONS

Given that COVID-19 spreads easily from person to person and can be transmitted by asymptomatic individuals, controlling COVID-19 may require more robust contact tracing capacity than existed in many jurisdictions prior to the pandemic. In addition, given the lack of available vaccines or prophylaxis for COVID-19, health departments usually request that exposed individuals voluntarily self- quarantine and may conduct regular follow-up and/or facilitate housing and other support programs for quarantine. Experts generally advocate two approaches to expanding U.S contact tracing—expanding the contact tracing workforce and the use of new technologies to help identify and notify potential contacts. Some domestic COVID-19 contact tracing efforts have faced initial challenges with individuals refusing to share information with health departments, indicating potential individual liberty and privacy considerations.

Workforce Considerations

Depending on the design of its contact tracing program, jurisdictions may require an expanded workforce to conduct interviews and manage contact tracing efforts. Johns Hopkins University and the Association of State and Territorial Health Officials have recommended between 4 and 81 tracers per 100,000 population, based on level of illness in a given region.

Recruitment

Given the need to augment existing capacity, several states have recruited paid and volunteer contact tracing staff from state employees, public health and medical schools, AmeriCorps volunteers, and other institutions. Some states have also worked with private entities to manage contact tracing efforts. For example, Indiana contracted with a private company, Maximus, to manage a call center for contact tracing efforts.

Training

Contact tracers need specialized education and skills, including an understanding of medical terms, knowledge of patient confidentiality requirements, and an ability to effectively interview and counsel patients. CDC has published online training for contact tracing programs. Several states have also implemented training programs in partnership with non-profit organizations and universities.

Contact tracing programs need individuals with varying skill levels, including established public health experts to help manage programs as well as skilled tracers to contact and interview individuals. Jurisdictions may also consider the need for cultural competence and ability to engage with diverse communities affected by COVID-19, such as skills in non-English language proficiencies.

TECHNOLOGY CONSIDERATIONS

A challenge in traditional contact tracing is the difficulty patients have comprehensively recalling close contacts, even with the assistance of trained public health workers. COVID-19 patients may be infectious long before receiving a positive test result, and thus may need to recall weeks of close contacts. Tools that usedigital technologies to automate this aspect of contact tracing have been developed, though their adoption in the United States has been uneven. CDC has issued guidance to aid jurisdictions in choosing and implementing these tools.

Location and Proximity Tracking

Technologists have been working to create smart phone-based applications (apps) to augment conventional contact tracing and notification. These use location or proximity tracking to identify who has had close contact with infected individuals during a specific window of time. Location tracking apps collect time and physical location data using Global Positioning System (GPS), cell tower, or Wi-Fi signals, while proximity tracking apps use the exchange of Bluetooth signals between devices to establish contact. Apple and Google have developed a protocol to allow apps developed by public health departments to work across both Android and Apple operating systems. They have chosen not to support location data collection to address privacy and security concerns. Contact tracing and notification apps have been adopted in several nations and some U.S. states, with mixed results.

Adoption

Contact tracing apps require broad adoption and self-reporting by infected individuals to be effective.

Researchers estimate that 80% of U.S. smartphone users (56% of the population) need to use an app to effectively control COVID-19. Various polls estimate a range of 50%- 60% of the U.S. population are willing to use a contact tracing app. One poll estimated that 29% of the U.S. population would be willing to share location data. Existing state app programs face adoption challenges. For example, as of June 24, 2020, 4% of North Dakota's population was using its tracking app.

Effectiveness

Some experts have argued that technologies relying on only "exposure notification" would not be adequate for slowing COVID-19 spread, as they may not allow for epidemiological analyses of cases necessary for public health interventions. Rather, they argue that location data is needed, along with building or improving states' data management systems. Some arguethat public health programs should consider other measures if digital technology solutions are not widely accepted.

Other Technologies

Several states currently use Sara Alert, an open-source automated tracking and reminder system. It allows public health departments to manage symptom and contact data provided by patients and provide automatic notification, follow-up, and symptom reporting.

Individual Liberty and Privacy Considerations

U.S. public health has long faced a tension between individual liberty considerations andmeasures required for population-level communicable disease control. Civil liberty and other groups have raised concerns that apps tying location data to health data could be obtained by malicious actors or used for broader government monitoring. A mistrust of government may also affect traditional contact tracing efforts to collect information.

Contact tracing data security and privacy (collected by both traditional means and by digital tools) is mostly governed by state rather than federal law. State law related to the privacy and security of data collected in the course of contact tracing efforts varies.

Funding

Congress has appropriated funding in several supplemental measures that can support contact tracing efforts by jurisdictions and the CDC. Funding available for grants/cooperative agreements with jurisdictions for public health programs (that can involve contact tracing as one component) include not less than $950 million P.L. 116- 123, not less than $1.5 billion in P.L. 116-136, and not less than $11 billion in P.L. 116-139. Additional CDC funding in the supplemental measures could also be used.

Issues for Congress

If Congress considers contact tracing an important component of the federal response to COVID-19, it may consider the following:

Leadership and Coordination

Currently, most contact tracing efforts—including workforce and technology components—are led by jurisdictions with guidance, assistance, and funding from CDC. Congress may consider whether the federal government should play a bigger role in coordinating contact tracing efforts across jurisdictions and helping standardize tools and practices.

Trust

Reports from existing efforts indicate difficulty obtaining needed information from individuals or encouraging technology adoption. Congress may consider how to facilitate public trust in contact tracing, such as by nationwide education and awareness efforts.

Privacy and Security

Congress may consider whether new federal authorities related to the privacy and security of data collected in the course of contact tracing are needed.

Evaluation

States are employing many different contact tracing strategies, some of which may be more effective in controlling disease spread than others. CDC has developed a *COVID Tracer* tool to aid in evaluating approaches. Congress may consider how to ensure strategies are adequately evaluated to help identify what works in the United States and disseminate findings.

In: Testing and Contract Tracing … ISBN: 978-1-53618-857-8
Editor: Ernesto M. Batista © 2020 Nova Science Publishers, Inc.

Chapter 8

HEALTH DEPARTMENT CHECKLIST: DEVELOPING A CASE INVESTIGATION AND CONTACT TRACING PLAN FOR CORONAVIRUS DISEASE 2019 (COVID-19)*

U.S. Department of Health and Human Services, Centers for Disease Control and Prevention

Case investigation and contact tracing are well-honed skills that adapt easily to new public health demands and are effective tools to slow the spread of COVID-19 in a community. Thoughtful planning can help ensure that these activities facilitate compassionate care for the people affected by COVID-19 and also prevent community transmission of the virus.

* This is an edited, reformatted and augmented version of U.S. Department of Health and Human Services publication No. CS317274, dated 05/29/2020.

Scaling Up Staffing Roles Involved in Case Investigation & Contact Tracing (Guidance Section II)			
Staffing Plan	Completed	In Progress	*Not Started*
Estimate # of case investigators/contact tracers needed	○	○	○
Recruit and hire surge workforce	○	○	○
- Include consideration for culturally and linguistically diverse populations that the jurisdiction serves	○	○	○
Develop organizational structure (identification of staff who will perform key roles identified in CDC guidance)	○	○	○
Training	Completed	In Progress	Not Started
Develop training plan for current and new case investigators and contact tracers, including supervisors/leads - Include knowledge-based and skills-based training as well as opportunities for continuous and peer-to-peer learning	○	○	○
Determine how training will be delivered	○	○	○
Determine how training will be tracked to ensure all staff are trained	○	○	○

Case Investigation & Contact Tracing Activities (Guidance Section IV & Guidance Section V)			
Case Investigation & Contact Tracing Strategy	Completed	In Progress	Not Started
Define close contact and contact elicitation window	○	○	○
Develop criteria for discontinuation of self-isolation and self-quarantine	○	○	○
Develop testing strategy for: - Suspected and probable cases	○	○	○
- Asymptomatic and symptomatic contacts	○	○	○
- Outbreaks in congregate settings	○	○	○
- Possibly for community at-large	○	○	○
Develop case investigation strategy to prioritize cases if unable to investigate all confirmed and probable cases (triaging protocol likely needed)	○	○	○
Develop close contact monitoring strategy to prioritize close contacts to monitor and/or modify intensity of monitoring depending on public health resources available	○	○	○
Program Workflow	Completed	In Progress	Not Started
Describe how cases are identified in your jurisdiction's data management system (case report CMR, lab test, other)	○	○	○
Describe how case interview assignments are made	○	○	○

Case Investigation & Contact Tracing Activities (Guidance Section IV & Guidance Section V)			
Diagram and/or describe in detail the program workflow with surge staff and their supervision incorporated	○	○	○
Procurement	Completed	In Progress	Not Started
Procure any needed supplies, including PPE, COVID-19 kits for patients and contacts, materials/equipment for case investigation and contact tracing staff (e.g., laptops, tablets, cell phones)	○	○	○
Laboratory Services	Completed	In Progress	Not Started
Establish linkage to testing sites	○	○	○
Develop understanding of statewide laboratory capacity and laboratory turnaround time for results reporting	○	○	○
Identify SARS-CoV-2 tests in use by laboratories serving the jurisdiction	○	○	○
Prototcols	Completed	In Progress	Not Started
Develop protocol for triaging cases	○	○	○
- Obtaining necessary information to inform triaging	○	○	○
- Determining case assignment	○	○	○
Develop case investigation protocol	○	○	○
- Can include interview guides, call scripts	○	○	○

Case Investigation & Contact Tracing Activities (Guidance Section IV & Guidance Section V) (Continued)			
Prototcols	Completed	In Progress	Not Started
- Protocol covers: › Confidential notification	○	○	○
› Risk assessment	○	○	○
› Self-isolation instructions including any daily monitoring	○	○	○
› Linkage to self-isolation support services and medical services (if needed)	○	○	○
› Linkage to testing (if needed and available)	○	○	○
› Close contact elicitation	○	○	○
› Discontinuation of self-isolation	○	○	○
- Specimen collection for testing (if applicable to role), proper PPE use	○	○	○
- Case investigation when patients are unable to participate (including minors); proxy interviews	○	○	○
- Use of data collection forms and tools	○	○	○

Case Investigation & Contact Tracing Activities (Guidance Section IV & Guidance Section V)			
- Establish timelines for 1st contact interviews	○	○	○
- Develop goals for timeliness of interviews	○	○	○
Develop contact tracing protocol	○	○	○
- Can include interview guides, call scripts	○	○	○
- Protocol covers: › Confidential notification	○	○	○
› Risk assessment	○	○	○
› Self-quarantine instructions including daily monitoring	○	○	○
› Linkage to self-quarantine support services and medical services (if needed)	○	○	○
› Linkage to testing (if available)	○	○	○
› Discontinuation of self-quarantine	○	○	○
- Contact tracing activities when contacts are minors	○	○	○

Case Investigation & Contact Tracing Activities (Guidance Section IV & Guidance Section V) (Continued)			
- Specimen collection for testing (if applicable to role), proper PPE use	○	○	○
- Use of data collection forms and tools	○	○	○
- Establish timelines for 1st contact interviews	○	○	○
- Develop goals for timeliness of interviews	○	○	○
Develop protocol for assessing need and eligibility of patients and contacts for support services, triaging requests, and providing linkage to needed services	○	○	○
Develop protocol for medical monitoring of patients with COVID-19 who are at higher risk for severe disease	○	○	○
Develop protocol for using interpretation services if case investigator/contact tracer is not fluent in primary language of patient with COVID-19 or close contact	○	○	○
Develop protocol for providing case investigation and contact tracing services to people who are deaf or who have hearing loss	○	○	○
Develop protocol for serving public health orders for isolation and quarantine, if applicable	○	○	○

Outbreaks (Guidance Section VI)			
Complex Investigations	Completed	In Progress	Not Started
Develop guidance for handling complex investigations (e.g., outbreaks in congregate living or workplace settings)	○	○	○
- Formation of interdisciplinary team(s)	○	○	○
- Triage protocol for handing over investigations to team	○	○	○
- Plan for surge staffing if needed	○	○	○

Special Considerations (Guidance Section VII)			
Prototcols	Completed	In Progress	Not Started
Develop protocol for managing case investigations when a patient is unable to participate (e.g., cognitively impaired, deceased, intubated, unconscious, a minor)	○	○	○
Develop protocol for interjurisdictional case investigation and contact tracing	○	○	○
Develop protocol for case investigation and contact tracing for flights (or other mode of public transportation) arriving in the US or between US states, or cruise ships arriving at US ports of entry	○	○	○

Building Community Support (Guidance Section VIII)			
Communications and Community Engagement Strategy	Completed	In Progress	Not Started
Develop a communications and community engagement strategy	○	○	○

Building Community Support (Guidance Section VIII) (Continued)			
- Engage local community leaders, public officials, and influencers	○	○	○
- Develop clear, empowering messages that create awareness of case investigation and contact tracing activities and encourage acceptance	○	○	○
› Also share messages that dispel misinformation and direct public to reliable sources	○	○	○
- Use all available communication channels to reinforce messages	○	○	○
Communications and Community Engagement Strategy	*Completed*	*In Progress*	*Not Started*
- Ensure messages and materials are culturally sensitive	○	○	○
- Tailor messages to reach specific audiences, including vulnerable populations in the community	○	○	○
- Develop or adapt existing health education materials to share with patients and close contacts	○	○	○
› Translate into primary languages of affected community members (also consider translating data collection instruments)	○	○	○
› Include materials for low literacy levels and that are graphics-based (more images than text)	○	○	○
- Identify communication avenues (social media, newspapers, TV news stories, billboards, TV ads)	○	○	○

Data Management (Guidance Section IX)			
Data Management Infrastructure	Completed	In Progress	Not Started
Develop and implement data management infrastructure	○	○	○
- Laboratory, provider, and contact case reports should be transmitted electronically and seamlessly imported into the system in an automated fashion	○	○	○
- Develop modules for: › Case investigations of confirmed and probable cases,	○	○	○
› Patient risk assessment (including contact elicitation),	○	○	○
› Contact investigation (including risk assessment)	○	○	○
› Should be editable without the need for vendors/contractors	○	○	○
› Should be able to link multiple individuals within the system	○	○	○
- Establish user roles in data management system	○	○	○
- Develop routine canned reports for feedback to staff	○	○	○
- Develop routine canned reports to review program successes and identify areas for improvement	○	○	○
- Develop interview forms for patients and close contacts that incorporate critical data elements	○	○	○

Data Management (Guidance Section IX) (continued)			
- Collaborate with healthcare providers for data sharing (e.g., access to electronic health records)	○	○	○
- Ensure that local data security and confidentiality standards are being met	○	○	○

Evaluating Success (Guidance Section X)			
Evaluation and Quality Improvement	Completed	In Progress	Not Started
Develop plan for evaluation and quality improvement	○	○	○
- Consider setting targets for select metrics	○	○	○
- Select process and outcome metrics to routinely review	○	○	○
- Use reports to identify areas for training and help leadership identify any necessary program adjustments	○	○	○
- Identify staff member who will run reports	○	○	○
- Identify staff who will receive reports	○	○	○
- Determine frequency reports will be run	○	○	○
Develop protocol for supervisory review and feedback on case and contact investigations	○	○	○

Confidentiality and Consent (Guidance Section XI)			
Security and Confidentiality	Completed	In Progress	Not Started
Develop plan addressing security and confidentiality	○	○	○
- Assess standards currently in place to protect patient information and determine if modifications are needed for COVID-19	○	○	○
Develop Protocols for: - Security of confidential case investigation and contact tracing information	○	○	○
- Maintaining confidentiality, including legal requirements for public health personnel	○	○	○

Support Services to Consider (Guidance Section XII)			
Support Services	Completed	In Progress	Not Started
Develop plan for providing support services	○	○	○
- Assess services available for patients, contacts, and their families	○	○	○
- Fill critical gaps in wraparound services	○	○	○
- Establish eligibility criteria	○	○	○
- Provide alternate housing to support the isolation of patients and quarantine of close contacts who are unable to do so safely at their home	○	○	○

Support Services to Consider (Guidance Section XII) (Continued)			
- Provide telemedicine safety net pool of providers for on-call clinical consult with patients and contacts who do not have a primary healthcare provider	○	○	○
- Partner with local community groups and organizations that can help support specific populations	○	○	○
- Establish processes for connecting patients and contacts to support services	○	○	○

This checklist is a supplement to CDC's Health Departments: Interim Guidance on Developing a COVID-19 Case Investigation & Contact Tracing Plan and is a tool that can assist health departments in developing a comprehensive plan. This tool does not describe mandatory requirements or standards; rather, it highlights important areas for consideration.

For additional information, users can access the corresponding section of the guidance document listed in each header (i.e., Guidance Section #).

COVID-19 case investigation and contact tracing activities will vary based on the level of community transmission, characteristics of the community and their populations, and the local capacity to implement both case investigation and contact tracing.

In: Testing and Contract Tracing … ISBN: 978-1-53618-857-8
Editor: Ernesto M. Batista © 2020 Nova Science Publishers, Inc.

Chapter 9

COVID-19 CASE INVESTIGATION AND CONTACT TRACING SUPERVISOR OR LEAD TRAINING: GUIDANCE, RESOURCES, AND SAMPLE TRAINING PLAN*

U.S. Department of Health and Human Services, Centers for Disease Control and Prevention

BACKGROUND

This document contains a sample training plan including training topics that may be helpful for state and local public health jurisdictions to consider when designing their own training plan for COVID-19 case investigation and contract tracing supervisors or leads. Each heading represents the learning objective for that section. Suggested training modalities/formats are

* This is an edited, reformatted and augmented version of U.S. Department of Health and Human Services, Publication No. CS 317134-A, dated May 20, 2020.

provided, as well as information about sample existing trainings and resources. This document may be updated as new resources become available.

For the purposes of this document, a case investigation and contact tracing supervisor or lead directly oversees the work of the case investigator and/or contact tracer and others who may work as part of a team. The supervision or leadership of these teams is combined into one position for the purposes of this sample training plan. This position coordinates between case investigators and contact tracers as an essential component of the quality oversight of the contact tracing program as part of the public health response.

Overall Training Goal

After completing all training below, learners should be able to be effective COVID-19 case investigation and contact tracing supervisors or leads. If seeking a sample training plan, trainings, and resources for other positions, refer to the contact tracing training plan here or the case investigation training plan here.

Target Audience

Public health professionals.

Identify Strategies to Reduce Spread of COVID-19

For this section, self-paced online training (e.g., curated reading list, videos, or eLearning course) is suggested. Inclusion of a post-test is strongly recommended. This section can be omitted if learners are up-to-date or have previously participated in other training that has provided an adequate overview of these content areas.

- Background
  - General
  - Epidemiology and surveillance principles
  - Update on current emergency response
- COVID-19 disease specific information
  - Signs/symptoms, and routes of transmission
  - Incubation period and infectious period
  - Testing
  - Diagnosis and current management
  - Prevention and control (including self-isolation for patients and self-quarantine for contacts)
- Ways to prevent spread of COVID-19
  - General precautions (e.g., social distancing)
  - Role of public health, case investigation, and contact tracing in reducing spread
  - Other ways to reduce spread

Identify the Primary Components of COVID-19 Case Investigation and Contact Tracing

A variety of modalities would be appropriate, including live webinar/teleconference, recorded webinar, or a self-paced eLearning course. Inclusion of a post-test is strongly recommended. This section can be omitted if learners are up-to-date or have previously participated in the contact tracing or case investigation training.

- Foundational principles of public health
  - General
- Relevant terminology

    - Case definition
    - Public health jurisdiction's case investigation and contact tracing terminology
    - Terms that may be used in other jurisdictions (e.g., other states, federal)
- Introduction to case investigation and contact tracing
    - General
    - Define case investigation
    - Describe basic steps of case investigation
        - Case identification and prioritization
        - Use of public health data sources such as surveillance to collect information about the case
        - Investigate case
        - Notification of positive test results
        - Interview including contact elicitation
        - Isolation vs quarantine
        - Follow-up and next steps
    - Define contact tracing
    - Describe basic steps of contract tracing
        - Test and test results information
        - Overview of case investigation and elicitation
        - Trace
        - Quarantine or isolate
        - Follow-up
    - Describe skills and qualities necessary for case investigators and contact tracers
    - Active listening skills, including the use of open-ended questions
    - Motivational interviewing skills
    - Risk communication, problem solving, emotional intelligence skills
    - Cultural sensitivity
    - Adaptations for cases with communication impairments and non-English speakers

List Requirements for Protecting Health Information

Self-paced online training (e.g., curated reading list, videos, or eLearning course) is suggested. Inclusion of a post-test is strongly recommended.

- Overview of health information privacy/security
    - Why it is important to protect health information
    - Potential consequences if information is not protected
- Health information privacy and confidentiality
    - Oath of confidentiality, if applicable in the jurisdiction
- Health information data security
- Ethics of data collection during an outbreak

Describe the Qualities, Skills, and Styles of Effective COVID-19 Case Investigation and Contract Tracing Leads

Live training or on the job learning and feedback (whether through videoconference or a live course on a learning management system) is suggested so that learners can receive real-time feedback and ask questions. Breakout sessions with smaller groups could be effective if multiple trainers or facilitators are available. Inclusion of a post-test is strongly recommended.

- Qualities and skills of effective team leads
    - General
    - Understands the duties and protocols of case investigators and contact tracers
    - Explains past experiences in contact tracing/DIS CDC work

- Demonstrates leadership in their supervision of staff:
  - Orients towards developing and improving case investigation and contact tracing staff on their team though CQI, feedback performance reviews and mentorship
  - Communicates successfully with all members of the team
  - Exhibits fairness and trustworthiness in interactions with staff
  - Focuses staff on the task at hand, intervening in the spread of COVID-19, through leading by example
  - Demonstrates resourcefulness and problem solving to accomplish necessary tasks

- Management styles
  - Importance of management style and the effectiveness of the team
  - Your unique management style and how it can be used to ensure success of the team
- Management of remote teams
  - General
  - Unique challenges of managing a team remotely
  - Importance of resiliency

Identify Time Management Practices for Case Investigation and Contact Tracing Leads

In the midst of an outbreak, time management is of particular importance. Self-paced online training (e.g., curated reading list, videos, or eLearning course) is suggested. Inclusion of a post-test is strongly recommended.

- Keys to time management
  - General

- Understand factors that will influence and interrupt your day to day including daily tasks, meetings, staff, emails, and the crisis of the day
- Set priorities, with patient care and interrupting disease transmission at the forefront
- Utilize technology to its full potential
- Delegate to staff in a systematic manner

Describe a Team Lead's Role in Training and Development

Even the best training course has little effect without supervisor leadership. Live training (whether through videoconference or a live course on a learning management system) is suggested so that learners can receive real-time feedback and ask questions. Breakout sessions with smaller groups could be effective if multiple trainers or facilitators are available.

- Team Lead's role in training and on the job learning
  - Assess training needs and conduct performance evaluations to guide training needs
  - Organize formal training opportunities initially and then supplemental training while on the job, as indicated by the performance evaluations
  - Adjust training to match participant skill-level
  - Facilitate learning opportunities through informal training on the job
  - Establish learning collaboratives
  - Establish an ad hoc or structured mentoring opportunities

Monitor Performance of Case Investigators and Contact Tracers

An electronic guide, job aids, self-paced asynchronous eLearning, or live training (whether through videoconference or a live course on a learning management system) describing jurisdiction-specific protocols for monitoring performance of case investigators.

- Importance of auditing
  - Set clear expectations
  - Assess how case investigator and contact tracer does key activities by observation and performance measurement
  - Identify individual strengths and weaknesses to provide developmental opportunities
  - Implement CQI systems with regular measurement and feedback loops for local outputs
  - Develop an audit schedule based on experience and expertise
  - Reference historical materials
- Indicators for individual supervision of Case Investigators
- Indicators for individual supervision of Contact Tracers
- Audit tools
  - Canned reports at the level of individual case investigators and contact tracers ensure that staff are meeting expectations
  - Patient interaction audits
  - Audit feedback form
- Feedback and follow-up

TRAINING CATALOGUE BY LEARNING OBJECTIVE

Identify Strategies to Reduce Spread of COVID-19

Making Contact: A Training for COVID-19 Contact Tracers: The Basics of Coronavirus Disease 2019 (COVID-19) – Lesson 1

Topic areas: Background, signs/symptoms, general precautions, testing, prevention and control, other ways to reduce spread

- Register: https://www.train.org/main/course/1091302/compilation
- Target audience: Contact tracers and new case investigators
- Description: Contact tracers must understand the basics of coronavirus disease transmission in order to perform contact tracing and disease intervention activities effectively. Lesson one (The Basics of Coronavirus Disease 2019 (COVID-19)) will provide an overview of coronavirus disease 2019 (COVID-19), including its incubation and infectious period, symptoms, and how to prevent it. Please note, lessons must be completed in order from one to four.

Lesson 1 learning objectives:

1) Describe what COVID-19 is
2) Describe how to prevent COVID-19 transmission
3) List symptoms of COVID-19
4) Define social distancing, quarantine, and isolation
5) Describe the incubation and infectious period

Emerging Respiratory Viruses, Including COVID-19: Methods for Detection, Prevention, Response and Control

Topic area: Background

- Register: https://www.train.org/main/course/1090092/
- Target audience: Public health professionals

- Description: This course provides a general introduction to COVID-19.

Learning objectives:

1) Describe the nature of emerging respiratory viruses, how to detect and assess an outbreak, strategies for preventing and controlling outbreaks due to novel respiratory viruses
2) Describe strategies that should be used to communicate risk and engage communities to detect, prevent and respond to the emergence of a novel respiratory virus

COVID-19 Public Health Strategy Basic Concepts – NDPHTN

Topic areas: Epidemiology and surveillance principles, signs/ symptoms, testing, prevention and control, general precautions

- Register: https://www.train.org/main/course/1090675/
- Target audience: Public health professionals
- Description: Provides a basic background to the COVID-19 pandemic and describe the important steps to flatten the curve of COVID-19. Also provides an overview of crisis communication strategies and coordinating crisis response.

Learning objectives:

1) Review coronavirus history
2) Review COVID-19 characteristics
3) Discuss 6 concepts to flatten the curve
4) Review the 10 social distancing recommendations
5) Review COVID-19 testing concepts
6) Discuss how cocooning protects high-risk individuals
7) Discuss key concepts of crisis communications in pandemics

Boots on the Ground Part 1: Foundational Epidemiology

Topic area: Epidemiology and surveillance principles

- Register: https://www.train.org/main/course/1076135/
- Target audience: Public health professionals and others without a background in epidemiology
- Description: Provides basic principles of epidemiology and public health practice. Includes key terms used in epidemiologic and explains types of epidemiology research.

Learning objectives:

1) Define epidemiology
2) Describe the key factors impacting the incidence and spread of disease, injury, or health outcome (i.e., agent, host, environment)
3) Describe basic key terms in epidemiology
4) Describe distribution of disease, injury, or health outcomes and understand bias, validity, and reliability in assessing public health problems
5) Identify bias, validity, and reliability
6) Identify research methods

COVID-19 Contact Investigation Training

Topic area: Signs/symptoms

- View: https://www.ncsddc.org/wp-content/uploads/2020/03/FINAL-COVID19-Contact-Training-03112020.pdf
- Target audience: Case and contact investigators
- Description: This course covers background information on COVID-19, tools that Washington State is using for case investigation, interviewing techniques, and resources for case and contact investigations.

Learning objectives:

1) Discuss COVID-19 background
2) Discuss case investigation tools
3) Identify investigation interview techniques
4) Discuss types of contact follow-up
5) Identify COVID case and contact investigation resources

COVID-19 Real-Time Legal Response: Focus on Quarantine, Isolation, and Other Social Distancing Powers

Topic area: General precautions, prevention and control

- Register: https://www.train.org/cdctrain/course/1090658/
- Target audience: Public health professionals
- Description: Following a brief series of COVID-19 legal updates, this real-time session will focus on an array of social distancing legal responses among federal, state, and local authorities, notably quarantine, isolation, school and other closures, and proposed "lockdowns." After an initial presentation, your questions and comments will be addressed.

Learning objectives:

1) Assess the legal bases for social distancing in response to COVID-19
2) Understand the core legal steps to engage quarantine and isolation
3) Consider varied powers of federal, state and local governments to institute school or other closures
4) Explore the constitutional limits of proposed lockdowns and other aggressive social distancing measures

COVID-19 Infection Prevention and Control in the Household (Microlearning)

Topic area: General precautions

- Register: https://www.train.org/main/course/1090934/
- Target audience: General public health staff
- Description: This microlearning is designed to take 15 minutes. You will learn about instructions to give your patients who are taking care of a probable or confirmed case of COVID-19 in the household.

Learning objectives:

1) Identify COVID-19 infection prevention and control measures for the household

CDC Coronavirus Disease 2019 (COVID-19) Webpages

Topic area: Epidemiology

- Cases, Data, and Surveillance

Topic area: Signs/symptoms

- Symptoms of Coronavirus

Topic area: Update on current emergency response

- CDC in Action

Topic area: Prevention and control

- Social Distancing, Quarantine, and Isolation

Topic areas: General precautions

- Prevent Getting Sick

Topic area: Testing

- Testing for COVID-19

Identify the Primary Components of COVID-19 Case Investigation and Contact Tracing

Emerging Respiratory Viruses, Including COVID-19: Methods for Detection, Prevention, Response and Control

Topic area: Foundational principles of public health, introduction to case investigation and contact tracing

- Register: https://www.train.org/main/course/1090092/
- Target audience: Public health professionals
- Description: This course provides a general introduction to COVID-19.

Learning objectives:

1) Describe the nature of emerging respiratory viruses, how to detect and assess an outbreak, strategies for preventing and controlling outbreaks due to novel respiratory viruses
2) Describe strategies should be used to communicate risk and engage communities to detect, prevent and respond to the emergence of a novel respiratory virus

Public Health 101 Series - Introduction to Public Health

Topic area: Foundational principles of public health

- Register: https://www.train.org/main/course/1059661/
- Target audience: Individuals new to public health
- Description: This course introduces learners to the mission of public health and key terms in the field. The course covers historical developments in public health, the roles of different stakeholders, public health's core functions and essential services, determinants of health, and the Health Impact Pyramid.

Learning Objectives:

1) Describe the purpose of public health
2) Define key terms used in public health
3) Identify prominent events in the history of public health
4) Recognize the core public health functions and essential services
5) Describe the role of different stakeholders in the field of public health
6) List determinants of health
7) Recognize how individual determinants of health affect population health

Making Contact: A Training for COVID-19 Contact Tracers: The Basics of Contact Tracing – Lesson 2

Topic area: Relevant terminology, define contact tracing, investigation and elicitation, trace, quarantine or isolate

- Register: https://www.train.org/main/course/1091302/compilation
- Target audience: Contact tracers
- Description: The goal of lesson 2 (The Basics of Contact Tracing) is to provide an overview of the principles that will guide your work as a contact tracer. You will have the opportunity to learn basic definitions of contact tracing, gain an understanding of the steps

involved, and become aware of the importance of confidentiality. Please note, lessons must be completed in order from one to four.

Learning objectives:

1) Define PUI, contact, and contact tracing
2) Describe the objectives of contact tracing
3) List four fundamentals of contact tracing
4) Describe the importance of privacy protections
5) Identify the four main steps involved in the contact tracing process

Making Contact: A Training for COVID-19 Contact Tracers: Case Monitoring and Resources – Lesson 4

Topic area: Relevant terminology, follow-up

- Register: https://www.train.org/main/course/1091302/compilation
- Target audience: Contact tracers and case investigators
- Description: Case investigators and contact tracers will follow-up and monitor cases (PUIs or their contacts) to ensure they are following appropriate isolation or quarantine instructions and to track the development of any potential COVID-19 symptoms. Lesson 4 (Case Monitoring and Resources) will provide information on the different types of case monitoring and the activities you might be involved in. Please note, lessons must be completed in order from one to four.

Learning objectives:

1) Explain the difference between the two types of case monitoring
2) Describe potential follow-up activities that may be required during monitoring

3) Identify the types of resources and services that may be provided during the monitoring period
4) Explain what it means to escalate or "refer up" a case that needs more help than you're able to provide

COVID-19 Epidemiology Grand Rounds

Topic area: Introduction to case investigation and contact tracing

- Watch: https://www.facebook.com/ucsfepibiostat/videos/275226896828213/
- Target audience: Public health professionals
- Description: Provides epidemiology updates on COVID-19, including impact of social distancing, health disparities, and comprehensive section on contact tracing (begins around 48:00).

Learning objectives: Not available

An Introduction to Follow-up for Positive COVID-19 Cases and their Close Contacts

Topic area: Introduction to case investigation and contact tracing

- View: http://www.maventrainingsite.com/maven-help/pdf/LBOH%20Presentation%20COVID-19%20Case%20Investigation%20Introductory%20Training%20Webinar_April8.pdf
- Target audience: Public health professionals
- Description: Provides an overview of COVID-19 transmission, testing, and common vocabulary. Describes contact tracing and interview tools.

Learning objectives: Not available

Making Contact: A Training for COVID-19 Contact Tracers: The Basics of Contact Tracing – Lesson 1

Topic area: Introduction to case investigation and contact tracing

- Register: https://www.train.org/main/course/1091302/compilation
- Target audience: Case investigators and contact tracers
- Description: Contact Tracers must understand the basics of coronavirus disease transmission in order to perform contact tracing and disease intervention activities effectively. This lesson will provide an overview of coronavirus disease 2019 (COVID-19), including its incubation and infectious periods, symptoms, and how to prevent it. Please note, lessons must be completed in order from one to four.

Learning objectives:

1) Describe what COVID-19 is
2) Describe how to prevent COVID-19 transmission
3) List symptoms of COVID-19
4) Define social distancing, quarantine, and isolation
5) Describe the incubation and infectious periods

Making Contact: A Training for COVID-19 Contact Tracers: Effective Communication and Interviews – Lesson 3

Topic area: Introduction to case investigation and contact tracing, motivational interview skills, risk communication, problem solving, and emotional intelligence skills, cultural sensitivity, adaptations for contacts with hearing impairments

- Register: https://www.train.org/main/course/1091302/compilation
- Target audience: Contact tracers and case investigators
- Description: As a contact tracer, you will conduct interviews with people who may have been exposed to COVID-19. Depending on how your team is organized, you may also conduct interviews with persons under investigation (PUIs). Lesson 3 (Effective Communication and Interviews) will provide information on how to use effective communication techniques, prepare for and conduct an interview, and approach your interactions with cultural humility. Some of these terms may be new to you, and we'll cover them as we move through the lesson. Please note, lessons must be completed in order from one to four.

Learning objectives:

1) Name at least three communication techniques for effective interviewing
2) Explain the importance of showing cultural humility during case interviews
3) Describe how to prepare for an interview
4) Explain the four parts of an interview

General Contact Tracing Phone Calls

Topic area: Define case investigation, define contact tracing

- Register: https://www.train.org/main/course/1091008/
- Target audience: Volunteer callers for Michigan
- Description: This training is a generalized contact tracing training to prepare volunteers for assisting and completing contact calls for

persons who have been exposed to COVID19. The training briefly describes why contact training is important and what the process of contact training calls entails.

Learning objectives:

1) Discuss what is contact tracing and why it is important
2) Discuss how to de-escalate difficult conversations
3) Discuss the script when calling someone exposed
4) Describe resources available to you to answer questions
5) Review how you will be receiving contacts, how you should be documenting and sharing the information you have gathered, to whom you should be reporting, and how often

Interviewing Unit 5: Cluster Interviews and Re-Interviews

Topic area: Motivational interviewing skills

- Register: https://www.train.org/main/course/1089364/
- Target audience: STD partner services providers
- Description: Provides elements of cluster interviews for STD partner services providers. Includes the format of the interview and tips for providing risk reduction messages.

Learning objectives:

1) Identify the reasons and conditions for conducting a Cluster Interview, including planning
2) Identify the elements of the Cluster Interview format and the difference in formats between a Cluster Interview and an Original Interview
3) Explain the process for choosing a Cluster candidate

COVID-19 Contact Investigation Training

Topic area: Motivational interviewing skills

- View: https://www.ncsddc.org/wp-content/uploads/2020/03/FINAL-COVID19-Contact-Training-03112020.pdf
- Target audience: Case and contact investigators
- Description: This course covers background information on COVID-19, tools that Washington State is using for case investigation, interviewing techniques, and resources for case and contact investigations.

Learning objectives:

1) Discuss COVID-19 background
2) Discuss case investigation tools
3) Identify investigation interview techniques
4) Discuss types of contact follow-up
5) Identify COVID case and contact investigation resources

Effective Interviewing for Contact Investigation: Self-Study Modules

Topic area: Motivational interviewing skills

- View: https://www.cdc.gov/tb/publications/guidestoolkits/interviewing/tbinterviewing_ssmodules.pdf
- Target audience: TB interviewers
- Description: This resource will offer guidance to both new and experienced TB interviewers about how to communicate clearly with patients under various circumstances. Consists of 4 modules, including an overview of the TB interview for contact investigations, basics of communication and patient education, cultural competency, and special interview circumstances.

Learning objectives:

1) Define a TB interview
2) Formulate a TB interview strategy
3) Identify who requires a TB interview and for what reasons
4) Prioritize TB interviews based on various factors
5) Determine an infectious period for contact identification
6) Conduct a TB interview in a logical and productive manner
7) Conduct a re-interview asking the appropriate follow-up questions
8) Explain why patient education is important in the TB interview process
9) Define communication
10) Identify verbal and nonverbal patient cues and their meanings
11) Use closed, open-ended, and focused questions to gather descriptive, yet targeted information
12) Utilize the techniques of reflection, paraphrasing, and summarizing to affect the course of the interview
13) Address and overcome communication barriers
14) Select, and communicate through, an appropriate interpreter
15) Apply effective communication concepts to patient education
16) Describe the concepts of culture and cultural competency
17) Identify various factors that contribute to an individual's culture
18) Understand why cultural competency is essential in TB interviewing
19) Assess the communication process based on a patient's verbal and nonverbal cues
20) Limit the barriers of language, dialect, lifestyle, and belief differences during an interview
21) Describe how TB interviews may vary depending on the patient's life circumstances
22) Decide when to use, how to choose, and how to interview a proxy
23) Conduct a source case interview by selecting an appropriate interviewee and eliciting appropriate contact and exposure setting information
24) Conduct interviews in outbreak circumstances

25) Understand social network analysis and the role the interviewer plays

Introduction to Telephone Interviewing for DIS

Topic areas: Motivational interviewing skills

- Watch: https://www.train.org/main/course/1090632
- Target audience: STD partner services providers
- Description: This module will introduce partner services providers (i.e., DIS) to the basic principles and best practices for conducting telephone interviews. It covers professionalism, confidentiality and cultural competency. Learners also learn how to prepare for and conduct a telephone interview.

Learning objectives:

1) Demonstrate confidence when planning and conducting telephone interviews
2) Understand principles and best practices for conducting telephone interviews
3) Improve communication skills and maximize interviewing effectiveness

TB Contact Investigation Interviewing Skills Course: Introduction to Contact Investigation Process

Topic areas: Motivational interviewing skills

- View: https://www.cdc.gov/tb/education/skillscourse/default.htm
- Target audience: Public health professionals

- Description: The TB Contact Investigation Interviewing Skills Course is designed as an interactive, skill-building training. The course provides an overview of the contact investigation process, basic communication and interviewing skills, and opportunities to apply those skills in role play activities.

Learning objectives:

1) Explain the purpose of a TB contact investigation
2) Describe core concepts and skills that are required to conduct a TB contact investigation
3) Determine when to initiate a TB contact investigation
4) Describe the systematic approach to conducting a TB contact investigation

COVID-19 Public Health Strategy Basic Concepts – NDPHTN

Topic areas: Risk communication, problem solving, and emotional intelligence skills

- Register: https://www.train.org/main/course/1090675/
- Target audience: Public health professionals
- Description: Provide a basic background to the COVID-19 pandemic and describe the important steps to flatten the curve of COVID-19. Also provides an overview of crisis communication strategies and coordinating crisis response.

Learning objectives:

1) Review coronavirus history
2) Review COVID-19 characteristics
3) Discuss 6 concepts to flatten the curve
4) Review the 10 social distancing recommendations

5) Review COVID-19 testing concepts
6) Discuss how cocooning protects high risk individuals
7) Discuss key concepts of crisis communications in pandemics

Introduction for Trauma Informed Care for DIS

Topic area: Risk communication, problem solving, and emotional intelligence skills

- Register: https://cdc.train.org/cdctrain/course/1090752/
- Target audience: Public health professionals
- Description: This course is designed to introduce Disease Intervention Specialists (DIS) to the principles and strategies of trauma-informed care, so they are equipped with the knowledge and tools necessary to support clients who have experienced trauma. This course includes many printable resources to refer back to and to include in your DIS toolkit.

Learning objectives:

1) Summarize the definition of trauma and its impact on the brain
2) Describe the conceptual framework for trauma-informed care
3) Provide at least two examples of applying trauma-informed care in the DIS context

CERC Overview for COVID-19

Topic area: Risk communication, problem solving, and emotional intelligence skills

- Watch: https://emergency.cdc.gov/cerc/training/webinar_20200406.asp

- Target audience: Public health professionals
- Description: Provide an overview of crisis and emergency risk communication (CERC) principles and their application to COVID-19 messages.

Learning objectives:

1) Define the six crisis and emergency risk communication (CERC) principles
2) Describe the lifecycle of CERC and how communication works at each phase of a crisis
3) Describe how emergency risk communication is different from regular communication
4) Describe the psychology of a crisis
5) Describe the process for gathering audience feedback
6) Describe how to tailor messages to target audiences
7) Develop a crisis communication plan
8) List best practices of a spokesperson
9) Explain best practices for engaging stakeholders through communication during an emergency

Communication Skills

Topic area: Risk communication, problem solving, and emotional intelligence skills

- Register: https://www.train.org/main/course/1089357/
- Target audience: STD partner services providers
- Description: Provides learners with an understanding of the basic communication skills necessary for partner services providers, and to give them opportunities to practice those communication skills. This module also focuses on various problem solving techniques, and the importance of maintaining an assertive stance.

Learning objectives:

1) Describe factors associated with good communication
2) Identify barriers to communication
3) Define assertive, non-assertive, and aggressive communication and explain the distinctions between them

Disaster Health Core Curriculum: Competency 4: Communication

Topic area: Risk communication, problem solving, and emotional intelligence skills

- Watch: https://emergency.cdc.gov/cerc/training/webinar_20200406.asp
- Target audience: Public health professionals
- Description: Provides relevant, actionable guidance on applied principles and practices of crisis risk communication in public health emergencies and disasters.

Learning objectives:

1) Explain the operational relevance of the following concepts in the context of public health crisis risk communication: risk perception, mental noise, trust determination, and negative dominance
2) Explain the relevance of cultural competency in the context of public health emergency risk communication
3) Identify strategies to communicate in a culturally competent fashion in public health emergencies and disaster events
4) Identify authoritative sources for information gathering in a public health crisis and disasters that can inform effective emergency risk communication during and after these events

5) Demonstrate the features and utility of a message map as a tool for public health emergency risk communication

TB Contact Investigation Interviewing Skills Course: Communication Skills for Building Rapport during Contact Investigation Interviewing

Topic areas: Risk communication, problem solving, emotional intelligence skills

- View: https://www.cdc.gov/tb/education/skillscourse/default.htm
- Target audience: Public health professionals
- Description: The TB Contact Investigation Interviewing Skills Course is designed as an interactive, skill-building training. The course provides an overview of the contact investigation process, basic communication and interviewing skills, and opportunities to apply those skills in role play activities.

Learning objectives:

1) Describe how to build rapport
2) List at least six effective communication skills
3) Describe assertive, passive, and aggressive behavior

TB Contact Investigation Interviewing Skills Course: Special Circumstances

Topic areas: Risk communication, problem solving, emotional intelligence skills

- View: https://www.cdc.gov/tb/education/skillscourse/default.htm
- Target audience: Public health professionals

- Description: The TB Contact Investigation Interviewing Skills Course is designed as an interactive, skill-building training. The course provides an overview of the contact investigation process, basic communication and interviewing skills, and opportunities to apply those skills in role play activities.

Learning objectives:

1) Decide when to use a proxy for an interview
2) Explain how to work with the management of congregate settings
3) List two strategies for working with the media during a contact investigation

Receiving Feedback

Topic area: Risk communication, problem solving, emotional intelligence skills

- Register: https://www.train.org/main/course/1059257/
- Target audience: Public health professionals
- Description: Explores the reactions that typically occur when a person receives corrective feedback or criticism. Learn an approach to receive feedback in a productive manner and practice receiving feedback using that approach.

Learning objectives: Not available

Health Literacy for Public Health Professionals

Topic area: Cultural sensitivity

- Register: https://www.train.org/main/course/1078759/
- Target audience: Public health professionals

- Description: The purpose of this web-based training program is to educate health professionals about public health literacy and their role in providing health information and services and promoting public health literacy. The course uses a 508-compliant template, knowledge checks, scenario-based interactions, video clips, and a post-test to engage learners. The course includes an evaluation, glossary, and resource list.

Learning objectives:

1) Define public health literacy
2) List factors that influence public health literacy
3) Identify who is affected by public health literacy
4) Identify consequences of limited public health literacy
5) Determine who the stakeholders in public health literacy are
6) Recognize the role of public health literacy in meeting core public health services
7) Apply lessons learned to improve public health literacy

COVID-19 Case and Contact Investigations Training for Tribes

Topic area: Cultural sensitivity

- Watch: https://register.gotowebinar.com/recording/9127662154523742734
- View slides: https://secureservercdn.net/50.62.172.232/tvl.3bf.myftpupload.com/wp-content/uploads/2020/03/Slides-Case-and-Contact-Investigations-Training-for-Tribes-03-27-2020.pdf
- Target audience: Native American tribes
- Description: This course provides information for Tribes to help them determine whether they will conduct case and contact investigations for COVID-19 or defer to Washington State.

Additionally, the course provides training for tribal staff to conduct case and contact investigations.

Learning objectives:

1) Describe why case and contact investigation is important for Tribes
2) Discuss COVID-19 background
3) Identify investigation interview techniques
4) Discuss case investigation tools
5) Discuss public health recommendations for contacts
6) Discuss types of contact follow-up
7) Identify COVID case and contact investigation resources

TB Contact Investigation Interviewing Skills Course: Cultural and Diversity Considerations

Topic area: Cultural sensitivity

- View: https://www.cdc.gov/tb/education/skillscourse/default.htm
- Target audience: Public health professionals
- Description: The TB Contact Investigation Interviewing Skills Course is designed as an interactive, skill-building training. The course provides an overview of the contact investigation process, basic communication and interviewing skills, and opportunities to apply those skills in role play activities.

Learning objectives:

1) Define cultural competency
2) State of the four elements of cross-cultural communication

The Guide to Providing Effective Communication and Language Assistance Services

Topic area: Cultural sensitivity, adaptations for contacts with communication impairments

- Register: https://thinkculturalhealth.hhs.gov/education/communication-guide
- Target audience: Health care providers
- Description: The Guide will help your organization communicate in a way that considers the cultural, health literacy, and language needs of your patients.

Learning objectives:

1) Cross-cultural communication skills
2) Verbal communication strategies
3) Written communication strategies
4) Notice of communication and language assistance services

Cultural Competency Program for Disaster Preparedness and Crisis Response

Topic area: Cultural sensitivity

- Register: https://thinkculturalhealth.hhs.gov/education/disaster-personnel
- Target audience: Any disaster or emergency response personnel interested in learning more about culturally and linguistically appropriate services
- Description: Research shows that cultural minority groups suffer disproportionately during every phase of a disaster. This e-learning

program will equip you with the knowledge, skills, and awareness to best serve all individuals, regardless of cultural or linguistic background.

Learning objectives:

1) Course 1 provides an introduction to CLAS and its relevance to disaster preparedness and crisis response
2) Course 2 covers how to provide CLAS during the preparation phase of a disaster, including conducting a community needs assessment
3) Course 3 covers how to provide CLAS during the response phase of a disaster, including meeting physical and mental health needs
4) Course 4 covers how to provide CLAS during the recovery phase of a disaster, including rebuilding neighborhoods

Implicit Bias in Public Health Practice

Topic area: Cultural sensitivity

- Register: https://www.mitrainingcenter.org/courses/ibpha1219
- Target audience: Public health professionals
- Description: The field of public health increasingly focuses on health equity and population health outcomes. While systemic factors are major drivers of inequities, what is the role of the individual? This recorded webinar will introduce the idea of implicit bias and how it is relevant to all public health professionals, regardless of discipline or role in an agency. Participants will learn key definitions, examine data showing the implications of implicit bias in public health, and discuss some strategies to prevent it. Ultimately, no matter how well-intended, we all have some biases we can address to improve our positive impact on population health and on each other.

Learning objectives:

1) Define implicit bias and its relation to public health practice
2) Reflect on personal and professional biases
3) Introduce bias busting techniques

Cross-Cultural Communications Cognition and Linguistics – NDPHTN

Topic area: Cultural sensitivity

- Register: https://www.train.org/main/course/1087168/
- Target audience: Public health professionals
- Description: This training is facilitated through the North Dakota Public Health Training network to explain cross-cultural communications, cognition and linguistics.

Learning objectives:

1) Describe the process of developing meaning in message respondents
2) Explain how meaning transfer relates to the communications model
3) Recognize the importance of the seven dimensions of cultural distance in cross-cultural communications
4) Describe the tri-systemic model of cognition and how that model applies to public health communications
5) Demonstrate the importance of stories for transmitting meaning in relationship cultures
6) Describe the breadth of worldwide languages and dialects
7) Describe the role of languages
8) Describe three basic steps to overcome language barriers
9) Explain the importance of horizontal communicators in effective community messaging

10) Briefly explain the importance of the semantic differential and language impact on culture

Cultural Humility: People, Principles, and Practice

Topic area: Cultural sensitivity

- Watch: https://www.youtube.com/watch?v=SaSHLbS1V4w
- Target audience: Public health professionals
- Description: "Cultural Humility: People, Principles and Practices," is a 30-minute documentary by San Francisco State professor Vivian Chávez, that mixes poetry with music, interviews, archival footage, and images of community, nature and dance to explain what Cultural Humility is and why we need it. The film describes a set of principles that guide the thinking, behavior and actions of individuals and institutions to positively affect interpersonal relationships as well as systems change.

Learning objectives:

1) Lifelong learning and critical self-reflection
2) Recognizing and changing power imbalances
3) Developing institutional accountability

Culturally Competent Public Health Practice for Deaf and Hard of Hearing Populations

Topic area: Adaptations for contacts with communication impairments

- Register: https://www.train.org/cdctrain/main/1087468/external icon

- Target audience: Public health and healthcare professionals
- Description: This training will present tools and knowledge for working with the deaf and hard of hearing community, as well as common misconceptions about deaf culture and sub-cultures within the community.

Learning objectives:

1) Create awareness of deaf culture and sub-cultures within the deaf community
2) Discuss the benefits and importance of working with a sign interpreter
3) Identify gaps in health literacy among the deaf community
4) Formulate best methods for working with deaf and hard of hearing community

Other Files and Webpages

Topic area: Foundational principles of public heath

- The Public Health System & the 10 Essential Public Health Services
    - Agency name: CDC

Topic area: Notification of exposed individuals (contacts)

- Coronavirus – Known Contact to a Confirmed Case of Coronavirus Messaging Guide
    - Agency name: Public Health Madison and Dade County

COVID-19 Contact Investigation Interim Script

- Agency name: Washington Department of Health Resource

LIST REQUIREMENTS FOR PROTECTING HEALTH INFORMATION

Emerging Respiratory Viruses, Including COVID-19: Methods for Detection, Prevention, Response and Control

Topic area: Foundational principles of public health

- Register: https://www.train.org/main/course/1090092/
- Target audience: Public health professionals
- Description: This course provides a general introduction to COVID-19.

Learning objectives:

1) Describe the nature of emerging respiratory viruses, how to detect and assess an outbreak, strategies for preventing and controlling outbreaks due to novel respiratory viruses
2) Describe strategies that should be used to communicate risk and engage communities to detect, prevent and respond to the emergence of a novel respiratory virus

IDPH Office of Health Protection Data Security & Confidentiality Guideline Training

Topic areas: Health information privacy/security, health information data security

- Register: https://www.train.org/main/course/1058826/
- Target audience: Local public health staff who have access to confidential information

- Description: The purpose of this training is to provide an overview of the Data Security and Confidentiality Guidelines developed by the Illinois Department of Public Health Office of Health Protection and review the federal and state statutes, rules, and regulations that address the legal protection of confidential health information. This course also outlines the standards and requirements for state and local health department staff as well as community based organizations in the collection, transmission, storage, and maintenance of confidential information.

Learning objectives:

1) Provide an overview of the Data Security and Confidentiality Guidelines
2) Review federal and state statutes, rules, and regulations regarding health information
3) Outlines the standards and requirements for state and local health department staff as well as community-based organizations in the collection, transmission, storage, and maintenance of confidential information
4) Understand your role in keeping data secure in terms of: data collection, data sharing and release, and physical security

HIPAA Awareness – Module 1

Topic areas: Health information privacy and confidentiality

- Register: https://www.train.org/main/course/1047429/
- Target audience: Public health and healthcare professionals
- Description: This 20-minute HIPAA Awareness Training was developed by the Kansas Department of Health and Environment and is provided for the convenience of Kansas public health and healthcare agencies. We recommend this course for new employees,

employees who have not had HIPAA training in the past or as a refresher course.

Learning objectives:

1) Explain the source of HIPAA
2) Identify two HIPAA rules
3) Indicate two on-site HIPAA information sources
4) Identify two violation consequences

ADH HIPAA Privacy and Security Training

Topic areas: Health information privacy and confidentiality

- Register: https://www.train.org/main/course/1009552/
- Target audience: General Public Health Staff
- Description: This training is designed to help educate Arkansas Department of Health (ADH) staff concerning HIPAA legislation, the proper use and disclosure of protected health information (PHI), the proper safeguards for confidential information including electronic protected health information (ePHI) or other confidential information), and highlights from ADH HIPAA Policies and Procedures. It is not intended to replace ADH Policies.

Learning objectives:

1) Describe HIPAA
2) Discuss the proper use and disclosure of protected health information
3) Identify safeguards for confidential information including electronic protected health information
4) Explain ADH HIPAA Policies and Procedures

Health Information Privacy and Confidentiality

Topic areas: Health information privacy and confidentiality

- Register: https://www.train.org/main/course/1065718/
- Target audience: Allied health professionals, nurses, general public health staff, information systems professionals
- Description: Medical records are subject to privacy and confidentiality. This webinar will explore existing regulations and Health Insurance Portability and Accountability Act (HIPAA) as it relates to patient information. As we embark on the age of highly efficient technological capabilities, the ability to protect medical records has many challenges. Building public trust brings awareness to how privacy and confidentiality are properly handled through the course of research or student projects. We will discuss general aspects centered on the sensitive subject of cyberspace and medical record security. Recommendations based on the laws that govern privacy, along with research findings, will be shared.

Learning objectives:

1) Explain patient privacy and confidentiality as it relates to HIPAA
2) Discuss who has rights to patient records
3) Assess advantages and disadvantages of electronic records
4) Discuss APUS and HIPAA

COVID-19: Data Sharing for Public Health Surveillance, Investigation and Intervention

Topic areas: Health information privacy and confidentiality, ethics of data collection during an outbreak

- Register: https://www.train.org/main/course/1090857/

- Target audience: Public health professionals
- Description: Public health's COVID-19 surveillance, investigation and intervention balances an individual's right to privacy against the public's and other's right to know. Amid the COVID-19 outbreak, questions about data sharing under a national emergency have surfaced. Is HIPAA still fully in effect during this public health emergency? How does HIPAA apply to public health departments? What COVID-19 information may public health share with the media, emergency responders, law enforcement and others? This webinar will identify various federal and state laws, including HIPAA, that impact public health's ability to share COVID-19 information.

Learning objectives:

1) Review current data sharing questions facing your peers
2) Understand HIPAA's data sharing limitations and opportunities
3) Provide an awareness of other federal and state law considerations

Information Privacy & Security (IPS)

Topic area: Health information data security

- Register: https://about.citiprogram.org/en/series/information-privacy-and-security-ips/
- Target audience: Teachers, educators, IRB administrators, administrators, IRB members, individuals working with identifiable health data (HIPAA-defined "PHI"), researchers, instructors, students
- Description: IPS covers the principles of data protection, focusing on the healthcare-related privacy and information security requirements of the Health Insurance Portability and Accountability Act (HIPAA) and the educational records and data-related

requirements of the Family Educational Rights and Privacy Act (FERPA).

Data Management in Disasters & Public Health Emergencies Recording

Topic area: Ethics of data collection during an outbreak

- Register: https://www.train.org/main/course/1080061/
- Target audience: Researchers, analysts, public health professionals, information systems professionals
- Description: Nicole Strayhorn, National Library of Medicine Associate Fellow, discussed the results of her project to identify open data sources and data sharing policies used during disasters and public health emergencies. For the purposes of this short-term project, she narrowed her research to the data needs of stakeholders, and the challenges of sharing and accessing data around the ongoing Zika virus outbreak.

Describe the Qualities, Skills, and Styles of Effective Case Investigator Supervisors

TB Contact Investigation Interviewing Skills Course—Providing Feedback

Topic areas: Qualities and skills of effective supervisors

- View: https://www.cdc.gov/tb/education/skillscourse/day3/day-3-providing-feedback_final.pptx
- Target audience: Trainers and supervisors

- Description: The TB Contact Investigation Interviewing Skills Course is designed as an interactive, skill-building training to improve the abilities of both new and experienced staff who are responsible for conducting TB contact investigation interviews. The course provides an overview of the contact investigation process, basic communication and interviewing skills, and opportunities to apply those skills in role play activities.

Learning objectives:

1) Why is feedback important?
2) Components of constructive feedback
3) Order of feedback
4) Receiving feedback

Leadership Introduction – NDPHTN

Topic areas: Qualities and skills of effective team leads

- View: https://www.train.org/main/course/1086530/
- Target audience: Public health professionals
- Description: The goal of this course is to define why leadership is important is for public health.

Learning objectives:

1) Define leadership
2) Explain why adaptive leadership is important for public health
3) Define the difference between social marketing and community engagement
4) Discuss some basic concepts of extreme leadership

Principles and Practices of Public Health Management – NDPHTN

Topic areas: Qualities and skills of effective team leads, management styles

- Register: https://www.train.org/main/course/1086536/
- Target audience: Public health professionals
- Description: The goal of this course is to learn about some principles and practices for public health management.

Learning objectives:

1) Review Fayol's 14 principles of management
2) Discuss how the 4 leadership styles relate to centralization and decentralization
3) Briefly introduce and discuss informal groups, the quality improvement process, organizational planning, negotiations, dispute resolution, and measuring a manager's performance

Leadership Management Communication

Topic areas: Qualities and skills of effective team leads, management styles

- Register: https://www.train.org/main/course/1012711/
- Target audience: Public health professionals
- Description: No matter how effective a leader/manager you already are, this course is designed to refresh and refine the skills needed to lead your teams to success in today's fast-paced and stressful health care environment. By exploring effective leadership styles and

strategies, this course provides specific tools to enhance leadership/ management communication.

Learning objectives:

1) Identify the differences between leadership and management, describe the tasks and essentials of effective leadership, and identify the difference between dissonant and resonant leadership styles
2) Understand how and why well-intentioned management strategies sometimes backfire, and how to keep that from happening
3) Apply strategies that enable you to think, react, communicate, and lead with higher levels of emotional intelligence
4) Identify the major reasons for low employee motivation and utilize strategies that motivate and inspire the workforce to maximize individual and group performance
5) Understand ways to identify morale problems and apply strategies that ameliorate or rectify morale problems as well as negative mood contagion
6) Increase your ability to promote ideas and plans through the application of specific persuasion and influence strategies
7) Understand the qualities of an effective change manager
8) Understand the characteristics and components of successful teams and apply strategies to enhance team communication

Volunteer Management for Emergency Response

Topic area: Qualities and skills of effective team leads

- Register: https://u-m-canvas.it.umich.edu/courses/354/pages/course-details?module_item_id=3057
- Target audience: Public health professionals responsible for working with volunteers of different professional backgrounds during times of emergency response.

- Description: This live webinar will provide examples of ways in which local health departments are mobilizing and training volunteers to respond to COVID-19, along with best practices for training and managing volunteers for short-term and long-term activities related to emergency response in general.

Learning objectives:

1) Discuss best practices for managing volunteers during rapidly changing situations
2) Identify strategies for training volunteers for short-term and simple volunteer opportunities
3) Recognize different approaches needed to train volunteers for long-term and more complex volunteer opportunities

Leading at a Distance

Topic areas: Management of remote teams

- Register: https://www.linkedin.com/learning/leading-at-a-distance/remote-workers-are-the-future-of-business
- Target audience: Remote supervisors
- Description: Technology has enabled many former office workers to work from home or anywhere remotely. As the overall job landscape shifts, the number of remote workers will likely continue to increase. For the managers and leaders spearheading these remote teams, as well as teams that consist of remote and in-person employees, making the jump from in-person to virtual leadership can be challenging. In this course, instructor Kevin Eikenberry lays out how to lead effectively from a distance. He dives into the basics of remote leadership, such as how working remotely changes interpersonal dynamics. Plus, he shares tips for getting results at a distance—including how to provide remote coaching and

feedback—as well as how to build trust, set reasonable boundaries as a long-distance leader, and more.

Learning objectives:

1) How did we get to remote teams?
2) The remote leadership model
3) What success looks like at a distance
4) Providing coaching and feedback
5) How remote politics works
6) Building trust at a distance
7) Communicating effectively
8) Leveraging technology as a remote leader
9) Getting honest feedback

Managing a Virtual Team

Topic areas: Management of remote teams

- Register: https://www.linkedin.com/learning/managing-virtual-teams-4/managing-people-at-a-distance
- Target audience: Remote supervisors
- Description: Working remotely has been on the rise for many years now, with research showing that hiring managers expect nearly half of all their workers to be working remotely over the next decade. While many trends feed into this way of organizing work, managing the work effectively will be key to the success of organizations globally. In this course, instructor Phil Gold provides managers with a clear approach for getting the most out of their remote teams. He zeros in on the key factors that will ensure productivity, engagement, and growth, as well as a manager's role in building trust, removing roadblocks, nurturing connections with team members, and setting clear goals.

Learning objectives:

1) Providing consistency and structure in a remote team
2) Managing mixed remote and onsite teams
3) Fostering equality and transparency
4) Creating opportunities for in-person interactions
5) Maintaining regular contact with remote team members
6) Managing workloads and deliverables

Leading Virtual Meetings

Topic areas: Management of remote teams

- Register: https://www.linkedin.com/learning/leading-virtual-meetings/welcome-to-better-virtual-meetings
- Target audience: Remote professionals
- Description: Leading virtual meetings is a critical competency for leaders who manage a remote or blended team. Join leadership and management expert Kevin Eikenberry as he identifies the challenges to holding a productive meeting online, and shares tactics for making these meetings successful. Learn about how to choose the right platform, set expectations for conduct, clarify roles, create a great agenda, and more.

Learning objectives:

1) The challenges of virtual meetings
2) Choosing the right platform to meet virtually
3) Setting clear behavioral expectations
4) Innovating in a virtual meeting
5) Pre-determining a desired outcome
6) Creating a great meeting agenda

7) Facilitating virtual meetings
8) Encouraging participation
9) Keeping on track in the moment
10) Ending a meeting with an action plan

Time Management: Working from Home

Topic areas: Management of remote teams

- Register: https://www.linkedin.com/learning/time-management-working-from-home/welcome
- Target audience: Remote professionals
- Description: Working from home is a wonderful opportunity, but time management can be a challenge. With so many demands on your time and attention, it's a tricky balancing act to stay productive. In this course, bestselling author and productivity expert Dave Crenshaw offers best practices for anyone who works full- time or occasionally from home. Dave begins by showing how to set up a dedicated workspace for maximum productivity, including tips on setting up your computer to ensure you stay focused. Then Dave walks through how to craft your daily schedule for peak productivity and plan meaningful breaks to avoid burnout. He explains how to collaborate with remote coworkers, including how to use virtual meetings productively. Finally, Dave offers advice for working parents and other caregivers who might be balancing professional and personal responsibilities in the home.

Learning objectives:

1) Create a productive environment by limiting distractions
2) Evaluate and choose the best technology to increase your productivity
3) Differentiate between constant effort and a healthy working rhythm

4) Define expectations around communication while remaining responsive
5) Identify the benefits of relationship building
6) Learn how to manage interruptions and emergencies at home

Thriving in an Online Work Environment

Topic area: Management of remote teams

- Register: https://rmphtc.org/thriving-in-an-online-work-environment/index.html#/
- Target audience: Trainers of case investigators and/or contact tracers in State and local health jurisdictions.
- Description: In early 2020, when the COVID-19 pandemic hit the U.S., much of the public health workforce suddenly shifted to full-time remote work and service delivery. These professionals immediately faced a number of critical challenges, from managing the stress of the crisis while maintaining productivity to converting in- person meetings and trainings to online settings. This course is full of tips, videos, and resources to help public health professionals stay productive and connected in an online environment.

Learning objectives:

1) Explore the various videos, tips, and resources provided to help you stay connected and motivated in an online environment
2) Recognize how stress can influence productivity during uncertain times and how to manage
3) Consider the various ways you can now facilitate online meetings
4) Recognize the various tools available to you if you need to convert in-person trainings

Building Resilience

Topic areas: Importance of resiliency

- Register: https://www.linkedin.com/learning/building-resilience/what-why-and-how-to-become-resilient
- Target audience: Working professionals
- Description: Have trouble getting by when the going gets tough? Everyone wants to perform well when the pressure's on, but a lot of us withdraw in times of stress or adversity. If you can build your resilience, you'll have an easier facing new challenges and earn a valuable skill to offer employers. In this course, Kelley School of Business professor and professional communications coach Tatiana Kolovou explains how to bounce back from difficult situations, by building your "resiliency threshold." She outlines five training techniques to prepare for difficult situations, and five strategies for reflecting on them afterward. Find out where you are on the resilience scale, identify where you want to be, and learn strategies to close the gap.

Learning objectives:

1) Define the term resilience
2) Identify strategies for facing rejection in your day to day life
3) Recognize the skills you can practice to increase your resilience
4) Explore reflection strategies you can use during a situation in order to build resilience
5) Examine five post-event resilience building strategies using real-world examples

Managing Stress for Positive Change

Topic areas: Importance of resiliency

- View: https://www.linkedin.com/learning/managing-stress-for-positive-change/welcome
- Target audience: Supervisors and managers
- Description: In the workplace, stress is often viewed in purely negative terms. It's seen as a response that should simply be minimized or pushed aside; however, it's possible to use stress to fuel positive change. In this course, join instructor Heidi Hanna, PhD as she discusses what stress is, exactly; how you can train yourself to use stress in more effective ways; and what managers can do to reduce employee stress when an organization experiences difficult times. She covers how individuals can use stress for good by assessing and adjusting it, as well as what you-as a manager-can do to create an environment and communication style that helps connect employees to the bigger picture.

Learning objectives:

1) Define "stress" and explain why it often occurs in the workplace
2) Recognize the differences between acute and chronic stress
3) List the three steps for managing stress
4) Name three things the brain craves
5) Identify the differences between primary stress reactions
6) Recall the benefits of rhythmic breathing

Identify Time Management Practices for Case Investigation and Contact Tracing Leads

Time Management: Working from Home

Topic areas: Time management

- Register: https://www.linkedin.com/learning/time-management-working-from-home/welcome
- Target audience: Remote professionals
- Description: Working from home is a wonderful opportunity, but time management can be a challenge. With so many demands on your time and attention, it's a tricky balancing act to stay productive. In this course, bestselling author and productivity expert Dave Crenshaw offers best practices for anyone who works full- time or occasionally from home. Dave begins by showing how to set up a dedicated workspace for maximum productivity, including tips on setting up your computer to ensure you stay focused. Then Dave walks through how to craft your daily schedule for peak productivity and plan meaningful breaks to avoid burnout. He explains how to collaborate with remote coworkers, including how to use virtual meetings productively. Finally, Dave offers advice for working parents and other caregivers who might be balancing professional and personal responsibilities in the home.

Learning objectives:

1) Create a productive environment by limiting distractions
2) Evaluate and choose the best technology to increase your productivity
3) Differentiate between constant effort and a healthy working rhythm
4) Define expectations around communication while remaining responsive
5) Identify the benefits of relationship building
6) Learn how to manage interruptions and emergencies at home

MONITOR PERFORMANCE OF CASE INVESTIGATORS

TB Contact Investigation Interviewing Skills Course—Providing Feedback

Topic areas: Feedback and follow-up

- View: https://www.cdc.gov/tb/education/skillscourse/day3/day-3-providing-feedback_final.pptx
- Target audience: Trainers and supervisors
- Description: The TB Contact Investigation Interviewing Skills Course is designed as an interactive, skill-building training to improve the abilities of both new and experienced staff who are responsible for conducting TB contact investigation interviews. The course provides an overview of the contact investigation process, basic communication and interviewing skills, and opportunities to apply those skills in role play activities.

Learning objectives:

1) Why is feedback important?
2) Components of constructive feedback
3) Order of feedback
4) Receiving feedback

Other Files and Webpages

Topic area: Historic references

- CDC Methods for Implementing and Managing Contact Tracing for Ebola virus Disease in Less-affected Countries
    - Agency name: CDC

- WHO Implementation and Management of Contact Tracing for Ebola Virus Disease
    - Agency name: WHO
- Guidelines for the Investigation of Contacts of Persons with Infectious Tuberculosis Recommendations from the National Tuberculosis Controllers Association and CDC
    - Agency name: CDC
- Performance Guidelines for Contact Investigation: The TB Interview—A Supervisor's Guide for the Development and Assessment of Interviewing Skills
    - Agency name: New Jersey Medical School Global TB Institute

In: Testing and Contract Tracing … ISBN: 978-1-53618-857-8
Editor: Ernesto M. Batista © 2020 Nova Science Publishers, Inc.

Chapter 10

CONTACT TRACING: PART OF A MULTIPRONGED APPROACH TO FIGHT THE COVID-19 PANDEMIC*

U.S. Department of Health and Human Services, Centers for Disease Control and Prevention

COVID-19 CONTACT TRACING FOR HEALTH DEPARTMENTS

This document highlights basic principles of *contact tracing* to stop COVID-19 transmission; detailed guidance for health departments and potential contact tracers is forthcoming.

Contact tracing, a core disease control measure employed by local and state health department personnel for decades, is a key strategy for preventing further spread of COVID-19. Immediate action is needed. Communities must scale up and train a large contact tracer workforce and

* This is an edited, reformatted and augmented version of Department of Health and Human Sevices publication, No. 316704A, dated April 29, 2020.

work collaboratively across public and private agencies to stop the transmission of COVID-19.

Certain core principles of contact tracing must always be adhered to:

- Contact tracing is part of the process of supporting patients with suspected or confirmed infection.
- In contact tracing, public health staff work with a patient to help them recall everyone with whom they have had close contact during the timeframe while they may have been infectious.
- Public health staff then warn these exposed individuals (contacts) of their potential exposure as rapidly and sensitively as possible.
- To protect patient privacy, contacts are only informed that they may have been exposed to a patient with the infection. They are not told the identity of the patient who may have exposed them.
- Contacts are provided with education, information, and support to understand their risk, what they should do to separate themselves from others who are not exposed, monitor themselves for illness, and the possibility that they could spread the infection to others even if they themselves do not feel ill.
- Contacts are encouraged to stay home and maintain social distance from others (at least 6 feet) until 14 days after their last exposure, in case they also become ill. They should monitor themselves by checking their temperature twice daily and watching for cough or shortness of breath. To the extent possible, public health staff should check in with contacts to make sure they are self-monitoring and have not developed symptoms. Contacts who develop symptoms should promptly isolate themselves and notify public health staff. They should be promptly evaluated for infection and for the need for medical care.

Contact Tracing Is a Specialized Skill

To be done effectively, it requires people with the training, supervision, and access to social and medical support for patients and contacts. Requisite knowledge and skills for contact tracers include, but are not limited to:

- An understanding of patient confidentiality, including the ability to conduct interviews without violating confidentiality (e.g., to those who might overhear their conversations)
- Understanding of the medical terms and principles of exposure, infection, infectious period, potentially infectious interactions, symptoms of disease, pre-symptomatic and asymptomatic infection
- Excellent and sensitive interpersonal, cultural sensitivity, and interviewing skills such that they can build and maintain trust with patients and contacts
- Basic skills of crisis counseling, and the ability to confidently refer patients and contacts for further care if needed
- Resourcefulness in locating patients and contacts who may be difficult to reach or reluctant to engage in conversation
- Understanding of when to refer individuals or situations to medical, social, or supervisory resources
- Cultural competency appropriate to the local community

Contact Tracing Is Part of the Process of Supporting Patients and Warning Contacts of Exposure in Order to Stop Chains of Transmission

Given the magnitude of COVID-19 cases and plans to eventually relax mitigation efforts such as stay at home orders and social distancing, communities need a large number of trained contact tracers. These contact tracers need to quickly locate and talk with the patients, assist in arranging for patients to isolate themselves, and work with patients to identify people with whom the patients have been in close contact so the contact tracer can locate them. The actual number of staff needed is large and varies depending on a number of factors including but not limited to:

- The daily number of cases
- The number of contacts identified
- How quickly patients are isolated, and contacts are notified and advised to stay home, self-monitor, and maintain social distance from others

THE TIME TO START BUILDING THE TRAINED WORKFORCE IS NOW

Time is of the Essence

Identifying contacts and ensuring they do not interact with others is critical to protect communities from further spread. If communities are unable to effectively isolate patients and ensure contacts can separate themselves from others, rapid community spread of COVID-19 is likely to increase to the point that strict mitigation strategies will again be needed to contain the virus.

Contact tracers need to:

- Immediately identify and interview people with SARS CoV-2 infections and COVID-19 (i.e., disease)
- Support isolation of those who are infected
- Warn contacts of their exposure, assess their symptoms and risk, and provide instructions for next steps
- Link those with symptoms to testing and care

Based on our current knowledge, a close contact is someone who was within 6 feet of an infected person for at least 15 minutes starting from 48 hours before illness onset until the time the patient is isolated. They should stay home, maintain social distancing, and self-monitor until 14 days from the last date of exposure.

Contact Investigation in Care Facilities, Other Congregate Living Settings and Households with Many People Living in One House Is a Priority

Contact investigation of patients with COVID-19 potentially exposed at work and patients in health care facilities, congregate living settings or housing with many people is complex. Appropriate engagement with infection control and occupational health programs is recommended. Priority settings include:

- Health care facilities including long-term care facilities
- Group home/board
- Homeless shelters
- Federal, state and local correctional facilities
- Crowded, multigenerational housing

In addition to health care workers, it is important to assess interactions between residents and all staff, including but not limited to activity coordinators, food service staff, and sanitation management. Transitional case management plans should be put in place for patients in isolation and contacts who are separated for monitoring. Management plans should also be created for transitioning from one setting to another, such as transitions from hospitals to acute or long-term care facilities or home isolation, or from prison and jail to parole and probation.

Social Services and Housing Will Be Needed for Contacts Unable to Separate Themselves from Others in Their Current Living Situation

Separating contacts from people who are not exposed is critical to the success of any contact tracing effort and requires social supports for individual compliance and medical monitoring. First and foremost is the assessment of an individual's ability to stay in home and maintain social distance from others, a safe environment that provides the necessary supports (private room and bathroom, adequate food and water, and access to medication) and the ability to practice adequate infection control. For a portion of the U.S. population this will be a challenge, particularly for some of the most vulnerable populations.

Support services for consideration include but may not be limited to housing, food, medicine, and economic supports. For contacts without a primary care provider, linkage to clinical care may be needed. Support for medical monitoring includes patient care packages (e.g., thermometers, sanitizers, mask, gloves) and technological supports for medical monitoring (e.g., mobile phone apps). If possible, contacts should be asked to voluntarily stay home, monitor themselves, and maintain social distancing from others.

However, health departments have the authority to issue legal orders of quarantine, should the situation warrant that measure.

Communication with the Public Is Crucial

Engagement of the public with contact tracers must be widely accepted in order to protect friends, family, and community members from future potential infections.

Key public officials and community leaders will need to be engaged and supportive of contact tracing efforts. Consider reaching out to community leaders as part of the neighborhood-level contact tracing team. To be successful, a community will need public awareness, and understanding and acceptance of contact tracing and the need for contacts to separate themselves from others who are not exposed. Community members need to take responsibility to follow the guidance from public health agencies.

Data Management and Technology Will Be Needed

Case investigation, contact tracing, and contact follow-up and monitoring will need to be linked with timely testing, clinical services, and agile data management systems to facilitate real-time electronic transmission of laboratory and case data for public health action.

Technology partners are key in the modification of existing systems and the development of new user-friendly data interfaces to manage multiple data streams with seamless interoperability. Case management tools can help automate key pieces of the contact tracing process, making the overall process more efficient. Ideally, data systems would also include automated reports to aid in monitoring progress and outcomes of contact tracing. Data sharing agreements between local, tribal and state, and federal jurisdictions need to be established or augmented to ensure timely and accurate data collection and sharing. The adoption of emerging technologies that can assist private and public health practitioners with client communication, medical monitoring, and strategies to amplify contact tracing may greatly help with scaling up contact tracing as needed.

Ongoing Monitoring and Assessment of Contact Tracing Efforts Will Be Needed

Public health agencies and their partners will need to monitor some key components of their programs to improve performance as needed. Potential metrics routinely reviewed could include the following process and outcome measures:

- Case interviewing: Time to interview from symptom onset and from diagnosis; proportion interviewed; median number of contacts elicited; proportion with no contacts elicited.
- Contact notification: Proportion of contacts notified; time from first potential exposure to notification.
- Contact follow-up: Daily proportion of contacts whose status is evaluated; proportion of contacts with symptoms evaluated within 24 hours of onset of symptoms; proportion of contacts who complete their full self-monitoring period.
- Contact tracing efficacy: Percent of new COVID-19 cases arising among contacts during self-monitoring period.

In: Testing and Contract Tracing … ISBN: 978-1-53618-857-8
Editor: Ernesto M. Batista © 2020 Nova Science Publishers, Inc.

Chapter 11

CONTACT TRACING – CDC'S ROLE AND APPROACH*

U.S. Department of Health and Human Services, Centers for Disease Control and Prevention

OVERVIEW

Contact tracing is an effective disease control strategy that involves investigating cases and their contacts and then interrupting disease transmission—typically by asking cases to isolate and contacts to quarantine at home voluntarily. Contact tracing is a key strategy to prevent the further spread of COVID-19.

Case investigation is the identification and investigation of patients with confirmed and probable diagnoses of COVID-19 (cases). *Contact tracing*, also referred to as contact investigation, is the identification, monitoring, and support of the individuals (contacts) who have been exposed to the patient

* This is an edited, reformatted and augmented version of Department of Health and Human Services publication, No. CS 317432-A, dated 06/11/2020.

and possibly infected themselves. This process prevents further transmission of disease by separating people who have (or may have) an infectious disease from people who do not.

> Prompt identification, voluntary isolation or quarantine, and monitoring of a person diagnosed with COVID-19 and their contacts can effectively break the chain of disease transmission and prevent further spread of the virus. Case investigation and contact tracing are core disease control measures that have been used by state and local health departments for decades to slow or stop the spread of infectious diseases.

Core Principles of Contact Tracing During the COVID-19 Pandemic

Contact tracing should be conducted for close contacts of confirmed or probable COVID-19 patients.

Contact tracing steps include:

1. Case investigation: Public health staff work with a patient to help them recall everyone with whom they have had close contact during the time when they may have been infectious. For COVID-19, a close contact is defined as any individual who was within 6 feet of an infected person for at least 15 minutes starting from 48 hours before the person began feeling sick until the time the patient is isolated.
2. Contact tracing: Public health staff begin contact tracing by notifying exposed individuals (contacts) of their potential exposure as rapidly and sensitively as possible, not revealing the infected patient's identity.
3. Contact support: Contacts are provided with education, information, and support to help them understand their risk, what they should do to separate themselves from others who are not exposed, and how to monitor themselves for illness. In addition, they are informed of the

possibility that they could spread the infection to others even if they themselves do not feel ill.

4. Self-quarantine: Contacts are encouraged to stay home and maintain social distance from others (at least 6 feet) until 14 days after their last exposure to the infected patient, in case they also become ill.

Every effort should be made to interview the patient and contacts by telephone, text, or video conference instead of in person. Contact tracing is a labor-intensive process that requires a well-trained workforce of effective communicators who can approach individuals with compassion and build trust.

CDC's Role in COVID-19 Contact Tracing

Communities must scale up and train a large case investigation and contact tracer workforce and work collaboratively across public and private agencies to stop the transmission of COVID-19. As the nation's public health agency and the primary resource for State, Tribal, Local, and Territorial (STLT) health departments on managing disease outbreaks, CDC's primary role in contact tracing is to provide guidance and support to help STLT health departments launch effective contact tracing programs. The ultimate goal is for STLT jurisdictions to have robust public health systems that include a fully developed contact tracing workforce.

In support of this goal, CDC is providing STLTs with guidance, training, and technical assistance on contact tracing.

CDC also provides COVID-19 assistance directly to STLT health departments through over 300 CDC field assignees embedded in health departments across the nation. Moreover, CDC links STLTs with other federal agencies, academia, and other organizations that offer contact tracing/case management staffing solutions.

To support surge staffing needs in health departments and tribal communities, CDC has funded the CDC Foundation to hire local staff to augment STLT jurisdictions' COVID response efforts, including contact tracing. The CDC Foundation will work with health departments and Area Indian Health Boards (AIHBs) to hire and place 665 public health professionals, including contact tracers, in health departments and AIHBs.

IMPORTANT CONSIDERATIONS FOR CONTACT TRACING

There are several key considerations for developing STLT jurisdictional contact tracing plans:

- Expanding staffing resources. Contact tracing in the United States will require that states, tribes, localities and territories recruit and hire adequate levels of well-trained case investigators and contact tracers.
- Training staff. Successful case investigation and contact tracing for COVID-19 depends on a robust and well-trained public health workforce. Contact tracing requires staff with adequate training, excellent and tactful interpersonal skills, cultural sensitivity, and language and interviewing skills that allow them to build and maintain trust with clients and contacts.
- Investigating cases and identifying contacts. Case investigators must be able to advise people with probable or confirmed COVID-19 infection to self-isolate immediately, if they are not doing so already. Case investigators also must be prepared to interview cases and ask them to identify people who may have been exposed (contacts). Investigators then need to provide support to help cases self-isolate and determine if they need social services.
- Tracing and monitoring contacts of infected people. Contact tracers must be able to notify contacts of their exposure, advise them to self-quarantine, and to self- monitor for COVID-19 symptoms. They need to be able to determine what support services contacts need to effectively self-quarantine.

- Monitoring the effectiveness of contact tracing. Public health officials should be prepared to monitor the completeness and timeliness of contact tracing activities, including the number of cases identified among contacts.
- Using digital tools. Adoption and evaluation of digital case management or contact tracing tools may make the traditional contact tracing process faster and more efficient.

CDC continues to engage with each state health department to review these key areas and address barriers that could prohibit them from effectively conducting contact tracing.

TOOLS AND RESOURCES

As many states face the need to rapidly scale up their staff capacity, CDC is providing programmatic guidance, technical assistance, and resources to help them hire and train new and existing staff. CDC has developed a range of guidance documents and is facilitating access to a variety of case investigation and contact tracing training products and tools for a diverse and evolving public health workforce. These products and tools are available through the Get and Keep America Open website, which is continuously updated. A wealth of information is available, including the Interim Guidance on Developing a COVID-19 Case Investigation & Contact Tracing Plan, resources on how to train a workforce, and guidance on using digital tools for contact tracing. CDC also partners with national organizations and other partners to identify and share lessons learned and promising practices associated with surge staffing and continuous improvement in contact tracing and case investigation practices.

In: Testing and Contract Tracing …
Editor: Ernesto M. Batista
ISBN: 978-1-53618-857-8
© 2020 Nova Science Publishers, Inc.

Chapter 12

CONTACT TRACING: DO YOUR PART TO KEEP YOUR FAMILY, FRIENDS, AND COMMUNITY SAFE*

U.S. Department of Health and Human Services, Centers for Disease Control and Prevention

WHAT YOU CAN EXPECT TO HAPPEN DURING CONTACT TRACING IF YOU HAVE BEEN DIAGNOSED WITH COVID-19

1. If you have been in close contact with someone who has COVID-19, a public health worker will call you to inform you that you may have been exposed to COVID-19.

---

* This is an edited, reformatted and augmented version of U.S. Department of Health and Human Services, Centers for Desease Control and Prevention publication CS317837-A.

Any information you share with public health workers is CONFIDENTIAL. This means that your personal and medical information will be kept private.

2. You should stay at home and self-quarantine for 14 days, starting from the last day you were possibly exposed to COVID-19.

Self-quarantine means staying home, monitoring your health, and maintaining social distancing (at least 6 feet) from others at all times.

3. The public health worker can provide information about COVID-19 testing in your area.

If you need support or assistance with self-quarantine, your health department or community organizations may be able to provide assistance.

4. If you become ill during the 14 days of self-quarantine, you should notify the health department and seek medical care if your symptoms worsen or become severe. Emergency warning signs include trouble breathing, persistent pain or pressure in the chest, confusion, inability to wake or stay awake, or bluish lips or face.

We can all work together to help slow the spread of COVID-19.

Do your part to keep your family and your community safe: Answer the call to slow the spread.

In: Testing and Contract Tracing … ISBN: 978-1-53618-857-8
Editor: Ernesto M. Batista © 2020 Nova Science Publishers, Inc.

Chapter 13

CONTACT TRACING APPS*

United States Government Accountability Office

WHY THIS MATTERS

Contact tracing can help reduce transmission rates for infectious diseases like COVID-19 by identifying and notifying people who may have been exposed. Contact tracing apps, notably those using proximity tracing, could expedite such efforts. However, there are challenges, including accuracy, adoption rates, and privacy concerns.

THE TECHNOLOGY

What is it? Contact tracing is a process in which public health officials attempt to limit disease transmission by identifying infected individuals,

* This is an edited, reformatted and augmented accessible version of the United States Government Accountability Office Publication, Science, Technology Assessment, and Analytics, No. GAO-20-666SP Contact Tracing Apps, dated July 2020.

notifying their "contacts"—all the people they may have transmitted the disease to—and asking infected individuals and their contacts toquarantine, if appropriate (see figure 1). For a highly contagious respiratory disease such as COVID-19, a contact could be anyone who has been nearby. Proximity tracing applications (apps) can expedite contact tracing, using smartphones to rapidly identify and notify contacts.

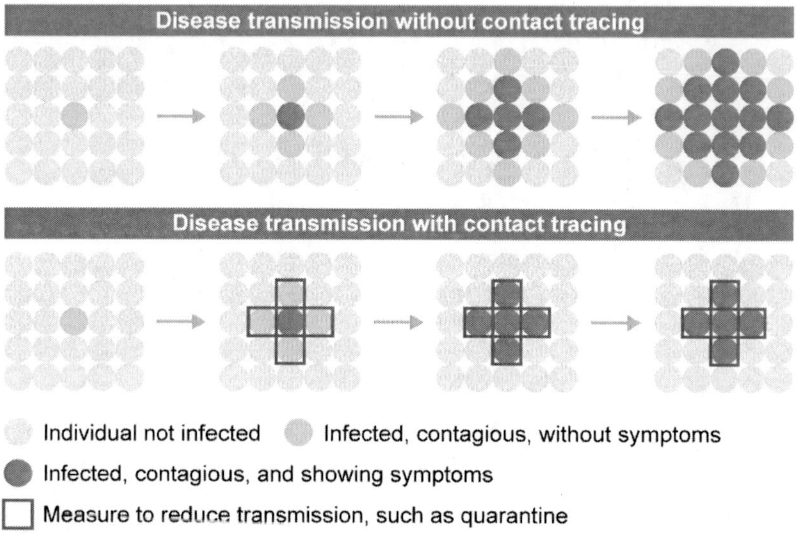

Source: Marcel Salathe and Nicky Case.| GAO-20-666SP.

Figure 1. A simplified depiction of disease transmission. Through contact tracing, an infected individual's contacts are notified and may be asked to quarantine. (In reality, some contacts may not become infected, and some of those infected may not show symptoms.)

How does it work? In traditional contact tracing, public health officials begin by identifying an infected individual. They then interview the individual to identify recent contacts, ask the individual and their contacts to take containment measures, if appropriate (e.g., a 14-day quarantine for COVID-19), and coordinate any needed care and testing. Proximity tracing apps may accelerate the process by replacing the time-consuming interviews needed to identify contacts. Apps may also identify more contacts than interviews, which rely on interviewees' recall and on their being acquainted with their contacts.

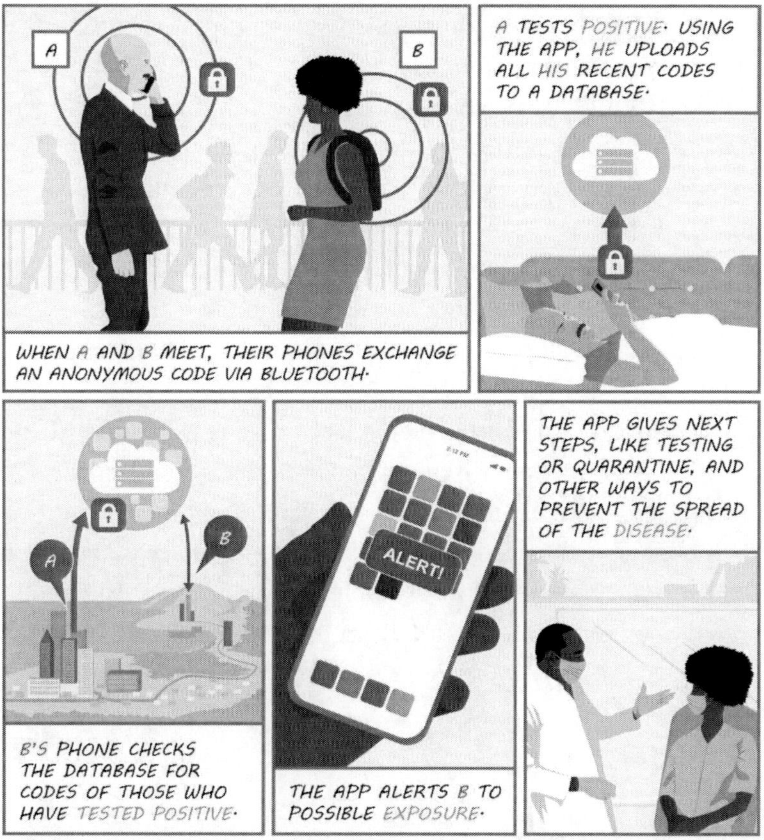
A
B
WHEN A AND B MEET, THEIR PHONES EXCHANGE AN ANONYMOUS CODE VIA BLUETOOTH.
A TESTS POSITIVE. USING THE APP, HE UPLOADS ALL HIS RECENT CODES TO A DATABASE.
A
B
B'S PHONE CHECKS THE DATABASE FOR CODES OF THOSE WHO HAVE TESTED POSITIVE.
ALERT!
THE APP ALERTS B TO POSSIBLE EXPOSURE.
THE APP GIVES NEXT STEPS, LIKE TESTING OR QUARANTINE, AND OTHER WAYS TO PREVENT THE SPREAD OF THE DISEASE.

Source: GAO analyysis of literature related to various proximity tracing apps. | GAO-20-666SP.

Figure 2. Bluetooth-based proximity tracing apps exchange information, notify contacts exposed to an infected person, and provide follow-up information.

Public health authorities provide the apps, often using systems developed by companies or research groups. Users voluntarily download the app for their country or region and opt in to contact tracing. In the U.S., state or local public health authorities would likely implement proximity tracing apps.

Proximity tracing apps detect contacts using Bluetooth, GPS, or a combination of both. Bluetooth-based apps rely on anonymous codes shared between smartphones during close encounters. These codes contain no information about location or user identity, helping safeguard privacy. The apps allow public health authorities to set a minimum time and distance threshold for someone to count as a contact.

Contact tracing can be centralized or decentralized. With a centralized approach, contacts identified by the app are often saved to a government server, and an official notifies contacts of possible exposure. For a decentralized approach, contact data are typically stored on the user's device at first. When a user voluntarily reports infection, the user's codes are uploaded to a database that other app users' phones search. Users who have encountered the infected person then receive notifications through the app (see Figure 2).

How mature is it? Traditional contact tracing is well established and has been an effective infectious disease response strategy for decades. Proximity tracing apps are relatively new and not as well established.

Their contact identifications could become more accurate as developers improve app technology, for example by improving Bluetooth signal interpretation or using information from other phone sensors.

Opportunities

- Reach more people. For accurate COVID-19 contact tracing using traditional methods, public health experts have estimated that the U.S. would require hundreds of thousands of trained contact tracers because of the large number of infections. Proximity tracing apps can expedite and automate identification and notification of the contacts, reducing this need.
- Faster response. Proximity tracing apps could slow the spread of disease more effectively because they can identify and notify contacts as soon as a user reports they are infected.
- More complete identification of contacts. Proximity tracing apps, unlike traditional contact tracing, do not require users to recall or be acquainted with people they have recently encountered.

Challenges

- Technology. Technological limitations may lead to missed contacts or false identification of contacts. For example, GPS-based apps may not identify precise locations, and Bluetooth apps may ignore barriers preventing exposure, such as walls or protective equipment. In addition, apps may overlook exposure if two people were not in close enough proximity long enough for it to count as a contact.
- Adoption. Lower adoption rates make the apps less effective. In the U.S., some states may choose not to use proximity tracing apps. In addition, the public may hesitate to opt in because of concerns about privacy and uncertainty as to how the data may be used. Recent scams using fake contact tracing to steal information may also erode trust in the apps.
- Interoperability. Divergent app designs may lead to the inability to exchange data between apps, states, and countries, which could be a problem as travel restrictions are relaxed.
- Access. Proximity tracing apps require regular access to smartphones and knowledge about how to install and use apps. Some vulnerable populations, including seniors, are less likely to own smartphones and use apps, possibly affecting adoption.

POLICY CONTEXT AND QUESTIONS

Although proximity tracing apps are relatively new, they have the potential to help slow disease transmission. But policymakers will need to consider how great the benefits are likely to be, given the challenges. If policymakers decide to use proximity tracing apps, they will need to integrate them into the larger public health response and consider the following questions, among others:

- What steps can policymakers take to build public trust and encourage communities to support and use proximity tracing apps, and mitigate lack of adoption by some populations?
- What legal, procedural, privacy, security, and technical safeguards could protect data collected through proximity tracing apps?
- What can policymakers do to improve coordination of contact tracing efforts across local, state, and international jurisdictions?
- What can policymakers do to expedite testing and communication of test results to maximize the benefits of proximity tracing apps?
- What can policymakers do to ensure that contact identification is accurate and that its criteria are based on scientific evidence?

Selected References

Centers for Disease Control and Prevention. *Guidelines for the Implementation and Use of Digital Tools to Augment Traditional Contact Tracing*. June 16, 2020.

Congressional Research Service. *Digital Contact Tracing Technology: Overview and Considerations for Implementation.* IF11559. Washington, D.C.: May 29, 2020.

Ferretti, L., et al. "Quantifying SARS-CoV-2 transmission suggests epidemic control with digital contact tracing." *Science*, vol. 368, no. 6491 (2020).

World Health Organization, *Digital tools for COVID-19 contact tracing.* WHO/2019-nCoV/ Contact_Tracing/Tools_Annex/2020.1. June 2, 2020.

In: Testing and Contract Tracing …
Editor: Ernesto M. Batista
ISBN: 978-1-53618-857-8
© 2020 Nova Science Publishers, Inc.

Chapter 14

CONTACT TRACING WORKFLOW (COVID-19)*

U.S. Department of Health and Human Services, Centers for Disease Control and Prevention

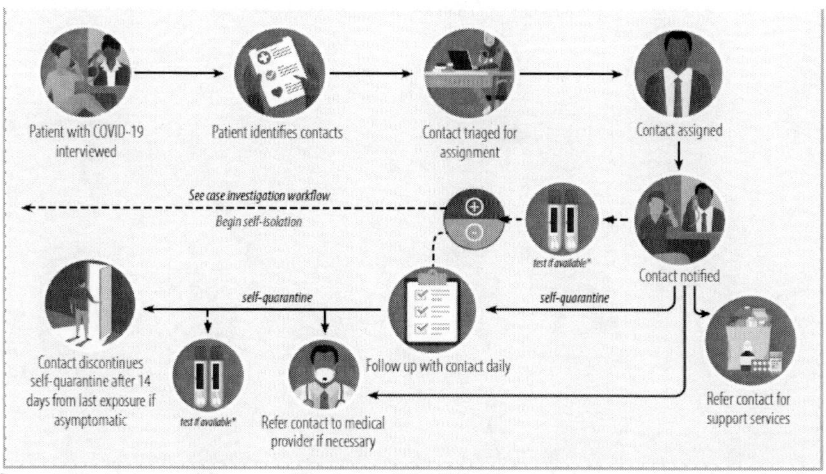

* If contact tests positive or develops COVID-19 symptoms, case investigation is necessary.

---

* This is an edited, reformatted and augmented accessible version of Department of Health and Human Services publication, No. CS 317008-A, dated 06/15/2020.

In: Testing and Contract Tracing … ISBN: 978-1-53618-857-8
Editor: Ernesto M. Batista © 2020 Nova Science Publishers, Inc.

Chapter 15

CDC-Funded Training for the COVID-19 Contact Tracing Workforce*

U.S. Department of Health and Human Services, Centers for Disease Control and Prevention

Background

Contact tracing is a key strategy to prevent the further spread of COVID-19. Contact tracing in the United States requires states, tribes, localities, and territories to recruit, hire, and train adequate levels of case investigators and contact tracers. Successful case investigation and contact tracing for COVID-19 depends on a robust and well-trained public health workforce, with staff who have excellent and tactful interpersonal skills, cultural sensitivity, and language and interviewing skills that help them to build and maintain trust with clients and contacts.

* This is an edited, reformatted and augmented version of Department of Health and Human Services publication CS 317984-A 07/13/2020.

The CDC COVID-19 Response and the CDC Division of STD Prevention are supporting two cooperative agreements to train the COVID-19 contact tracing workforce. The newly funded National Network Disease Intervention Training Centers (NNDITC) and the Association of State and Territorial Health Officials (ASTHO) in partnership with the National Coalition of STD Directors (NCSD) are leading a nationwide, coordinated training effort to build a well-trained public health COVID-19 contact tracing workforce, including case investigators, contact tracers, and contact tracing supervisors.

KNOWLEDGE-BASED TRAINING

ASTHO and NCSD are collaborating with CDC and NNDITC to expand existing training and develop new knowledge-based COVID-19 contact tracing trainings. ASTHO is a national nonprofit organization representing public health agencies in the United States and over 100,000 public health professionals. NCSD is a national public health membership organization representing health department STD directors, their support staff, and community-based partners across 50 states, seven large cities, and eight U.S. territories.

These trainings are available online. The trainings incorporate a variety of learning approaches including online instructional modules, recorded videos of sample interviews with cases and contacts, and other interactive online components.

The initial goals of the partnership are to:

- Expand the existing ASTHO training, Making Contact: A Training for COVID-19 Contact Tracers.
- Develop additional modules to build the knowledge about COVID-19 that case investigators and contact tracers need.
- Develop a training course for contact tracing supervisors.

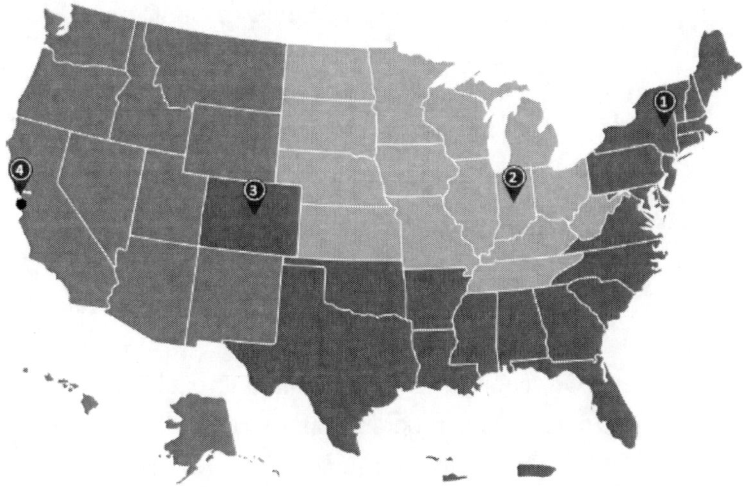

Skills-Based Training

Once contact tracers and case investigators complete online knowledge-based training, they need additional skills to be effective. CDC is partnering with NNDITC to scale up virtual skills-based training for contact tracers, case investigators, and their managers. This instructor-led training will be delivered virtually. The NNDITCs have a long history of training Disease Intervention Specialists, the key workforce in health departments who investigate infectious disease outbreaks, including STDs, HIV, tuberculosis (TB), and any emerging infectious disease threats.

NNDITC comprises a national skills-based curricula development and coordination center — the University of California, San Francisco (UCSF) Disease Intervention Training Centers (DITC) — and four regional centers that will provide the virtual skills-based interactive trainings:

- Region 1: Health NY DITC in Albany, New York
- Region 2: Health Care Education and Training (HCET) DITC in Indianapolis, Indiana
- Region 3: Denver Public Health DITC in Denver, Colorado

- Region 4: UCSF DITC in San Francisco, California

Curriculum Development Center in San Francisco, California.
The partnership is aimed at training three initial COVID-19 cohorts:

- State and local health department staff
- Individuals hired as part of the CDC Foundation COVID-19 Corps
- CDC's Public Health Associate Program (PHAP) trainees

These trainees will continue to be supported through necessary on-the-job trainings, such as mentorship programs and virtual learning collaboratives, offered by the NNDITC to hone the trainees' skills while they are working at a health department.

Impact

The trainings planned by the NNDITC, ASTHO, and NCSD will enhance the knowledge and skills of the contact tracing workers essential to the COVID-19 pandemic response in the United States. Specifically, the trainings will 1) ensure that U.S. contact tracers have a standard set of skills and knowledge needed to do their jobs well, 2) bolster health departments' ability to work across jurisdictions to reduce the spread of COVID-19 in the United States, and 3) build a highly proficient public health workforce that can reduce the spread of other current and future health threats. These cooperative agreements contribute to the national COVID-19 response while sustainably strengthening the public health workforce for the future.

Additional Information

To access the knowledge-based training from ASTHO, please visit TRAIN: https://www.train.org/main/course/1091302/compilation.

In: Testing and Contract Tracing … ISBN: 978-1-53618-857-8
Editor: Ernesto M. Batista © 2020 Nova Science Publishers, Inc.

Chapter 16

DIGITAL CONTACT TRACING TOOLS FOR COVID-19*

U.S. Department of Health and Human Services, Centers for Disease Control and Prevention

Digital contact tracing tools *vary in purpose, features, and complexity,* but they can add value to traditional contact tracing efforts by:

- Improving the efficiency and accuracy of data management and *automating tasks;*
- Reducing the burden of data collection on public health staff by allowing electronic self-reporting by cases and contacts;
- Using location data to *identify community contacts unknown to the case* to look at possible exposure.

---

* This is an edited, reformatted and augmented version of Department of Health and Human Services publication CS 316626-A 04/20/2020.

Public health staff may have different contact tracing challenges, making a one-size-fits-all solution unlikely. Below are some items to consider when selecting the best tool for contact tracing.

Primary Purpose			
		Case Management Tools to capture data on cases and contacts; some allow for automated notification and follow-up	Proximity Tracking Tools that use Bluetooth or GPS to track an individual's exposure to cases; used in addition to contact tracing case management tools
Primary User	PHAs	• PHAs collect information on cases and contacts and follow up when necessary	• PHAs receive information that users choose to share to enhance contact tracing
	Cases and Contacts	• Users report symptoms and contacts and can receive information	• Users elect to share data and are alerted if they have been close to a COVID-19 case
	Key Points	• Ability to receive information from COVID-19 data systems through importation or automated means • Allow for automated notifications and follow-up	• Proximity-sensing technologies that preserve personal privacy are still under development by many groups across the country • Requires community-wide adoption

What Is CDC Doing?

- Conducting a landscape analysis and evaluation of contact tracing tools;
- Generating preliminary tool recommendations for piloting tracing in areas with limited introduction of COVID-19;
- Coordinating with public health agencies, healthcare organizations, academic institutions, non-profit organizations, and private companies to maximize contact tracing effectiveness.

In: Testing and Contract Tracing … ISBN: 978-1-53618-857-8
Editor: Ernesto M. Batista © 2020 Nova Science Publishers, Inc.

Chapter 17

GUIDELINES FOR THE IMPLEMENTATION AND USE OF DIGITAL TOOLS TO AUGMENT TRADITIONAL CONTACT TRACING*

U.S. Department of Health and Human Services, Centers for Disease Control and Prevention

COVID-19 CONTACT TRACING FOR HEALTH DEPARTMENTS, VERSION 1

INTRODUCTION

This document describes two broad categories of digital contact tracing tools, how and where they can improve timeliness and efficiency in the contact tracing process, and defines their minimum and preferred features.

---

* This is an edited, reformatted and augmented version of Department of Health and Human Services publication, updated on June 16, 2020.

This document is based on research and ongoing discussions with contact tracing and informatics experts across local, state, territorial, tribal, and federal government agencies; national public health associations; academic consortia; and nongovernmental organizations.

This document builds on previous guidance; it is a living body of knowledge and will be revised frequently in response to new information and the evolving needs of state, local, tribal, and territorial health departments.

Use of trade names and commercial sources is for identification only and does not imply endorsement by the U.S. Department of Health and Human Services or the Centers for Disease Control and Prevention.

TOOLS OVERVIEW

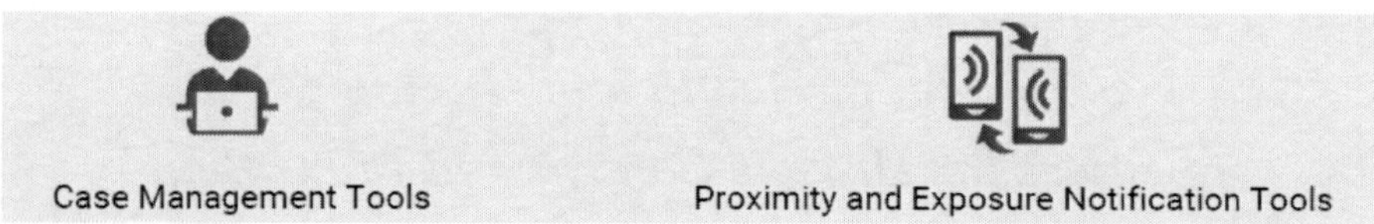

Tools That Make the Traditional Contact Tracing Process Faster and More Efficient

- These tools can streamline the electronic capture and management of data on patients and contacts by enabling automation of contact notification and follow-up, and by allowing patients and contacts to electronically self-report (e.g., demographic and clinical data, contacts, services needed).

- Workflows may integrate with surveillance systems or other workforce management tools (e.g., virtual call centers, test scheduling, support services).

Tools That May Help Identify More Contacts and Notify Them of Exposure Faster Than Traditional Contact Tracing Alone

- Voluntary, opt-in tools using Bluetooth or GPS technologies (most commonly via smartphone apps) can be used to estimate the proximity and duration of an individual's exposure to patient(s) diagnosed with COVID-19.
- More data (from pilots and limited implementations) are needed to quantify the public health value of these tools.

Technology can support case investigation and contact tracing but cannot take the place of a trained public health workforce for interviewing, counseling, and providing support for those impacted by COVID-19.

IMPORTANT FEATURES

Tables 1 and 2 define minimum and preferred features for case management tools and for proximity and exposure notification tools, organized by contact tracing task and crosscutting theme, respectively. A minimum feature is defined as one that all health departments should invest in. A preferred feature is defined as an enhancement that makes the contact tracing process timelier and/or more efficient. When only one category is listed, this indicates that additional functionality may not be needed.

Table 1. Minimum and preferred features of digital contact tracing tools, by contact tracing task

	For health departments[1] that choose to use only case management tools for contact tracing, the tools should:	For health departments that choose to supplement contact tracing with the use of voluntary, opt-in proximity or exposure notification tools, the tools should:[2]
	Patient Identification	
Minimum	• Enable manual import of existing case investigation / patient data from health department and/or laboratory information systems	• Enable patients diagnosed with COVID-19 to electronically self-report confirmed test results, data facilitating connection with services needed to support 14-day self- quarantine period (e.g., safe housing, food, medicine), and best means of communication • Enable health departments or laboratories to authenticate self-reported test results as a precondition for automated contact notification
Preferred	• Enable real-time automated synchronization of case investigation / patient data from health department and/or laboratory information systems • Provide electronic reporting feature for patients with positive lab results to self-identify, report test results, relevant demographic and clinical data (e.g., date of symptom onset), data facilitating connection with services needed to support 14-day self-quarantine period (e.g., safe housing, food, medicine), and best means of communication • Enable health departments or laboratories to authenticate self-reported test results	• Enable automatic integration of minimum data above from consenting patient with validated test result into the health department's surveillance system or case management tool

[1] Local, state, tribal, and territorial public health departments.

[2] Health departments choosing to supplement traditional contact tracing with the use of proximity or exposure notification tools should still select case management tools that meet at least the minimum functionality for each contact tracing task. Proximity or exposure notifications do not need to meet the minimum or preferred functionality of the case management tools.

	Contact Elicitation / Identification	
Minimum	• Enable health department to perform manual data entry of contacts of patients reported during phone calls with patients	• Enable health department to define different exposure risk levels used to identify contacts based on how close and how long their exposure was (e.g., within 6 feet of patient for 15 minutes or more)
Preferred	• Provide electronic means for patients to securely self- report contacts and their best means of communication	• Enable automatic modification of exposure risk level based on self-reported protective behaviors (e.g., mask use), events (e.g., recovery from illness, vaccination) or mass gathering detected by multiple exposure alerts received in quick succession
	• For health departments that choose to use only case management tools for contact tracing, the tools should:	• For health departments that choose to supplement contact tracing with the use of voluntary, opt-in proximity or exposure notification tools, the tools should:
	Contact Notification	
Minimum	• Allow customizable manual, anonymous, and automated notifications[3] to elicited contacts in the following order of priority: recorded voice message, email, and text message • Enable messaging to be tailored to the likelihood of exposure, include links to health information resources and services to support 14-day self-quarantine period, and provide next steps (e.g., testing, self-quarantine) •	• Enable anonymous[4] automated notification to contacts who opt-in to being notified, while also preserving anonymity of patient • Enable notified contacts to voluntarily report relevant demographic data, data facilitating connection with supportive services, and best means of communication • Allow messaging to be tailored to the likelihood of exposure based on the risk level, include links to health information resources and services to

[3] Health departments should consider prioritizing resource allocation to calling contacts or conducting in-person interviews as necessary; when personnel capacity is limited, the case management tool should employ automated messaging that incorporates rapport-building human elements (e.g., delivered in audio or video by trusted local or national health figure)

[4] For tools using geolocation-based proximity tracing, we recommend participatory sharing methods that require health departments to validate case status and protect the privacy of patients, contacts, and local businesses. For Bluetooth-enabled exposure notification tools, we recommend decentralized, bidirectionally anonymous methods. For an example of a protocol that employs this method, see the PACT protocol.

Table 1. (Continued)

	Enable logging date and time of notification to be used in measurements of time between patient identification and contact notification	support 14-day self-quarantine period, and provide next steps (e.g., testing, self-quarantine)
Preferred	• Integrate with telephone services to allow health department to call contacts using elicited information and log timestamp of call to be used in measurements of time between patient identification and contact notification	• Fully automate enrollment of contacts into follow-up and monitoring module of health department information system/case management tool (upon contact consent), instruct contact on follow-up and monitoring process, and direct them to health department's electronic platform for self-reporting
	Patient / Contact Follow up and Monitoring	
Minimum	• Enable health department to perform manual data entry of daily symptom and temperature data reported during phone calls with patients and contacts, as well as data facilitating connection of patienand contacts with supportive services (including instructions for medical assistance) • Enable seamless restart of workflow upon confirmation of case status among any contact	• Enable automated dispatch of reminders to elicited contacts for 14 days and provides link to platform to electronically self-report symptoms, temperature, and other information facilitating the connection with supportive services (if not supported by the health department's case management tool)
Preferred	• Enable automated dispatch of reminders to elicited contacts for 14 days and provides link to platform to electronically self-report symptoms, temperature, and other information facilitating the connection with supportive services • Enable automated analytics of patient and contact check-in logs and notifies health department personnel of patients and contacts who have missed daily check- ins	• Enable automatic prioritization and classification of self- reported symptom and temperature data, immediate contact notification to suggest testing, and immediate health department notification to provide support to the contact (if not supported by the health department's case management tool) • Be able to receive authentication of patient convalescence from health department to clear case status

Table 2. Minimum and preferred features of digital contact tracing tools, by crosscutting theme

	For health departments that choose to use only case management tools for contact tracing, the tools should:	For health departments that choose to supplement contact tracing with the use of voluntary, opt-in proximity or exposure notification tools, the tools should:
	Personal Privacy and Data Security	
Minimum	• Require consent of both patient and contact before collection and use of personally identifying information (PII) • Transparently inform patients and contacts of which data is collected, how it is used, and how long it will be retained • Authorize data access on a need-to-know basis for health department personnel • Use secure means of data transfer for any information that is shared between information systems within and between jurisdictions • Encrypt patient and contact data in transit and at rest Additionally, tools providing patients and/or contacts an electronic option for voluntarily self-reporting test results, symptoms, temperature, and other sensitive health data should: Implement measures to prevent introduction of false data Enable patients and contacts to opt-out of daily check- ins	• Require user consent before their data is shared with health department and contact notifications are initiated • Require that sharing location data, proximity data, or sensitive health data with a health department is not necessary for the user to benefit from the tool's exposure notification features • Allow user to revoke consent and delete the application from their device at any time • Require that data is encrypted and only stored locally on user's device prior to voluntary sharing with health department • Require that any willingly shared user data stored on a central server is encrypted in transit and at rest, and only accessible by authorized health department personnel • Undergo independent security and privacy assessment that addresses issues of trustworthiness, security, and privacy, and publicly provide results • Include safeguards to prevent introduction of false data • Use programmatic means of secure data transfer for any information that is shared between tool and health department information systems
Preferred	• Use programmatic means of secure data transfer[5] for any information that is shared between information	

[5] E.g., RESTful API transferring data over HTTPS or SSH.

Table 2. (Continued)

	• systems within and between jurisdictions Additionally, tools providing patients and/or contacts an electronic option for voluntarily self-reporting test results, symptoms, temperature, and other sensitive health data should: Automatically unsubscribe consenting patients and contacts from daily symptom and temperature monitoring after 14 days	
	Localization	
Minimum	• Provide self-reporting features in patient's and contact's language of choice and use plain language terms that can be easily understood	• Provide user interfaces and all content therein in user's language of choice and use plain language terms that can be easily understood
Preferred	• Provide voice messages, emails, text messages, and user interfaces shared with patient and contact in patient's and contact's language of choice and use plain language terms that can be easily understood	
	For health departments that choose to use only case management tools for contact tracing, the tools should:	For health departments that choose to supplement contact tracing with the use of voluntary, opt-in proximity or exposure notification tools, the tools should:
	Workflow Management and Reporting	
Minimum	Use a structured, electronic means of assigning, tracking, and closing out patient and contact follow-up and monitoring activities that can integrate into reporting workflows	Enable tagging of contacts by source (i.e., identified by patient or identified by proximity or exposure notification tool)
Preferred	• Possess configurable, robust reporting and analytics functionality (e.g., dashboards containing various configurable visual widgets)	
	User Experience	

Minimum	• Be easy to learn for both contact tracing workforce and IT system administrators • Be easily used within web browser on mobile and desktop environments	• Be easy to learn for both contact tracing workforce and general public
Preferred	• Support offline data entry and caching across platforms • Support efficient response to cross-jurisdiction case and contact investigation by being interoperable with tools used by health departments in neighboring states	• Be open source and interoperable with tools used by health departments in neighboring states
	Development, Operations, and Maintenance	
Minimum	• Be easily scalable to accommodate increases in cases and contacts • Use open architectures and open standards • Be developed and supported by vendors that can provide initial setup and comprehensive, rapid technical support and tool customization	• Provide cross-platform functionality (Android, and iOS, with reasonable backwards compatibility for older operating system versions) • Receive regular usability and feature updates as exposure risk levels are calibrated and use cases are refined
Preferred	• Be open source and provide cross-platform functionality (Android and iOS, with reasonable backwards compatibility for older operating system and web browser versions) • Be developed and supported by a vendor that has experience working in public health settings • Allow health department staff to perform some of their own customizations (e.g., adding new data elements, implementing data validation and business rules, developing reports)	

In: Testing and Contract Tracing … ISBN: 978-1-53618-857-8
Editor: Ernesto M. Batista © 2020 Nova Science Publishers, Inc.

Chapter 18

PRELIMINARY CRITERIA FOR THE EVALUATION OF DIGITAL CONTACT TRACING TOOLS FOR COVID-19*

U.S. Department of Health and Human Services, Centers for Disease Control and Prevention

COVID-19 CONTACT TRACING FOR HEALTH DEPARTMENTS, VERSION 1.2

INTRODUCTION

The following preliminary[1] criteria define minimum and preferred characteristics of digital contact tracing tools to help health departments overcome one or more obstacles in the COVID-19 contact tracing

* This is an edited, reformatted and augmented version of COVID-19 publication, updated on May 17, 2020.

[1] This document should be viewed as a living body of knowledge. It will be updated as more is learned.

workflow.[2] They are based on preliminary research and targeted discussions with contact tracing and informatics experts across county, state, and federal government; national public health associations; academic consortia; and nongovernmental organizations.

The table below lists minimum and preferred criteria for two categories of contact tracing technology: those for case management,[3] and those for proximity tracing.[4] Minimum and preferred criteria of the tools' technical and general attributes are described in Table 2.

= case management = proximity tracing

Table 1. Minimum and Preferred Capabilities of Digital Contact Tracing Tools

	Criteria	
Contact Tracing Task	Minimum	Preferred
Patient Identification / Follow-up	• Enables public health authorities (PHAs)[5] to import existing data (e.g., from PHA information systems)	• Can be configured for real-time synchronization of data from PHA information systems
	• Enables confidential collection of data (via PHA manual input) facilitating the connection of laboratory-confirmed patient with services needed to support a 14-day self-isolation process (e.g., safe housing, food)	• Enables patients to report their validated testing status, relevant demographic data, data facilitating the connection with supportive services, and the best means of communication

[2] This includes each task included in the first column of Table 1.

[3] Tools to streamline the electronic capture and management of data on cases and contacts; may also provide means of automating communication and follow up with contacts of an infected individual. Workforce management software (e.g., for orchestrating virtual call centers) is currently beyond the scope of this document.

[4] Tools that use Bluetooth or GPS technologies to estimate the proximity and duration of an individual's exposure to an infected person; used in addition to contact tracing case management tools.

[5] Local, state, tribal, and territorial public health departments.

	Criteria	
Contact Tracing Task	Minimum	Preferred
Contact Elicitation / Identification	• Enables PHAs to manually record data on contacts of patients	• Enables patients to self-report contacts • Can seamlessly import proximity data from patient once consent is received
Contact Notification	• Enables manual and automated notifications[6] to known contacts in the following order of priority: recorded voice message, email, and SMS • Messaging can be tailored to the likelihood of exposure, include links to health information resources, and provide next steps (e.g., testing, self-isolation)	• Enables automated notification to community contacts who opt in to being notified, based on history of proximity to patient (i.e., within 6 feet for 30 minutes or more) while also preserving anonymity of patients[7]
Contact Follow-up	• Enables PHA to initiate direct, manual follow-up with known contacts and collect longitudinal data and data facilitating the connection of contacts with services needed to support a 14-day self-isolation process Enables seamless restart of logic model / workflow upon confirmation of case status among any known contact	• Enables automated dispatch of reminders to known contacts and community contacts for 14 days with directions to call PHA or electronically self-report symptoms and other information facilitating the connection with supportive services Self-reported data are used for automatedprediction of case classification and provide immediate notification to contacts and PHA when infection is likely

[6] We recommend that automated messaging incorporate rapport-building human elements (e.g., delivered in audio or video by trusted local or national health figure).

[7] For tools using geolocation-based proximity tracing, we recommend participatory sharing methods that require health departments to validate case status. For tools with Bluetooth-enabled proximity tracing, we recommend decentralized, bidirectionally anonymous methods. For an example of a protocol that employs this method, see the PACT protocol. Inclusion does not indicate endorsement.

Table 2. Minimum and Preferred Attributes of Digital Contact Tracing Tools

Attribute	Minimum	Preferred
Technical		
Platform Support	• Can be easily used within web browser on mobile and desktop environments	• Provides cross-platform functionality (Android, and iOS, with reasonable backwards compatibility for older Android and iOS versions)
	• Supports offline data entry and caching	• Supports offline data entry and caching across platforms
Data Interoperability	• Supports manual data import from PHA information systems • Supports manual data export in common formats	• Use programmatic means of secure data transfer[8] between information systems within and between jurisdictions
Trustworthiness	• Uses open architectures and open standards	• Is open source
Users	• User access for PHAs	• User access by patients and their contacts
Availability	• Ready to use and rapidly deployable	• Already being used successfully by jurisdictions
Customizability	• Requires vendor to perform all customizations for PHAs	• Allows PHAs to perform some of their own customizations (e.g., adding new data elements, implementing data validation rules)
Privacy	• Transparently informs users of which data is collected, how it is used, and how long it will be retained • Implements measures to prevent introduction of false data • Requires consent of both index patient and contact before using of personally-identifying information (PII)	• Provides individuals the ability to delete their own data

[8] E.g., RESTful API transferring data over HTTPS or SSH.

Attribute	Minimum	Preferred
Technical		
	• Encrypts data in transit and at rest • Provides individuals access to their own data and ability to revoke consent at any time	
	• Provides publicly available independent security and privacy assessment that address issues of trustworthiness, security, and privacy	
	• Authorized data access only for PHAs and must be limited to need-to- know basis	
General		
Technical Support	Developer / vendor provides comprehensive technical support for PHAs	
Vendor Experience	The developer / vendor has experience working in public health settings	
Technical		
Localization	Self-reporting features are available in patient's and contact's language of choice	

In: Testing and Contract Tracing …
Editor: Ernesto M. Batista
ISBN: 978-1-53618-857-8
© 2020 Nova Science Publishers, Inc.

Chapter 19

DIGITAL CONTACT TRACING TECHNOLOGY: OVERVIEW AND CONSIDERATIONS FOR IMPLEMENTATION*

Patricia Moloney Figliola

BACKGROUND

"Contact tracing" is a public health measure used to control disease spread. Trained public health workers assist patients with an infectious disease recall their close contacts within a given timeframe, notify them of potential exposure, and provide advice to patients and contacts. Given the scale of the COVID-19 pandemic, some public health authorities are automating part of the tracing process with smartphone applications (apps). Some apps take advantage of Bluetooth signals to track individuals

* This is an edited, reformatted and augmented version of Congressional Research Service Publication No. IF11559, dated May 29, 2020.

proximity to one another, otherwise known as "digital exposure notification (DEN)" Bluetooth allows short-range wireless communications between electronic devices. Apps may also be used by public health authorities to enable "digital contact tracing" (DCT), which may also use location data.

DEVELOPMENT OF DCT AND DEN APPS IN THE UNITED STATES

In response to the COVID-19 pandemic, several countries have developed nationwide apps to support contact tracing among their citizens. Singapore developed and adopted both the BlueTrace protocol and TraceTogether app.

Although the app is used only in Singapore, its Government Technology Agency has made the BlueTrace protocol available to other countries; Australia has adopted the protocol for its app. South Korea, Bulgaria, Iceland, Germany, and France are among the countries that have released or are developing nationwide apps.

The United States has taken a decentralized approach, with states engaging the private sector to develop tracing tools. North Dakota, South Dakota, and Utah have independently deployed DCT apps using both location data and Bluetooth signals. Companies such as PricewaterhouseCoopers and Salesforce are developing apps to allow corporate clients to track the proximity of their employees within an office or on a campus. In both contexts, if a citizen or employee tests positive for COVID-19, other individuals who may be at risk can be identified and contacted. The possibility of widespread, and perhaps mandatory, monitoring, whether by the public or private sector, has drawn scrutiny from privacy advocates.

Apple-Google Collaboration

On April 10, 2020, Apple and Google, which develop the iOS and Android mobile phone operating systems, respectively, announced a partnership to develop a protocol to support the development of digital exposure notification apps that use a smartphone's Bluetooth signal. The protocol will work on both operating systems, which account for nearly the entire share of the U.S. mobile phone market. It was released to developers on May 20, 2020. *Figure 1* illustrates how apps built using the Apple-Google protocol are planned to work.

In the United States, users must download and opt in to an appropriate state or regional tracing app as well as opt in to the Apple-Google tracking feature in the operating system. Once enabled, a person's smartphone will exchange anonymous identifier beacon keys with nearby smartphones using the Bluetooth signal. According to both companies, personally identifiable information will not be collected.

The anonymous identifier beacon keys remain on a person's phone unless that person reports a positive COVID-19 diagnosis through the app. At that point, the phone uploads the last 14 days of proximate contact data to a server, which sends automated alerts to the individuals whose beacon keys are in the dataset. The alert provides recipients with public health information and what actions to take without revealing the identity of the infected person.

Considerations for Implementation

Discussion of U.S. digital contact tracing has identified a number of challenges related to its use, including Bluetooth limitations, app effectiveness versus personal privacy, interoperability, and coverage. Each poses a different challenge to effective use of digital tracing capabilities.

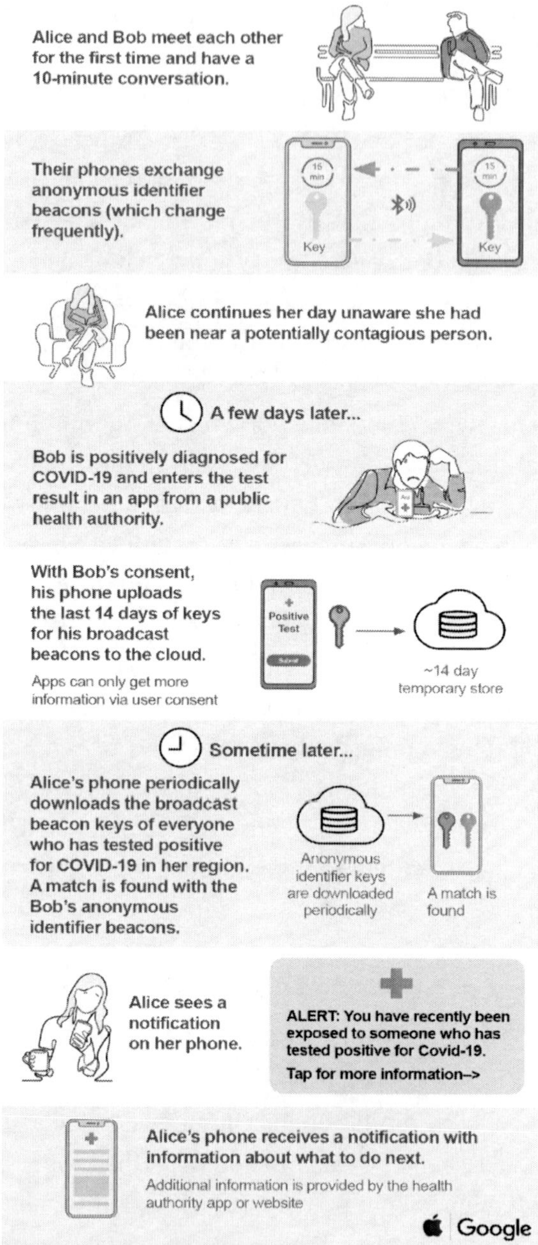
Alice and Bob meet each other for the first time and have a 10-minute conversation.
Their phones exchange anonymous identifier beacons (which change frequently).
15 min
Key
Key
Alice continues her day unaware she had been near a potentially contagious person.
A few days later...
Bob is positively diagnosed for COVID-19 and enters the test result in an app from a public health authority.
With Bob's consent, his phone uploads the last 14 days of keys for his broadcast beacons to the cloud.
Apps can only get more information via user consent
Positive Test
~14 day temporary store
Sometime later...
Alice's phone periodically downloads the broadcast beacon keys of everyone who has tested positive for COVID-19 in her region. A match is found with the Bob's anonymous identifier beacons.
Anonymous identifier keys are downloaded periodically
A match is found
Alice sees a notification on her phone.
ALERT: You have recently been exposed to someone who has tested positive for Covid-19.
Tap for more information–>
Alice's phone receives a notification with information about what to do next.
Additional information is provided by the health authority app or website
Google

Source: https://blog.google/documents/57/Overview_of_COVID-19_Contact_Tracing_Using_BLE.pdf.

Figure 1. Apple-Google Digital Exposure Notification Using Bluetooth.

Bluetooth Limitations

The Bluetooth signal strength and attenuation are variable and affected by numerous factors. Distance between smartphones, smartphone type, and object interference affect signal strength, which will be stronger when a smartphone is carried by hand and weaker from the bottom of a purse. Signal variation will make distance sensitivity calibration difficult, affecting the accuracy of the app.

Observers have noted that if the calibration is too sensitive, there would be a risk of false positives, but if it is not sensitive enough, some interactions would go undetected.

App Effectiveness Versus Personal Privacy

Bluetooth data cannot provide the location of possible contacts, only that two users have been proximate. Global Positioning System (GPS) data, and to a lesser extent cell tower signal and Wi-Fi data, can provide location information. Apps collecting both Bluetooth and location data provide greater detail to health officials than apps using only Bluetooth tracking, which may better support manual contact tracing efforts by identifying where exposure may have occurred. Apple and Google, though, have explicitly banned the collection of location data by apps built using their protocol to protect individual privacy.

State public health officials will need to decide to either use a Bluetooth-only app that will only identify encounters or use another app that will identify encounters and collect more detailed location data. They will also need to determine whether to make the use of digital contact tracing apps mandatory. Privacy advocates have raised concerns surrounding apps using location data, fearing the data may be used for punitive purposes, such as individual quarantine enforcement, or used for purposes unrelated to fighting the pandemic, such as law enforcement.

Interoperability

As of May 20, 2020, Apple and Google have reported that 22 countries across 5 continents and many U.S. states have decided to base their apps on its protocol. As noted earlier, though, some countries and U.S. states developed their digital contact tracing apps before Apple and Google made their announcement. Since Apple and Google disallow the collection of location data in apps using their protocol, the state apps already in use, and any new apps that use location data, will not be interoperable with those using the Apple-Google protocol. The inability to exchange data among some proximate app users will impact the effectiveness of digital contact tracing efforts.

Coverage: Public Attitudes and Tech Availability

Many epidemiologists have stated that apps will be effective in halting the spread of COVID-19 nationwide if between 60% and 80% of the population downloads and uses them. However, it may not be possible to reach even the low end of this estimate. A recent Washington Post-University of Maryland poll found that nearly 60% of Americans would be either unable or unwilling to use a digital contact tracing smartphone app. Differences in state digital contact tracing requirements and uneven adoption across states may further complicate efforts to reach the required number of users nationwide.

U.S. smartphone ownership rates will affect the ability to reach the estimated number threshold needed for effective digital contact tracing. The Pew Research Center found that in 2019, 81% of Americans had a smartphone, but that figure is lower for the elderly and those making less than $50,000. Those without smartphones will not benefit from public health interventions enabled by digital tracing apps.

RELATED LEGISLATIVE PROPOSALS

As of May 22, 2020, three bills have been introduced that address privacy issues related to digital contact tracing apps, one proposal from the Senate and a second proposal that has been introduced in both the House and the Senate:

- The Public Health Emergency Privacy Act (H.R. 6866, S. 3749) was introduced in the House by Representative Anna Eshoo on May 14, 2020, and referred to the Committee on Energy and Commerce the same day. The bill was introduced in the Senate by Senator Richard Blumenthal the same day and referred to the Committee on Health, Education, Labor, and Pensions.
- The COVID-19 Consumer Data Protection Act of 2020 (S. 3663) was introduced in the Senate by Senator Roger Wicker on May 7, 2020, and referred to the Committee on Commerce, Science, and Transportation the same day. A House version has not been introduced.

The three bills aimed at securing the data collected by digital contact tracing apps differ significantly in their approaches, such as:

- how and to what extent the legislation would ensure government transparency and consumer privacy;
- the scope of entities covered (private, or public and private);
- whether to preempt state laws that might require more robust consumer protections; and
- whether to provide a private right of action to individuals against companies if their data is used in an unauthorized manner.

In: Testing and Contract Tracing … ISBN: 978-1-53618-857-8
Editor: Ernesto M. Batista © 2020 Nova Science Publishers, Inc.

Chapter 20

COVID-19: Digital Contact Tracing and Privacy Law*

Eric N. Holmes and Chris D. Linebaugh

Many states, territories, and localities have implemented public health orders to limit the spread of Coronavirus Disease 2019 (COVID-19) in their respective communities, including stay-at-home orders, orders temporarily closing schools and businesses, and orders limiting the size of public gatherings. In preparation for the eventual relaxation and lifting of these orders, the Centers for Disease Control and Prevention (CDC) have advocated that public health authorities use robust "contact tracing" procedures to prevent the reoccurrence of widespread infections after communities reopen. While federal entities may advise on these procedures, state and local authorities are responsible for contact tracing operations, as provided by state law.

The term "contact tracing" generally refers to identifying and monitoring people who have been in contact with someone diagnosed with

* This is an edited, reformatted and augmented version of Congressional Research Service Publication No. LSB10511, dated July 9, 2020.

an infectious disease, in order to locate other potentially infected individuals quickly and take targeted control measures (such as quarantines) to prevent the broader spread of the illness. Contact tracing is standard procedure in public health investigations, and historically involves officials interviewing and contacting infected and potentially-exposed persons. However, some of the contact tracing proposals aimed at controlling the spread of COVID-19 suggest supplementing traditional contact tracing procedures with technology to collect data electronically. These proposals raise questions about how federal laws governing health information privacy may apply to electronic or digital contact tracing. One such provision is the "HIPAA Privacy Rule," which refers collectively to regulations promulgated by the Department of Health and Human Services (HHS) under the Health Insurance Portability and Accountability Act (HIPAA). This Sidebar discusses the HIPAA Privacy Rule's application to digital contact tracing and briefly discusses other federal laws that regulate data privacy.

HIPAA Privacy Rule Overview

The HIPAA Privacy Rule regulates the use and disclosure of protected health information (PHI) by "covered entities" and their "business associates." Covered entities include health plans, health care clearinghouses, and "health care providers" who transmit electronic health information in connection with a HIPAA-covered transaction (such as billing). A health plan is an "individual or group plan that provides, or pays the cost of, medical care." This includes health insurance companies, health maintenance organizations (HMOs), and government programs, such as Medicaid and Medicare, that pay for healthcare. Health care clearinghouses are defined as entities that process health information in a nonstandard format into a standard format, or vice versa. Lastly, health care providers include providers of services covered by Sections 1861(u) or 1861(s) of the Social Security Act (which includes, among other things, physicians' services, hospital services, physical therapy services, and skilled nursing facility services) or any person who otherwise "furnishes, bills, or is paid for health care in the normal course of business." Health care is defined as "care, services, or supplies related to the health of an individual." A business associate is one who, among other actions, "creates, receives, maintains, or transmits protected health information" on behalf of a covered entity for an activity regulated under HIPAA generally (not simply the Privacy Rule), such as claims processing, data analysis, processing or administration, utilization review, quality assurance, billing, benefit management, practice management, and repricing.

The HIPAA Privacy Rule recognizes that entities may engage in conduct that makes them covered entities ("covered functions"), while, at the same time, performing other functions that would not render them covered entities. For instance, institutions of higher learning may, in addition to providing education, run a health clinic that provides healthcare for students. Such an entity may become a "hybrid entity" by complying with organizational requirements that include designating a specific component of its organization as the "health care component." In such situations, only the designated health care component of a hybrid entity is required to comply with the HIPAA Privacy Rule.

As noted, the obligations of covered entities and their business associates under the HIPAA Privacy Rule revolve around the use and disclosure PHI. PHI includes information that (1) "identifies," or can reasonably "be used to identify," an individual; (2) is "created or received by a health care provider, health plan, employer, or health care clearinghouse"; (3) relates to an individual's past, present, or future physical or mental health, health care provision, or payment for the provision of health care; and (4) is transmitted by or maintained in electronic or any other form or medium. The HIPAA Privacy Rule, among other things, limits covered entities from using PHI or sharing it with third parties without valid patient authorization, unless the use is for purposes of treatment, payment, or "health care operations," or falls within a specific statutory exception.

One such exception that is particularly relevant to contact tracing allows covered entities to use or disclose PHI—without individual patient authorization or the opportunity for the patient to agree or object—to "a public health authority" that is legally authorized to collect the information "for the purpose of preventing or controlling disease, injury, or disability," including "the conduct of public health surveillance." A "public health authority" includes any agency or authority of the "United States, a State, a territory, a political subdivision of a State or territory, or Indian tribe," that is "responsible for public health matters as part of its official mandate," as well as "a person or entity acting under a grant of authority from or contract with" such an agency. This definition encompasses the CDC as well as state and local public health departments, among others. State and local health departments may engage in both covered and non-covered activities, and many choose to designate themselves as a "hybrid entity," so that their non-covered components need not comply with the HIPAA Privacy Rule's requirements.

Violations of the HIPAA Privacy Rule can lead to civil or criminal enforcement. The HHS Office of Civil Rights is responsible for investigating and enforcing civil violations of HIPAA's requirements and may impose monetary penalties, which vary depending on the violator's culpability. The U.S. Department of Justice has criminal enforcement authority under HIPAA and may seek fines or imprisonment against a person who "knowingly" obtains or discloses "individually identifiable health information" or "uses or causes to be used a unique health identifier" in violation of HIPAA's requirements.

MOBILE APPLICATION CONTACT TRACING OVERVIEW

Among the many challenges public health authorities face in tracking and controlling the spread of COVID-19 is that the disease is highly infectious and appears to be transmissible by people who do not show symptoms of COVID-19 and thus may not know that they are infected. In this environment, mobile applications (apps) may facilitate public health authorities' gathering data on potential exposures to use in contract tracing. As explained in this CRS In Focus, governments and technology companies have explored two schemes for gathering device data through contact tracing apps: location tracking and proximity tracking. *Location tracking* schemes collect location information from individuals' mobile devices, including global positioning system (GPS) and cell site location information, to map their locations over time. *Proximity tracking* schemes use Bluetooth technology to determine when two devices remain within a particular distance of each other for a specified amount of time, without collecting location data. Apps built using either scheme relate information to a unique identifier associated with a particular mobile device. For location tracking apps, these identifiers are mapped to particular locations, while proximity tracking apps broadcast identifiers over Bluetooth so app users may anonymously log encounters with other app users. In certain app configurations, an app user may report a positive COVID- 19 diagnosis within the app, which then could relay a report of that diagnosis—anonymously—to those app users who had been in proximity to the diagnosed person, and/or to public health authorities undertaking contact tracing investigations.

North Dakota and South Dakota have both deployed a location tracking system, while Google and Apple have changed their mobile operating systems to allow developers to create proximity tracking apps. Some apps may use both location and proximity tracking, such as an app previously deployed by Norway's government. In each case, app functionality may rely on several types of information with different sources, including information from the app user's device (such as the device's unique identifier) and information the app user voluntarily provides (such as a positive COVID-19 diagnosis).

INTERACTION OF THE HIPAA PRIVACY RULE WITH MOBILE APPLICATION CONTACT TRACING

As noted, the HIPAA Privacy Rule's protections do not apply to all health-related data. Only PHI held by covered entities and their business associates is subject to the Rule. Thus, the extent to which the Rule applies to digital contact tracing applications depends on whether the parties developing the apps and processing app information fall within the definitions of covered entities or business associates and whether the app uses PHI.

Are Public Health Authorities or App Developers Covered Entities or Business Associates?

Because state and local public health authorities are the primary users of data collected through contact tracing, a critical threshold issue is whether they are *covered entities* subject to the HIPAA Privacy Rule. This issue is complicated by the fact that a public health authority may perform various functions within one agency. For example, a public health authority may provide clinical care (e.g., diagnostic testing), and thus qualify as a health care provider subject to HIPAA's requirements. The same agency might also engage in community-wide or state-wide disease control activities, such as contact tracing, that do not appear to be among the functions by which HIPAA defines covered entities.

Thus, a health department that engages in both health care activities and disease control functions may choose to operate as a "hybrid entity." In so doing, state and local health departments may limit their obligations under the HIPAA Privacy Rule solely to their performance of discrete covered healthcare functions. Any information the "hybrid" agency obtains for use in disease control activities such as contact tracing would not be subject to HIPAA's privacy protections. Moreover, under the public health authority exception to the HIPAA Privacy Rule, this would include PHI received by the public health authority from a covered entity, such as a healthcare provider.

Third-party software developers standing alone are not generally covered entities subject to the HIPAA Privacy Rule. Moreover, a third-party software developer that creates, maintains, or administers an app used in a public health authority's contact tracing operations would not qualify as a business associate subject to the HIPAA Privacy Rule if the public health authority is not a covered entity when performing its disease control functions. That is because, as explained above, HIPAA defines a business associate as one who "creates, receives, maintains, or transmits protected health information" on behalf of a covered entity.

Do Contact Tracing Apps Use PHI?

Even if an entity is a covered entity or a business associate under HIPPA, HIPAA's Privacy Rule only applies to PHI. To be sure, contact tracing apps rely on health-related information (e.g., information that shows whether individuals have been diagnosed with, or exposed to, COVID-19). Thus, for any entities involved in the development and operation of a contact tracing app that might be covered entities or business associates, the applicability of the HIPAA Privacy Rule to them would largely depend on whether the information used for digital contact tracing is *individually identifiable*.

HIPAA deems health information not identifiable if the covered entity takes either of two steps. One option is that the covered entity can de-identify the information by ensuring that eighteen specific types of identifiers have been removed (including, for example, "all geographic subdivisions smaller than a State," "telephone numbers," and "device identifiers"). Alternatively, the covered entity may obtain documentation showing that an expert has determined that there is a "very small" risk of identification from the information. If this approach is chosen, the HHS Office of Civil Rights may assess the expert's qualifications in the course of an audit or investigation.

It is difficult to conceive how covered entities could de-identify the information required for contract tracing apps to function. Contact tracing apps will necessarily depend on information that accurately tracks individual movements and contacts. Both location tracking and proximity tracking apps function by associating a person who has tested positive for a disease with a device identifier generated by the app. In the case of location tracking apps, this includes GPS or cell site location information, which provides geographic information much smaller than a state. Apps also could request additional identifying information: Singapore's app, for example, requires app users to provide phone numbers. Accordingly, the most likely option by which a covered entity could establish that the health information used for digital contact tracing is not identifiable would be to obtain an expert determination that the risk of identification from the information is "very small."

Any such determination would likely assess the steps taken by the app to make identification more difficult. Google and Apple's proximity tracking framework provides for apps that use randomly generated identifiers, which cycle every 10-20 minutes to reduce the risk of linking any group of identifiers to an individual. Location tracking apps may take similar measures to mitigate tracking risk.

For example, North Dakota's app associates location information with a random ID number and only stores location information when a device remains at a location for more than ten minutes. However, even apps that associate information with randomly generated identifiers may be susceptible to "linkage attacks" in which an entity might be able to identify a particular device, and apps that collect more detailed information may pose even greater risks.

OTHER RELEVANT PRIVACY LAWS

Even when HIPAA does not apply, other federal privacy laws may come into play. As discussed in this CRS report, HIPAA is just one part of the "patchwork" of federal laws governing companies' privacy obligations. In particular, the companies that develop and maintain contact tracing apps must comply with the Federal Trade Commission Act's prohibition on unfair or deceptive acts or practices (UDAPs). The Federal Trade Commission (FTC), which enforces this prohibition, regularly brings enforcement actions against persons or companies for collecting or using personal information in a deceptive or unfair manner, such as when a company's privacy practices contradict its posted privacy policy. It is unclear, however, whether the FTC could bring a UDAP action against state health departments or app developers acting on their behalf. For example, courts have applied the state action doctrine—which provides immunity for certain state actions that might otherwise violate federal antitrust laws—to FTC suits brought under the FTC Act's prohibition of "unfair methods of competition." This doctrine may also apply to the FTC's UDAP authority. At least one district court has applied the state action doctrine to bar the FTC from using its UDAP enforcement power against a state entity, although that decision was later vacated on other grounds. However, the case law on this issue is relatively sparse.

Along with the FTC Act, the Communications Act may limit tracing apps' ability to gather cellphone GPS data. The Communications Act prohibits telephone carriers from using or disclosing "customer proprietary network information" (CPNI) unless the customer consents or a specific exception applies.

The Act defines CPNI to include information relating to the "location" of a customer's "telecommunications service" that is available to the carrier by "virtue of the carrier-customer relationship." However, CPNI excludes "aggregate" customer information from which "individual customer identities and characteristics have been removed," similar to how companies like Google and Apple claim they are endeavoring to de-identify information with their contact tracing frameworks.

Considerations for Congress

In summary, no single federal law creates consistent, clearly-applicable privacy protections for the information that likely would be gathered and used in contact tracing activities. In the context of digital contact tracing, state and local health departments conducting contact tracing and the app developers that assist them in that activity may not qualify as covered entities or business associates subject to HIPAA's requirements. Other federal laws, such as the FTC Act and Communications Act, may provide some privacy protections when HIPAAdoes not apply. Yet the reach of these laws is also limited. The FTC does not require entities to adopt particular privacy practices; it only takes enforcement action against corporate and private actors that it believes are engaged in unfair or deceptive conduct. The Communications Act's CPNI protections apply only to telephone carriers.

Members of the 116th Congress have proposed several COVID-19-related privacy bills. While an in- depth discussion of these bills is beyond the scope of this Sidebar, the Public Health Emergency Privacy Act (PHEPA), COVID–19 Consumer Data Protection Act of 2020 (CCDPA), and Exposure Notification Privacy Act (EPNA) would generally provide additional privacy rights and obligations related to entities' collection and use of personal information for contract tracing and exposure notification purposes. While the CCDPA and PHEPA would apply specifically to COVID-19, the EPNA would not be limited to the current pandemic.

In: Testing and Contract Tracing … ISBN: 978-1-53618-857-8
Editor: Ernesto M. Batista © 2020 Nova Science Publishers, Inc.

Chapter 21

"TRACING PAPERS": A COMPARISON OF COVID-19 DATA PRIVACY BILLS*

Jonathan M. Gaffney

As COVID-19 continues to spread, many public health authorities are turning to *contact tracing*— measures to identify, notify, and monitor infected individuals' contacts—to track potential COVID-19 exposure. Along with conventional techniques, technology companies, including Google and Apple, are developing digital contact-tracing and exposure notification tools. In addition, Congress has appropriated emergency funds to help facilitate contact-tracing efforts. But the idea of using personal information— including cell phone and location data—to track COVID-19 exposure has prompted groups such as the ACLU to raise privacy concerns and call for the protection of individuals' privacy and anonymity.

In response, Members of Congress have introduced four data privacy bills addressing digital contact- tracing and exposure notification:

---

* This is an edited, reformatted and augmented version of Congressional Research Service Publication No. LSB10501, dated June 26, 2020.

- the COVID-19 Consumer Data Protection Act of 2020 (CCDPA), S. 3663, introduced by Senators Roger Wicker, John Thune, Jerry Moran, Marsha Blackburn, and Deb Fischer on May 7, 2020;
- the Public Health Emergency Privacy Act (PHEPA), companion bills S. 3749 and H.R. 6866, introduced, respectively, by Senators Richard Blumenthal and Mark Warner and Representatives Anna Eshoo, Janice Schakowsky, Suzan DelBene, Yvette Clarke, G.K. Butterfield, and Tony Cardenas on May 14, 2020; and
- the Exposure Notification Privacy Act (ENPA), S. 3861, introduced by Senators Maria Cantwell and Bill Cassidy on June 1, 2020.

This chapter describes the main components of each bill and examines key differences among the proposals before identifying several issues for Congress.

KEY PROVISIONS AND MAJOR DIFFERENCES

The CCDPA, PHEPA, and ENPA would each take a similar approach to regulating contact-tracing data. Under each bill, a *covered entity* would have to take certain steps before and after collecting *covered data*, and each bill would grant certain rights to individuals over collected data. In addition, each bill would create enforcement mechanisms to ensure covered entities comply with their obligations with respect to covered data. But the bills contain several major differences, including the types of entities they cover and the precise rights they afford to individuals. While the CCDPA and PHEPA apply specifically to the current COVID-19 pandemic, the ENPA is not limited to the current public health emergency. The ENPA, however, applies only to data collected by an *automated exposure notification service*, which it defines as a tool for "digitally notifying, in an automated manner, an individual who may have become exposed to an infectious disease." The key provisions of each bill are discussed below, and *Table 1* summarizes their main differences.

Covered Data

Each bill would generally protect specific categories of data collected or used for contact-tracing or exposure notification. The CCDPA would apply to the narrowest set of data: "precise geolocation data, proximity data, a persistent identifier"—information that can be used to identify a user over time—"and personal health information." In contrast, the ENPA would protect any information linked or reasonably linkable to any individual or device collected, processed, or transferred as part of an automated exposure notification service. Each of the bills would also exclude certain data, including aggregate data that cannot identify a specific individual. The CCDPA would also exclude data collected by a covered entity concerning anyone "permitted to enter a physical site of operation" of the entity, including employees, vendors, and visitors.

Covered Entities

Each bill generally applies to entities that engage in contact-tracing or exposure notification or that develop tools that other entities use for contact-tracing or exposure notification. Under the CCDPA and ENPA, for example, a *covered entity* would include any entity or person engaged in a covered activity that is (1) subject to regulation by the Federal Trade Commission (FTC), (2) a common carrier as defined in the Communications Act of 1934, or (3) a nonprofit organization. The CCDPA does not apply to *service providers* that transfer or process data on behalf of covered entities but do not themselves collect covered data. The PHEPA would cover a broader range of entities, including government entities, but excluding health care providers, public health authorities, service providers, and persons acting in their individual or household capacity.

Covered Entities' Obligations

The bills would each impose obligations on covered entities with respect to covered data. Each bill would require a covered entity to

- not disclose or transfer an individual's data for any purposes other than those enumerated in the bills (CCDPA § 3(a), (b); PHEPA § 3(a), (c); ENPA § 5);
- publish a privacy policy to provide notice as to the type of data the entity collects, the purpose of the collection, how the entity will use collected data, and an individual's rights with respect to the data (CCDPA § 3(c)(1); PHEPA § 3(e); ENPA § 4(b));
- obtain an individual's affirmative express consent before collecting that individual's data (CCDPA § 3(a); PHEPA § 3(d)(1); ENPA § 4(a));
- provide an individual with the right to opt out of collection by withdrawing consent (CCDPA § 3(d); PHEPA § 3(d)(2); ENPA § 4(a)(1)(B));
- delete an individual's data on request or after a set period, such as the end of the COVID- 19 emergency under the PHEPA or on a 30-day rolling basis under the ENPA (CCDPA § 3(e); PHEPA § 3(g); ENPA § 6); and
- safeguard an individual's data by adopting appropriate data security measures (CCDPA § 3(h); PHEPA § 3(b); ENPA § 7).

Along with these obligations present in all three bills, there are several additional protections common to two of the three bills. For example, both the CCDPA and PHEPA require covered entities to *minimize* the data they collect and to provide a mechanism for an individual to *correct* inaccurate data. Also of note, the PHEPA and ENPA prohibit discrimination against an individual based on covered data.

Enforcement

All three bills would vest enforcement with the FTC through agency and judicial proceedings. The bills would also allow state attorneys general to enforce the bills' provisions in court. The PHEPA would provide a new *private right of action* that would allow individuals to sue covered entities for violations. And the ENPA would preserve an individual's ability to use existing remedies under federal or state law to enforce its provisions.

Relationship to State Laws

Table 1. COVID-19 Data Privacy Bills: Comparison of Key Differences

Provision	CCDPA, S. 3663	PHEPA, S. 3749 and H.R. 6866	ENPA, S. 3861
Covered Data—			
In general	*Covered data*: "precise geolocation data, proximity data, a persistent identifier, and personal health information" (§ 2(6)(a))	*Emergency health data*: "data linked or reasonably linkable to an individual or device, including [derived] data . . . that concerns the COVID-19 health emergency" (§ 2(8))	*Covered data*: "any information that is . . . linked or reasonably linkable to an individual . . . collected, processed, or transferred in connection with an automated exposure notification service" (§ 2(6))
Exclusions	Aggregate data, business contact information, de-identified data, employee screening data, and publicly available information (§ 2(6)(b)); data related to individuals permitted to enter a covered entity's physical location (§ 2(12))	Data that is not "linked or reasonably linkable" to an individual or device (§ 2(8))	Data that is not "linked or reasonably linkable" to an individual or device, including aggregate data (§ 2(6))
Covered Entities—			
In General	Any entity or person engaged in contact tracing that is subject to the FTC Act, a common carrier, or a nonprofit (§ 2(7))	Any entity or person engaged in contact tracing, including government entities (§ 2(4)(A))	An operator of an automated exposure notification service that is subject to the FTC Act, a common carrier, or a nonprofit (§§ 2(11), 10(a)(4))

Table 1. (Continued)

Provision	CCDPA, S. 3663	PHEPA, S. 3749 and H.R. 6866	ENPA, S. 3861
Exclusions	Service providers (§ 2(7)(C))	Health care providers; persons engaged in de minimis collection; service providers; persons acting in their individual or household capacity; and public health authorities (§ 2(4)(B))	Public health authorities (§ 2(11))
Non-Discrimination	No protections	Covered entities must adopt reasonable safeguards against discrimination (§ 3(a)(3)); government entities may not use data to interfere with voting rights (§ 4)	Prohibits discrimination by any person or entity based on covered data (§ 8)
Enforcement	FTC; state attorneys general (§ 4(a), (c))	FTC; state attorneys general; new private right of action (§ 6)	FTC; state attorneys general; existing private rights of action (§ 10)
Preemption	Preempts state laws and regulations governing covered entities' use of covered data (§ 4(b)(3))	Adopts reasonable safeguards to prevent unlawful discrimination on the basis of emergency health data, but does not "preempt or supersede" other federal or state laws or regulations (§ 7)	Does not "preempt, displace, or supplant" state laws (§ 10(c))
Effective Period	Date of enactment through the last day of the COVID-19 public health emergency (§ 2(8))	Thirty days after enactment through the end of the COVID-19 public health emergency (§§ 2(13), 8)	Indefinitely, beginning on the date of enactment (§ 10(g))

Source: Created by CRS using information from CCDPA, S. 3663; PHEPA, S. 3749 and H.R. 6866; and ENPA, S. 3861.

Both the PHEPA and ENPA explicitly provide that their provisions would not preempt or supersede any state laws. In contrast, the CCDPA would prohibit states from adopting or enforcing any laws or regulations governing the use of covered data.

Considerations for Congress

As state and local authorities consider whether to implement digital contact tracing or exposure notification to combat the COVID-19 pandemic, Congress may consider whether to enact a law governing the use of contact-tracing data to ensure uniformity and safeguard individuals' personal data. If Congress takes no action, digital contact-tracing and exposure notification solutions may be subject to existing federal and state privacy protections, including the Health Insurance Portability and Accountability Act (HIPAA) regulations and the California Consumer Privacy Act (CCPA). But existing federal privacy laws do not protect all contact-tracing data, and state laws—where they exist—impose a patchwork of requirements.

The CCDPA, PHEPA, and ENPA share a number of common provisions, suggesting some level of accord on how to regulate entities engaged in contact tracing. But the differences among the bills could make it difficult to reach agreement on final legislation. Two of the biggest divergences among the bills—whether to include a private right of action and whether to preempt state law—mirror differences in general data privacy bills introduced at the end of 2019 and earlier this year. Those provisions were "key sticking point[s]" in the debate over general-applicability data privacy legislation, and Congress has yet to reach a consensus. To move forward with a contact-tracing privacy bill, Congress may have to reach a compromise with respect to these issues.

In: Testing and Contract Tracing … ISBN: 978-1-53618-857-8
Editor: Ernesto M. Batista © 2020 Nova Science Publishers, Inc.

Chapter 22

CONSTITUTIONAL AUTHORITY TO REGULATE THE PRIVACY OF STATE-COLLECTED CONTACT-TRACING DATA*

Edward C. Liu

Amid the ongoing COVID-19 pandemic, several states have developed and promoted contact-tracing mobile device apps to identify individuals who may have had contact with infected persons. Additionally, the two largest manufacturers of mobile device operating systems, Apple (iOS) and Google (Android), have announced plans to release application programming interfaces (APIs) to "enable interoperability between Android and iOS devices using apps from public health authorities."

Several bills in the 116th Congress would regulate the privacy of information collected through such contact-tracing apps.

- S. 3663, the COVID-19 Consumer Data Protection Act of 2020, would (1) require certain covered entities that collect contact-tracing

* This is an edited, reformatted and augmented version of Congressional Research Service Publication LSB10502, dated June 26, 2020.

information to provide individuals with prior notice of such collection and the opportunity to opt-in to such collection; (2) prohibit the use of such information for purposes unrelated to tracking the spread of COVID-19; and (3) require covered entities to publicize their privacy and data security practices.

- S. 3749 and H.R. 6866, the Public Health Emergency Privacy Act (PHEPA), would prohibit certain entities from disclosing contact-tracing information for purposes unrelated to public health. The bill would also prohibit such information from being used for commercial advertising or marketing purposes, or to discriminate against individuals with respect to "goods, services, facilities, privileges, advantages, or places of accommodations." Covered entities include state governmental entities, although PHEPA specifically exempts public health authorities.
- S. 3861, the Exposure Notification Privacy Act (ENPA), requires operators of "automated exposure notification systems" (AENS) to limit enrollment in such systems to individuals who have provided affirmative express consent, to publicize the system's privacy policy, and to limit transfers of covered data to the minimum necessary to notify other users or a public health authority of potential exposures. ENPA also requires operators of an AENS to establish data security practices to protect the confidentiality, integrity, availability, and accessibility of covered data.

In general, the bills above limit coverage to entities subject to the jurisdiction of the Federal Trade Commission or explicitly exempt state public health authorities. Nevertheless, during the debate surrounding this legislation, questions may arise over Congress's authority to regulate state governments' collection and dissemination of the relevant information. As context for that potential debate, this Legal Sidebar examines constitutional limitations on Congress's regulation of state activity, particularly in the context of applying federal privacy protections to state-held information.

FEDERALISM AND THE ANTICOMMANDEERING DOCTRINE

Unlike the state governments, which enjoy a general police power, the federal government is limited to those enumerated powers provided to it in the U.S. Constitution. One such power that is particularly relevant to the instant analysis is the Constitution's Commerce Clause, which allocates to Congress the power "[t]o regulate Commerce with foreign Nations, and among the several States, and with the Indian Tribes." The Supreme Court has interpreted the Commerce Clause as authorizing Congress to regulate "the channels of interstate commerce, persons or things in interstate commerce, and those activities that substantially affect interstate commerce."

Legislation that falls within the bounds of the Commerce Clause may still be unconstitutional if it breaches "the principles of federalism contained in the Tenth Amendment," which provides that "[t]he powers not delegated to the United States by the Constitution, nor prohibited by it to the States, are reserved to the States respectively, or to the people." Whether the Tenth Amendment restricts Congress's authority to impose generally applicable regulations on the activities of states and their instrumentalities has been an ongoing debate since the latter half of the 20th century.

Legal Background

In 1974, the Court decided *National League of Cities v. Usery*, holding that Congress may not use the Commerce Clause to dictate "how essential decisions regarding the conduct of integral governmental functions are to be made." But the Supreme Court expressly overruled *National League of Cities* in its 1985 decision in *Garcia v. San Antonio Metropolitan Transit Authority* after efforts to define the scope of "integral governmental functions" proved "both impracticable and doctrinally barren." On the other hand, following *Garcia*, the Court held in two cases that Congress violates the Tenth Amendment when it commandeers states to enact or administer a federal regulatory program. In *New York v. United States*, the Court struck down a federal law that compelled states "to provide for the disposal of the radioactive waste generated within their borders." Similarly, in *Printz v. United States*, the Court invalidated a provision of federal law that required "state and local law enforcement officers to conduct background checks on prospective handgun purchasers."

Regulating State Databases

After the *New York* and *Printz* decisions, the Supreme Court decided *Reno v. Condon* in 2000, a Tenth Amendment challenge to the Driver's Privacy Protection Act (DPPA). The DPPA generally restricts the sale and disclosure of personal information held by state motor vehicle departments (DMVs) without an individual's consent. The DPPA also restricts the resale and redisclosure of drivers' information by private parties who have obtained that information from a state DMV.

After first holding that the Commerce Clause properly encompassed the sale or disclosure of such personally identifiable information as a "thing in interstate commerce," the Court found no Tenth Amendment concerns with the federal statute. Distinguishing the DPPA from the statutes struck down in *New York* and *Printz*, the Court held that

> the DPPA does not require the States in their sovereign capacity to regulate their own citizens. The DPPA regulates the States as the owners of data bases. It does not require the South Carolina Legislature to enact any laws or regulations, and it does not require state officials to assist in the enforcement of federal statutes regulating private individuals. We accordingly conclude that the DPPA is consistent with the constitutional principles enunciated in New York and Printz.

Most recently, in 2018, the Court's decision in Murphy v. National Collegiate Athletic Association reaffirmed the principle set forth in Reno that "[t]he anticommandeering doctrine does not apply when Congress evenhandedly regulates an activity in which both States and private actors engage."

ANALYSIS

Questions about Congress's authority to regulate the privacy of information collected by state public health departments through contact-tracing apps are seemingly similar to those the Supreme Court addressed in *Reno v. Condon*. As noted above, the Court in *Reno* first concluded that pieces of personal information collected by state DMVs were "things in interstate commerce" that fell within the Commerce Clause's scope. Under this reasoning, courts would likely consider the information collected by state public health departments through contact-tracing apps to likewise be "things in interstate commerce" subject to federal regulation under the Commerce Clause.

In addition, *Reno* appears to suggest that the Tenth Amendment is generally not an obstacle to federal regulation of the sale and disclosure of personal information collected through contact-tracing apps if such regulation is applied "evenhandedly" to both state and private holders of this information. The rationale under which the *Reno* Court upheld the DPPA's privacy requirements—that the statute "does not require the States in their sovereign capacity to regulate their own citizens" but merely "regulates the States as the owners of data bases"—appears to be equally applicable to security and interoperability requirements imposed on public and private custodians of contact-tracing data. Consequently, applying the Court's reasoning in *Reno*, so long as such federal regulation of contact-tracing apps applies evenhandedly to both state and private actors, and does not also require states to enact legislation or refrain from enacting legislation, it would likely not raise constitutional issues under the Tenth Amendment.

INDEX

A

accuracy, x, xii, xvi, 1, 2, 4, 5, 12, 13, 17, 18, 19, 22, 98, 112, 119, 123, 125, 126, 127, 128, 321, 333, 355
active infection, x, 3, 9, 11, 13, 14, 82, 124, 126
administrators, 174, 175, 176, 188, 289, 343
agencies, xiii, xv, xvii, 5, 20, 30, 41, 44, 45, 49, 60, 65, 84, 85, 86, 88, 92, 98, 110, 176, 181, 191, 197, 218, 225, 286, 306, 311, 315, 330, 334, 336
antibodies, x, 3, 5, 7, 9, 11, 13, 14, 16, 18, 19, 45, 124, 125
antigen, 3, 12, 13, 14, 16, 17, 18, 22, 24, 28, 45, 82, 123, 124, 126
appropriations, 35, 63, 67, 70, 77, 78, 79, 84, 85, 86, 88, 89, 90
assessment, 142, 154, 157, 160, 168, 190, 223, 239, 240, 281, 310, 341, 349
asymptomatic, xii, 7, 15, 17, 28, 32, 51, 57, 59, 63, 67, 72, 110, 129, 140, 147, 156, 157, 162, 166, 167, 168, 171, 219, 228, 307
automate, 225, 230, 311, 324, 340
availability, xii, xx, 11, 12, 33, 34, 35, 49, 69, 78, 79, 80, 81, 82, 83, 84, 85, 89, 90, 122, 123, 127, 348, 356, 378
awareness, 181, 233, 243, 281, 284, 288, 289

B

background information, 43, 259, 269
barriers, 128, 270, 275, 317, 325
beneficiaries, 55, 56, 57, 60, 61, 64, 66, 67, 89
benefits, 41, 43, 47, 55, 56, 58, 59, 62, 63, 73, 284, 298, 300, 301, 325, 326
blood, 3, 13, 14, 15, 45, 82, 124
blood plasma, 15
blood supply, 82
budgetary resources, 77
businesses, xii, xviii, 123, 174, 339, 359

C

case investigation, v, vi, xii, xiii, xiv, xvi, 129, 130, 131, 132, 133, 136, 139, 140, 141, 142, 143, 144, 145, 146, 147, 148, 149, 154, 162, 164, 168, 171, 172, 173, 174, 175, 176, 177, 178, 179, 180, 181, 182, 184, 185, 186, 187, 188, 189, 190, 192, 193, 194, 195, 198, 200, 201, 210, 217, 218, 219, 222, 224, 225, 228, 235, 236, 237, 238, 239, 240, 241, 242, 243, 244, 246, 248, 249, 250, 251, 252, 253, 254, 259, 260, 262, 265, 266, 267, 269, 279, 300, 311, 313, 314, 315, 316, 317, 327, 329, 337, 338
Centers for Disease Control and Prevention (CDC), vi, x, xi, xiii, xiv, xvii, xviii, 2, 7, 12, 20, 30, 32, 33, 35, 50, 51, 66, 77, 78, 79, 81, 83, 84, 85, 86, 90, 91, 92, 93, 94, 95, 96, 99, 100, 103, 105, 108, 109, 110, 114, 115, 116, 117, 118, 119, 120, 121, 128, 131, 142, 143, 147, 152, 153, 156, 160, 165, 167, 170, 171, 173, 174, 175, 176, 177, 180, 193, 197, 211, 227, 230, 232, 233, 234, 236, 248, 253, 261, 284, 302, 303, 313, 315, 317, 326, 329, 330, 331, 332, 334, 336, 359, 362
chain of disease transmission, xii, 130, 314
challenges, x, xi, xii, xvi, 1, 2, 12, 33, 108, 109, 123, 126, 127, 155, 159, 166, 169, 194, 229, 231, 254, 288, 290, 296, 298, 299, 321, 325, 334, 353, 362
childcare, 155, 169, 176
children, 55, 56, 58, 59, 73, 75, 155, 169, 177
clients, xii, xvii, 73, 130, 131, 132, 133, 134, 137, 138, 140, 141, 143, 144, 147, 149, 150, 151, 152, 153, 154, 155, 156, 157, 158, 159, 160, 161, 162, 163, 164, 171, 172, 173, 176, 178, 179, 180, 182, 185, 186, 187, 188, 189, 190, 191, 192, 193, 194, 195, 199,205, 210, 211, 212, 213, 273, 316, 329, 352
clinical diagnosis, x, 4, 10, 11
commercial, x, xii, xvii, xx, 2, 4, 12, 20, 27, 35, 43, 83, 87, 91, 95, 108, 109, 110, 111, 113, 115, 118, 119, 121, 336, 378
communication, 130, 132, 133, 134, 137, 151, 158, 162, 170, 176, 179, 180, 181, 195, 243, 252, 258, 267, 269, 270, 271, 272, 274, 275, 276, 277, 279, 280, 283, 291, 298, 300, 301, 302, 326, 346
communication skills, 271, 274, 276, 280
communication strategies, 258, 272, 280
community-based settings, x, 10, 11, 33
compilation, 257, 263, 264, 266, 267, 332
complexity, 112, 113, 118, 121, 122, 333
compliance, 53, 63, 134, 135, 154, 158, 165, 168, 223, 310
complications, x, 10, 11
conference, 152, 153, 165, 174, 315
confidentiality, xx, 140, 143, 151, 152, 157, 166, 174, 175, 179, 184, 188, 192, 194, 196, 219, 229, 245, 246, 253, 264, 271, 286, 287, 288, 307, 378
consent, xx, 340, 341, 346, 348, 372, 378, 380
constitutional issues, 381
constitutional limitations, xxi, 378
constitutional principles, 380
containment, ix, x, xi, 1, 9, 10, 107, 108, 145, 322
contamination, 109, 117, 127
control measures, xiii, xviii, 227, 261, 314, 360
cooperative agreements, xvii, 78, 81, 83, 191, 232, 329, 332
coordination, x, 1, 61, 83, 87, 134, 143, 160, 233, 326, 331
coronavirus, v, vi, ix, xi, xiii, xviii, 9, 10, 11, 12, 13, 14, 15, 16, 18, 19, 21, 22, 23, 24, 25, 26, 27, 28, 29, 32, 33, 35, 36, 37, 38, 39, 40, 41, 42, 43, 44, 47, 48, 49, 52,

53, 54, 56, 57, 58, 61, 62, 63, 64, 67, 68, 69, 71, 78, 79, 80, 81, 82, 84, 86, 88, 89,90, 91, 92, 93, 95, 96, 99, 100, 101, 102, 103, 104, 105, 106, 107, 108, 109, 114, 116, 118, 119, 120, 121, 122, 124, 128, 156, 170, 197, 198, 199, 227, 235, 257, 258, 261, 266, 272, 284, 359
cost, 3, 14, 23, 28, 31, 33, 38, 44, 45, 46, 48, 53, 55, 56, 58, 59, 61, 63, 65, 66, 67, 69, 71, 72, 75, 76, 121, 184, 360
cough, xv, 161, 167, 198, 218, 306
coughing, 198
covering, 25, 75, 76, 155, 169
COVID-19 testing, v, ix, x, xi, xiii, 1, 3, 4, 5, 6, 9, 10, 11, 12, 15, 16, 18, 23, 24, 25, 28, 32, 33, 34, 35, 37, 40, 41, 43, 44, 45, 46, 47, 48, 50, 51, 52, 53, 54, 55, 56, 57, 58, 59, 60, 61, 63, 66, 67, 69, 72, 73, 74, 76, 77, 86, 87, 88, 89, 94, 98, 99, 105, 119, 123, 127, 128, 131, 147, 258, 273, 320
critical infrastructure, 33, 132, 147, 149, 150, 163, 167

D

data analysis, 184, 361
data collection, 85, 91, 142, 179, 184, 225, 231, 239, 241, 243, 253, 286, 288, 290, 311, 333
data transfer, 341, 348
deaths, ix, x, 1, 9, 10, 92, 93
democrats, 31, 36, 38, 39, 104
demographic characteristics, 93
demographic data, 339, 346
Department of Defense, 2, 20, 29, 65, 66, 67, 79, 84, 89, 96, 118
Department of Health and Human Services, v, vi, vii, xvi, xvii, xix, 6, 21, 24, 25, 30, 78, 86, 89, 96, 100, 104, 106, 109, 129, 217, 235, 249, 313, 319, 327, 329, 333, 335, 336, 360
Department of Homeland Security, 81
Department of Justice, 362
Department of Labor, 44, 96, 102
detection, 14, 19, 28, 45, 48, 50, 58, 72, 84, 114, 120
diagnostic testing, v, ix, x, xi, xiii, 1, 2, 3, 6, 9, 11, 12, 13, 15, 16, 17, 18, 20, 25, 26, 28, 32, 45, 46, 51, 52, 53, 57, 63, 72, 81, 107, 108, 109, 110, 113, 119, 128, 227, 364
disaster, 30, 65, 68, 70, 81, 84, 191, 275, 280, 281
disclosure, 176, 287, 360, 361, 380, 381
discrimination, 179, 372, 374
disease control measure, xii, xiii, xv, 130, 217, 305, 314
diseases, xiii, xvi, 65, 92, 111, 112, 131, 194, 228, 314, 321
distribution, ix, 1, 21, 31, 43, 82, 83, 109, 110, 111, 121, 126, 128, 259

E

education, xv, 176, 218, 229, 233, 269, 270, 271, 276, 279, 280, 290, 302, 306, 314, 361
emergency, xix, 2, 5, 12, 13, 14, 15, 16, 18, 19, 22, 28, 30, 36, 37, 43, 46, 47, 48, 51, 53, 54, 56, 57, 58, 59, 61, 63, 65, 67, 68, 72, 74, 75, 76, 77, 79, 81, 84, 86, 90, 102, 114, 115, 119, 124, 153, 155, 159, 191, 199, 251, 261, 273, 274, 275, 276, 280, 289, 293, 294, 369, 370, 372, 373, 374
emergency management, 199
emergency response, 65, 77, 84, 90, 251, 261, 280, 293, 294
Emergency Use Authorization (EUA), xii, 4, 5, 13, 18, 19, 20, 22, 28, 43, 96, 108,

109, 114, 115, 116, 117, 118, 119, 120, 121, 122, 124, 125
emotional intelligence, 134, 137, 252, 267, 272, 273, 274, 275, 276, 277, 293
employees, 15, 47, 62, 65, 144, 147, 174, 175, 188, 198, 229, 286, 294, 300, 352, 371
employers, 83, 87, 165, 168, 175, 188, 190, 299
enforcement, 5, 49, 113, 115, 119, 199, 355, 362, 366, 367, 370, 372, 380
enrollment, xx, 64, 66, 76, 340, 378
environment, 12, 42, 154, 168, 198, 224, 259, 292, 297, 298, 300, 301, 310, 362
equipment, 6, 25, 27, 40, 68, 77, 79, 82, 83, 110, 124, 126, 127, 151, 152, 199, 238, 325

F

false negative, 5, 17, 19, 22, 112, 115, 124, 126
false positive, 5, 17, 18, 19, 112, 126, 355
federal agency, 60, 65
federal assistance, 30
federal authorities, 233
federal government, xvii, 23, 32, 36, 38, 40, 43, 60, 70, 72, 81, 84, 233, 336, 345, 379
federal law, xviii, 232, 360, 366, 367, 380
financial support, 39
flatten the curve, ix, x, xii, 1, 9, 11, 123, 258, 272
flexibility, 5, 12, 40, 45, 58, 59, 110, 184
food, 84, 137, 149, 154, 160, 163, 168, 189, 190, 199, 223, 224, 309, 310, 338, 346
Food and Drug Administration (FDA), xii, 4, 5, 6, 12, 13, 14, 15, 16, 18, 19, 20, 21, 22, 26, 28, 29, 34, 41, 42, 43, 45, 56, 58, 65, 85, 86, 96, 102, 106, 108, 109, 110, 111, 112, 113, 114, 115, 116, 117, 118, 119, 120, 121, 122, 124, 125, 127, 128
funding, xi, xiii, 10, 11, 25, 35, 37, 40, 41, 53, 61, 63, 69, 70, 71, 76, 77, 78, 79, 80, 81, 82, 84, 85, 86, 87, 88, 89, 227, 232, 233
funds, xix, 36, 37, 53, 64, 69, 70, 71, 77, 79, 81, 84, 85, 86, 87, 88, 89, 90, 369

G

guidance, xii, xiii, xiv, xv, xvii, 4, 5, 16, 20, 21, 22, 23, 24, 28, 32, 33, 34, 38, 39, 43, 45, 46, 49, 50, 51, 54, 58, 59, 61, 64, 66, 68, 72, 94, 95, 98, 100, 102, 108, 109, 110, 113, 121, 122, 131, 143, 144, 147, 150, 152, 153, 155, 156, 160, 162, 164, 165, 167, 169, 171, 173, 174, 175, 176, 177, 181, 199, 217, 225, 227, 230, 233, 236, 242, 248, 269, 275, 305, 311, 315, 317, 336
guidelines, xii, 24, 33, 51, 55, 95, 100, 101, 108, 110, 157, 188

H

health care, ix, x, xii, 1, 9, 10, 11, 12, 20, 21, 28, 30, 33, 34, 35, 38, 42, 44, 46, 49, 50, 51, 54, 55, 56, 60, 62, 63, 64, 65, 66, 67, 71, 72, 75, 76, 77, 80, 83, 87, 88, 92, 93, 108, 110, 113, 122, 126, 127, 128, 292, 309, 360, 361, 364, 371
health care costs, 62
health care professionals, 38
health care programs, 55
health care system, ix, x, 1, 9, 11, 63, 65
health condition, 50, 134, 148, 156, 159, 178
health education, 155, 169, 171, 189, 243
health impact, ix, x, 9, 11, 263
health information, xviii, 91, 95, 195, 253, 278, 285, 286, 287, 339, 347, 360, 362, 365, 366, 371, 373

health insurance, 35, 43, 44, 46, 47, 51, 52, 54, 55, 59, 62, 72, 73, 75, 360
health services, 61, 63, 64, 65, 90, 155, 278
health status, 159, 170, 193
hearing impairment, 267
hearing loss, 151, 164, 241
history, 15, 32, 146, 152, 156, 160, 195, 258, 263, 272, 331, 347
homes, 28, 33, 49, 101, 138, 175, 191
housing, 137, 144, 155, 169, 191, 222, 223, 224, 229, 246, 309, 310, 338, 346

I

identification, xii, xvi, xvii, 32, 45, 130, 192, 195, 236, 252, 270, 313, 314, 324, 325, 326, 336, 340, 365, 366
identity, xv, 140, 156, 158, 164, 218, 228, 306, 314, 323, 353
immigrants, 74, 75, 76, 178, 190
immigration, 74, 75, 76, 141, 173, 174, 178
immune response, 3, 13, 14, 16
immune system, 3, 14, 124
immunity, 15, 16, 34, 366
infection, x, xv, xvi, 3, 5, 7, 9, 11, 13, 14, 15, 16, 17, 19, 56, 57, 73, 78, 81, 82, 124, 125, 132, 138, 140, 148, 151, 152, 153, 160, 165, 173, 175, 177, 199, 218, 219, 222, 224, 261, 306, 307, 309, 310, 315, 316, 324, 347
infectious disease, xii, xvi, xviii, 18, 42, 65, 79, 81, 96, 111, 112, 129, 131, 140, 194, 198, 314, 321, 324, 331, 351, 360, 370
infrastructure, xi, 3, 10, 12, 20, 65, 76, 77, 78, 80, 82, 83, 85, 86, 90, 109, 110, 138, 149, 163, 167, 182, 244
initiation, 40, 130, 137, 138, 148, 186
injury, iv, 56, 57, 259, 362
institutions, 176, 191, 229, 283, 334, 361
instructional materials, 153
insurance coverage, x, 10, 11, 37, 43, 44, 46, 47, 51, 54, 59, 72, 75
interoperability, xx, 139, 225, 311, 353, 377, 381
interpersonal relations, 283
interpersonal relationships, 283
interpersonal skills, xvi, 141, 142, 316, 329
isolation, 126, 130, 132, 134, 137, 138, 140, 141, 144, 146, 148, 150, 151, 152, 153, 154, 155, 156, 157, 158, 159, 160, 161, 166, 168, 170, 173, 179, 185, 186, 187, 189, 190, 191, 193, 194, 195, 198, 213, 221, 223, 237, 239, 241, 246, 251, 257, 260, 264, 266, 308,309, 314, 346, 347
issues, x, xi, xix, 1, 5, 6, 12, 18, 19, 22, 24, 25, 27, 28, 29, 31, 76, 86, 93, 108, 109, 120, 122, 127, 136, 161, 171, 174, 177, 184, 341, 349, 357, 370, 375

J

jurisdiction, xxi, 34, 35, 92, 95, 133, 145, 146, 152, 155, 156, 158, 159, 164, 165, 166, 168, 169, 170, 177, 179, 180, 181, 189, 228, 236, 237, 238, 252, 253, 256, 343, 378

L

laboratory tests, 56
language barrier, 282
language diversity, 181
language skills, 131, 134, 137
law enforcement, 38, 149, 163, 198, 289, 355, 380
laws, xiii, xix, 70, 103, 140, 152, 184, 227, 228, 288, 360, 366, 367, 374, 375, 380
laws and regulations, 184
leadership, xiv, 132, 173, 184, 186, 189, 245, 250, 254, 255, 291, 292, 293, 294, 295, 296

learners, 250, 251, 253, 255, 263, 274, 278
learning, xiv, 142, 236, 249, 253, 255, 256, 257, 280, 283, 294, 295, 296, 297, 299, 300, 301, 330, 332, 361
literacy, 195, 243, 278, 280, 284
liver disease, 203, 205, 209
living arrangements, 135, 191
living conditions, 178
local authorities, xviii, 95, 260, 359, 375
local community, 219, 243, 247, 307
local government, ix, x, 1, 9, 10, 30, 31, 38, 68, 69, 191, 260
lung disease, 202, 205, 209

M

marketing, xx, 4, 42, 45, 113, 118, 196, 291, 378
media, 6, 19, 20, 23, 26, 27, 30, 31, 36, 38, 42, 50, 58, 66, 67, 68, 69, 70, 104, 105, 109, 114, 116, 118, 119, 120, 121, 174, 175, 176, 181, 196, 200, 205, 243, 277, 289
medical assistance, 72, 75, 340
medical care, xvi, 64, 68, 69, 73, 125, 160, 166, 167, 190, 218, 306, 320, 360
medicine, 23, 161, 224, 310, 338
mental health, 149, 152, 163, 190, 191, 281, 361
messages, 181, 193, 212, 214, 243, 268, 274, 342
mitigation, ix, x, 1, 9, 10, 11, 15, 25, 78, 81, 145, 146, 197, 220, 221, 307, 308
mobile device, xix, 184, 194, 363, 377
mobile phone, 224, 310, 353
modernization, 82, 83, 85
modifications, 4, 6, 42, 246
modules, 182, 184, 244, 269, 330
molecular biology, 116
molecular weight, 26

N

national emergency, 29, 65, 66, 289
nursing, 33, 49, 57, 101, 138, 149, 152, 155, 163, 169, 175, 360

O

occupational health, 160, 173, 174, 175, 222, 309
officials, xviii, 24, 67, 92, 118, 160, 173, 176, 177, 181, 199, 317, 321, 322, 355, 360, 380
operating system, xx, 231, 343, 353, 363, 377
operations, xviii, 37, 40, 67, 80, 167, 175, 359, 361, 364
opportunities, 126, 182, 186, 236, 255, 256, 272, 274, 276, 277, 279, 289, 291, 294, 296, 302
outpatient, 36, 37, 57, 62, 86, 154
outreach, 22, 159, 171, 181, 192
oversight, xv, 41, 85, 112, 132, 250

P

pandemic, v, vi, ix, x, xiv, xviii, xix, 1, 2, 4, 9, 10, 22, 23, 26, 27, 28, 30, 35, 38, 39, 40, 41, 60, 67, 68, 69, 70, 84, 85, 93, 94, 100, 106, 128, 130, 211, 217, 228, 258, 272, 298, 305, 314, 332, 351, 352, 355, 368, 370, 375, 377
payment for testing, xi, 10
platform, 79, 82, 91, 95, 138, 296, 340, 343, 348
policy, x, xii, xiii, xx, 4, 10, 11, 16, 19, 43, 49, 75, 92, 95, 102, 108, 109, 114, 115, 121, 122, 127, 227, 366, 372, 378
population, x, 3, 5, 7, 9, 11, 15, 19, 23, 25, 33, 37, 38, 58, 75, 125, 154, 169, 180,

212, 213, 224, 229, 231, 232, 263, 281, 310, 356
preparation, iv, xviii, 58, 111, 173, 281, 359
prevention, 141, 151, 152, 165, 193, 257, 258, 260, 261
principles, ix, xiii, xv, 132, 140, 217, 219, 251, 258, 259, 262, 263, 271, 273, 274, 275, 283, 284, 285, 289, 292, 305, 306, 307, 379
problem solving, 252, 254, 266, 272, 273, 274, 275, 276, 277
professionals, xiii, 130, 174, 250, 257, 258, 259, 260, 262, 265, 271, 272, 273, 274, 275, 276, 277, 278, 279, 281, 282, 283, 284, 285, 286, 288, 289, 290, 291, 292, 293, 296, 297, 298, 299, 301, 316, 330

R

reagents, 6, 26, 27, 28, 58, 111, 119, 120
recall, xv, xviii, 218, 230, 306, 314, 322, 324, 351
recommendations, iv, 32, 33, 130, 132, 134, 135, 139, 140, 147, 166, 170, 171, 188, 198, 258, 272, 279, 334
regulations, xix, 175, 188, 286, 288, 360, 374, 375, 379, 380
resources, xiv, 10, 12, 25, 35, 40, 65, 81, 98, 101, 110, 127, 132, 141, 143, 147, 148, 149, 151, 155, 156, 159, 163, 164, 166, 169, 170, 171, 172, 174, 186, 189, 190, 192, 196, 197, 200, 210, 211, 213, 219, 237, 250, 259, 260, 265, 268, 269, 273, 279, 298, 307, 316, 317, 339, 347
response, ix, x, xi, xii, xv, xvii, xix, 2, 9, 10, 13, 14, 23, 30, 37, 40, 61, 68, 69, 70, 75, 78, 81, 82, 84, 86, 88, 93, 94, 108, 114, 115, 119, 120, 121, 124, 130, 139, 144, 178, 233, 250, 258, 260, 272, 281, 300, 315, 324, 325, 332, 336, 343, 352, 369

S

safety, 33, 50, 59, 67, 68, 72, 104, 110, 112, 132, 147, 175, 189, 190, 193, 199, 247
SARS-CoV-2 virus, ix, x, xi, 1, 6, 9, 11, 13, 14, 26, 108, 116
school, x, xviii, 9, 11, 15, 18, 21, 28, 42, 59, 126, 146, 176, 177, 229, 260, 359
scope, 2, 7, 49, 50, 55, 76, 110, 132, 346, 357, 368, 379, 381
security, xx, 184, 188, 192, 194, 196, 231, 232, 233, 245, 246, 253, 285, 286, 288, 289, 326, 341, 349, 372, 378, 381
security practices, xx, 378
self-monitoring, xvi, 159, 170, 171, 218, 226, 306, 312
self-quarantine, xii, 130, 132, 135, 137, 138, 140, 141, 144, 162, 165, 166, 167, 168, 169, 170, 171, 179, 185, 187, 188, 189, 190, 191, 193, 194, 237, 240, 251, 315, 316, 320, 338, 339, 340
sensitivity, xvii, 5, 17, 18, 19, 22, 23, 28, 119, 131, 141, 181, 194, 219, 252, 267, 277, 278, 279, 280, 281, 282, 283, 307, 316, 329, 355
serology, ix, x, 1, 3, 4, 7, 9, 11, 13, 14, 15, 16, 19, 45, 56, 104, 123, 124, 125
serology testing, ix, x, 1, 3, 7, 9, 11, 14, 15, 16, 45
services, iv, xx, 11, 21, 25, 30, 36, 37, 43, 44, 45, 46, 48, 50, 51, 52, 53, 55, 56, 57, 58, 59, 60, 61, 62, 63, 64, 65, 66, 67, 69, 71, 72, 73, 74, 75, 89, 90, 134, 147, 151, 153, 155, 156, 159, 164, 165, 166, 168, 169, 173, 175, 189, 190, 191, 199, 224, 225, 239, 240, 241, 246, 263, 265, 268, 271, 274, 278, 280, 310, 311, 336, 338, 339, 340, 346, 347, 360, 378
social distance, xv, 154, 167, 168, 218, 220, 224, 306, 308, 310, 315
social network, 271

social services, 200, 316
social support, 130, 137, 141, 142, 154, 159, 160, 168, 186, 187, 189, 190, 191, 223, 310
supervision, xiv, 131, 144, 185, 219, 238, 250, 254, 256, 307
supply chain, x, 1, 6, 20, 24, 25, 27, 28, 29, 76, 77, 82, 85, 98
support services, 137, 143, 144, 149, 150, 163, 189, 190, 239, 240, 241, 246, 247, 316, 337
surveillance, 15, 20, 21, 23, 24, 32, 43, 48, 50, 59, 67, 72, 78, 81, 83, 85, 87, 91, 92, 101, 104, 120, 133, 138, 141, 144, 148, 184, 251, 252, 258, 259, 289, 337, 338, 362
symptoms, xvi, 16, 17, 19, 22, 32, 35, 38, 51, 57, 126, 130, 132, 134, 135, 137, 138, 140, 148, 149, 153, 155, 157, 158, 159, 161, 162, 163, 165, 166, 167, 169, 170, 171, 175, 183, 193, 194, 198, 199, 212, 214, 218, 219, 221, 226, 251, 257, 258, 259, 261, 264, 266, 306, 307, 308, 312, 316, 320, 322, 327, 334, 340, 341, 342, 347, 362
synchronization, 138, 192, 338, 346

T

teams, xiv, 35, 191, 250, 254, 292, 293, 294, 295, 296, 297, 298
technical assistance, xiii, 87, 227, 315, 317
telephone, 152, 158, 159, 165, 170, 188, 212, 271, 315, 340, 365, 367, 368
temperature, xv, 19, 134, 135, 137, 155, 158, 167, 168, 169, 170, 194, 218, 306, 340, 341, 342
territorial, xiii, xvii, 34, 50, 68, 69, 131, 143, 177, 192, 227, 336, 338, 346
testing capacity, xi, 10, 20, 21, 24, 27, 28, 30, 37, 61, 62, 63, 77, 78, 85, 86, 87, 89, 108, 109, 116, 117, 121, 130, 147, 162
testing program, 23, 33, 34, 35, 77, 78, 79, 81, 86
treatment, 4, 15, 16, 17, 18, 38, 42, 46, 48, 50, 56, 57, 64, 66, 71, 75, 76, 125, 126, 190, 228, 361
tuberculosis, xiii, 73, 131, 211, 228, 303, 331

U

uninsured, xi, 10, 34, 35, 36, 37, 55, 58, 59, 64, 69, 70, 71, 72, 74, 75, 76, 85, 89, 98

V

vaccines, ix, x, 9, 11, 65, 79, 82, 228
viral gene, 3, 13, 18, 116, 125
viruses, 13, 19, 26, 258, 262, 285
voluntary quarantine, xii, 130

W

workers, xviii, 33, 35, 38, 49, 126, 127, 128, 132, 147, 149, 150, 163, 167, 168, 174, 175, 191, 198, 223, 230, 294, 295, 309, 320, 332, 351
workflow, xvii, 144, 152, 165, 214, 238, 340, 345, 347
workforce, xiii, xiv, xv, xvi, xvii, 25, 77, 82, 83, 87, 130, 131, 132, 140, 142, 143, 144, 195, 218, 228, 229, 233, 236, 293, 298, 305, 315, 316, 317, 329, 331, 332, 337, 343
working conditions, 174
workplace, 16, 18, 21, 50, 59, 132, 148, 158, 174, 183, 203, 206, 209, 242, 300